OXFORD MEDICAL PUBLICATIONS

Oxford Handbook of
Critical Care

THIRD EDITION

Published and forthcoming Oxford Handbooks

Oxford Handbook of
Critical Care

THIRD EDITION

Mervyn Singer

Professor of Intensive Care Medicine;
Director, Bloomsbury Institute of Intensive Care Medicine,
University College London
London, UK

Andrew R. Webb

Medical Director and Consultant Physician,
Department of Intensive Care,
University College London Hospitals,
London, UK

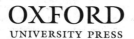

OXFORD
UNIVERSITY PRESS

OXFORD
UNIVERSITY PRESS

Great Clarendon Street, Oxford OX2 6DP

Oxford University Press is a department of the University of Oxford.
It furthers the University's objective of excellence in research, scholarship,
and education by publishing worldwide in

Oxford New York

Auckland Cape Town Dar es Salaam Hong Kong Karachi
Kuala Lumpur Madrid Melbourne Mexico City Nairobi
New Delhi Shanghai Taipei Toronto

With offices in

Argentina Austria Brazil Chile Czech Republic France Greece
Guatemala Hungary Italy Japan Poland Portugal Singapore
South Korea Switzerland Thailand Turkey Ukraine Vietnam

Oxford is a registered trade mark of Oxford University Press
in the UK and in certain other countries

Published in the United States
by Oxford University Press Inc., New York

British Library Cataloguing in Publication Data
Data available

Library of Congress Cataloging-in-Publication-Data
Data available

Typeset by Cepha Imaging Private Ltd., Bangalore, India
Printed in China
on acid-free paper by
C&C Offset Printing Co., Ltd.

ISBN 978–0–19–923533–9

22

Contents

Foreword

I am delighted, for several reasons, to write the foreword for the third edition of this handbook of critical care medicine. Firstly, both authors were former colleagues whose careers have blossomed very considerably since we all worked together. Secondly, the fact that three editions have been produced in the past 12 years with total sales of 30,000 reflects the rapidly emerging importance of intensive care as a specialty in its own right. Thirdly, the fact that about 20% of the material in this current edition is new reflects how quickly intensive care is changing.

Although this book is designed to fit the pocket it contains an enormous amount of clearly presented and important information. It is essential reading for nurses and doctors of all grades who are involved in looking after the critically ill.

Many acutely ill patients are still being cared for in general wards without ever being admitted to an intensive care unit. The popularity of the two previous editions of this book suggests it is being read by staff working in these non-critical care areas and I do believe this will assist them considerably in improving patient care.

The layout of the book lends itself extremely well to an electronic format, a move which I thoroughly endorse. I wish the book the success it thoroughly deserves.

David Bennett
Visiting Professor of Intensive Care Medicine
King's College London

foreword

Preface to the previous editions

Of all the medical specialities, few, if any, are as exacting and complex as critical care medicine. The required knowledge of physiology, pathophysiology, biochemistry, technology, and pharmacology; the unpredictability; the need to act and react decisively; the ability to communicate clearly with colleagues, patients, and relatives, often in stressful situations; the importance of working cohesively within an expanded team drawn from different backgrounds; and the regular occurrences of ethical and life-and-death dilemmas, all place heavy demands on the intensive care staff member.

This book does not aim to be a panacea; many areas of uncertainty in diagnosis and management remain. However, current best practice (at least as practised by us!) is described in succinct, concise, clinically orientated sections, covering therapeutic and monitoring, drugs and fluids, specific organ system disorders and complications, and general management philosophies. Ample space is provided to append or amend sections to suit your particular practice.

It will hopefully serve the consultant, junior doctor, nurse, or other paramedical staff as a reference book, aide memoire, and handy pocket book, providing rationales and solutions to most of the problems encountered.

Buoyed by the positive feedback we received after publication of the 1st edition of this book, we endeavoured to maintain the style and, where appropriate, changed the substance for the 2nd edition. This involved the addition of some new sections to describe recent innovations in either thought and/or process. However, many of the existing chapters were updated to reflect the rapid rate of change in ICU management that has occurred since we last put pen to paper.

Mervyn Singer
Andrew R. Webb
1996/2004

Preface to this edition

This new edition embraces the many recent developments occurring in critical care medicine, in particular the burgeoning number of randomised, multicentre trials and the increasing understanding of underlying basic science mechanisms. While not necessarily providing definitive answers, these studies have contributed significantly to our knowledge base and highlighted both the complexity of critical illness and the variation in individual response. They frequently demonstrate the need to recognise and treat deterioration promptly, and flag up the many detrimental effects of our current therapies and strategies. A balance needs to be sought between under- and over-treatment—be it for fluids, sedatives, antibiotics, pressors, ventilation, etc., and we will no doubt continue to refine this further in coming years, particularly with enhancements in monitoring and diagnostics.

These studies further demonstrate the 'one size fits all' paradigm on which traditional categorisation of patients is based, e.g. those with sepsis is, perhaps, overly simplistic. We should follow local, national, and international guidelines on patient management, yet still retain the flexibility of thought and action to diverge should an individual patient not follow the rules. We have thus provided a framework upon which a reasonable and rational practice can be based; this is clearly not the final word. We expect both healthy debate and continuing evolution!

In line with advances in critical care, other specialities have new treatments and management regimens for specific conditions that often bring affected patients to our attention. We gratefully acknowledge the input and advice received from Sheila Adam, Emma Morris, Alastair O'Brien, Marie Scully, Penny Shaw, and Simon Woldman.

Mervyn Singer
Andrew R. Webb
2009

Abbreviations

A&E	Accident and emergency
A–aDO$_2$	Alveolar–arterial oxygen difference
ABE	Arterial base excess
ACE	Angiotensin converting enzyme
ACMV	Assist control mechanical ventilation
ACT	Activated clotting time
ACTH	Adrenocorticotropic hormone
ADH	Antidiuretic hormone
AGE	Arterial gas embolism
AIDS	Acquired immunodeficiency syndrome
AIS	Abbreviated injury score
ALI	Acute lung injury
ALT	Alanine aminotransferase
ANCA	Anti-nuclear cytoplasmic antibodies
AP	Anteroposterior
APACHE	Acute physiology and chronic health evaluation
APTT	Activated partial thromboplastin time
ARDS	Acute respiratory distress syndrome
ASD	Atrio-septal defect
AST	Aspartate aminotransferase
ATP	Adenosine triphosphate
AV	Aortic valve
bd	Bis die (twice daily)
BiPAP	Bilevel positive airways pressure
BIS	Bispectral index
BNP	Brain natriuretic peptide
BOOP	Bronchiolitis obliterans with organising pneumonia
bpm	Beats per minute
Ca^{2+}	Calcium
CABG	Coronary artery bypass grafting
CaCl$_2$	Calcium chloride
Cal	Calorie
CAL	Chronic airflow limitation
CAM	Confusion assessment method
cAMP	Cyclic adenosine monophosphate
c-ANCA	Core anti-neutrophil cytoplasmic antibodies

CBF	Cerebral blood flow
CBV	Cerebral blood volume
CcO_2	End-capillary oxygen content
CD	Cluster of differentiation
CDI	Cranial diabetes insipidus
CFM	Cerebral function monitor
cGMP	Cyclic guanosine monophosphate
CJD	Creutzfeldt–Jacob disease
CI	Cardiac index
CK	Creatine kinase
Cl^-	Chloride
CLL	Chronic lymphocytic leukaemia
cm	Centimetre
cmH_2O	Centimetres of water
$CMRO_2$	Cerebral metabolic rate for oxygen
CMV	Controlled mandatory ventilation
CMV	Cytomegalovirus
CNS	Central nervous system
CO	Carbon monoxide
CO_2	Carbon dioxide
COHb	Carboxyhaemoglobin
COP	Colloid osmotic pressure
CPAP	Continuous positive airways pressure
CPK	Creatine phosphokinase
CPP	Cerebral perfusion pressure
CPR	Cardiopulmonary resuscitation
CRP	C-reactive protein
CSF	Cerebrospinal fluid
CT	Computerised tomography
CVA	Cerebrovascular accident
CVP	Central venous pressure
CVVH	Continuous veno-venous haemofiltration
CVVHD	Continuous veno-venous haemodiafiltration
CXR	Chest X-ray
d	Day
D	Dalton
DA	Dopamine
DDAVP	1-deamino-8-D-arginine vasopressin
DEAFF	Detection of early antigen fluorescent foci
deoxyHb	Deoxyhaemoglobin

DIC	Disseminated intravascular coagulation
dL	Decilitre
DNA	Deoxyribonucleic acid
DO_2	Oxygen delivery
DPG	Diphosphoglycerate
DS	Degree of substitution
DVT	Deep vein thrombosis
dyn.s	Dyne second
$ECCO_2R$	Extracorporeal carbon dioxide removal
ECF	Extracellular fluid
ECG	Electrocardiogram
ECMO	Extracorporeal membrane oxygenation
EEG	Electroencephalogram
EMG	Electromyogram
ENT	Ear, nose and throat
EPAP	Expiratory positive airway pressure
ERCP	Endoscopic retrograde pancreatography
ESBL	Extended spectrum beta-lactamase
FT	Endotracheal
EVLW	Extravascular lung water
$FADH_2$	Flavin adenine dinucleotide-H_2
FDP	Fibrin degradation product
FEV_1	Forced expired volume in 1 second
FFP	Fresh frozen plasma
FiO_2	Fractional inspired oxygen concentration
fL	Femptolitre
Fr	French gauge
FRC	Functional residual capacity
FTc	Corrected flow time
FVC	Forced vital capacity
g	Gram
GBM	Glomerular basement membrane
GCS	Glasgow coma score
G-CSF	Granulocyte-colony stimulating factor
GEDV	Global end-diastolic volume
GFR	Glomerular filtration rate
GI	Gastrointestinal
γGT	Gamma glutamyl transaminase
GMP	Guanosine monophosphate
GTN	Glyceryl trinitrate

GVHD	Graft versus host disease
h	Hour
H^+	Hydrogen ion
Hb	Haemoglobin
HCl	Hydrochloric acid
HCO_3^-	Bicarbonate
He	Helium
HELLP	Haemolysis, elevated liver enzymes & low platelets
HFJV	High frequency jet ventilation
HFO	High frequency oscillation
HITS	Heparin-induced thrombocytopaenia syndrome
HIV	Human immunodeficiency virus
HME	Head and moisture exchanger
H_2O	Water
hpf	High power field
HR	Heart rate
Hrly	Hourly
HUS	Haemolytic uraemic syndrome
Hz	Hertz
IABP	Intra-aortic blood pressure
ICP	Intracranial pressure
id	Internal diameter
I:E	Inspiratory : expiratory
ICP	Intracranial pressure
ICU	Intensive care unit
Ig	Immunoglobulin
IM	Intramuscular
IMV	Intermittent mandatory ventilation
INR	International normalised ratio
IPAP	Inspiratory positive airway pressure
IPPV	Intermittent positive pressure ventilation
IRS	Immune reconstitution syndrome
IS	Inspiratory support
ISS	Injury severity score
ITBV	Intrathoracic blood volume
ITP	Idiopathic thrombocytopaenic purpura
IU	International unit
IV	Intravenous
K^+	Potassium
KCl	Potassium chloride

kDa	Kilodalton
kg	Kilogram
kHz	Kilohertz
kIU	Kallikrein inhibitor units
kJ	Kilojoule
kPa	Kilopascal
kU	Kilounit
L	Litre
LA	Left atrium
L-NMMA	L-N^G-monomethyl arginine
LBBB	Left bundle branch block
LDH	Lactate dehydrogenase
LED	Light emitting diode
LFPPV	Low frequency positive pressure ventilation
LFT	Liver function test
L-NMMA	L-N-mono-methyl-arginine
LMW	Low molecular weight
LP	Lumbar puncture
LVEDP	Left ventricular end diastolic pressure
LVF	Left ventricular failure
LVOT	Left ventricular outflow tract
LVSW	Left ventricular stroke work
mcg	Microgram
μmol	Micromole
M,C&S	Microscopy, culture & sensitivity
mA	Milliamp
MAOI	Monoamine oxidase inhibitor
MAP	Mean arterial pressure
MARS	Molecular Adsorbent Recirculation System
MCA	Middle cerebral artery
MCV	Mean cellular volume
MDMA	3,4 methylenedioxy-methamphetamine
mEq	Milliequivalent
metHb	Methaemoglobin
Mg	Milligram
Mg^{2+}	Magnesium
MgSO$_4$	Magnesium sulphate
MI	Myocardial infarction
min	Minute
mL	Millilitre

mmHg	Millimetre of mercury
mmol	Millimole
MODS	Multiple organ dysfunction syndrome
MOF	Multiple organ failure
mOsm	Milliosmole
MPAP	Mean pulmonary artery pressure
MRSA	Meticillin-resistant *Staphylococcus aureus*
MSSA	Meticillin-sensitive *Staphylococcus aureus*
ms	Millisecond
MV	Mitral valve
μV	Microvolt
MW	Molecular weight
Na^+	Sodium
NAC	N-acetylcysteine
NaCl	Sodium chloride
NADH	Nicotinamide adenine dinucleotide-H
$NaHCO_3$.	Sodium bicarbonate
ng	Nanogram
NG	Nasogastric
NIRS	Near-infrared spectroscopy
nm	Nanometer
NMS	Neuroleptic malignant syndrome
NO	Nitric oxide
NSAID	Non-steroidal anti-inflammatory drug
NYHA	New York Heart Association
O_2	Oxygen
O_2ER	Oxygen extraction ratio
od	Once daily
OPS	Orthogonal polarisation spectroscopy
PA	Pulmonary artery
$PaCO_2$	Arterial partial pressure of carbon dioxide
PAF	Platelet activating factor
PAN	Polyarteritis nodosa
PAO_2	Alveolar partial pressure of oxygen
PaO_2	Arterial partial pressure of oxygen
PAWP	Pulmonary artery wedge pressure
$PaCO_2$	Partial pressure of carbon dioxide
PCI	Percutaneous coronary intervention
PCO_2	Partial pressure of carbon dioxide
PCR	Polymerase chain reaction

PDE	Phosphodiesterase
PEEP	Positive end expiratory pressure
PEEPi	Intrinsic positive end expiratory pressure (auto-PEEP)
PEG	Percutaneous enterogastrostomy
PEJ	Percutaneous enterojejunostomy
PGE_1	Prostaglandin E_1 (Alprostadil)
$PGI_{2\alpha}$	Prostaglandin $I_{2\alpha}$ (Epoprostenol)
pHi	Intramucosal pH
PI	Pulsatility index
PImax	Maximum inspiratory pressure
pKa	Acid dissociation constant
PO	Per os (by mouth)
PO_2	Partial pressure of oxygen
PO_4^{3-}	Phosphate
PP	Pulse pressure
ppm	Parts per million
PPV	Pulse pressure variation
PR	Per rectum
prn	Pro re nata (as required)
PSV	Pressure support ventilation
PT	Prothrombin time
PTCA	Percutaneous transluminal coronary angioplasty
PTLD	Post-transplant lymphoproliferative disorder
PTT	Partial thromboplastin time
PVL	Panton-Valentine Leukocidin
PVR	Pulmonary vascular resistance
qds	Quater die sumendum (take four times daily)
Q_s/Q_t	Shunt fraction
q.v.	Quod vide (which see)
RA	Right atrium
RAP	Right atrial pressure
RBBB	Right bundle branch block
RBC	Red blood cell
RCT	Randomised controlled trial
RDS	Respiratory distress syndrome
RQ	Respiratory quotient
rtPA	Recombinant tissue plasminogen activator
RTS	Revised trauma score
RV	Right ventricle
RVSW	Right ventricular stroke work

s	Second
SAH	Subarachnoid haemorrhage
SaO_2	Arterial oxygen saturation
SC	Subcutaneously
$ScvO_2$	Central venous saturation
SDF	Sidestream darkfield imaging
SI	Stroke index
SIADH	Syndrome of inappropriate antidiuretic hormone secretion
SIMV	Synchronised intermittent mandatory ventilation
SIRS	Systemic inflammatory response syndrome
SjO_2	Jugular bulb oxygen saturation
SL	Sublingually
SLE	Systemic lupus erythematosus
SpO_2	Pulse oximeter oxygen saturation
Spp	Species
SPV	Systolic pressure variation
Stat	Statim (immediately)
StO_2	Tissue oxyhaemoglobin concentration
SV	Stroke volume
SvO_2	Mixed venous saturation
SVR	Systemic vascular resistance
SVT	Supraventricular tachycardia
SVV	Stroke volume variation
TB	Tuberculosis
Tds	Ter die sumendum (take three times daily)
TED	Thromboembolic disease
TEN	Toxic epidermal necrolysis
TENS	Transcutaneous electric nerve stimulation
TF	Tissue factor
THAM	Tris-hydroxy-methyl-aminomethane
TIPSS	Transjugular intrahepatic portosystemic stented shunt
TISS	Therapeutic intervention scoring system
TPN	Total parenteral nutrition
TRALI	Transfusion-related acute lung injury
TRISS	Trauma injury severity score
TSH	Thyroid stimulating hormone
TSLC	Total static lung compliance
TT	Thrombin time
TTP	Thrombotic thrombocytopaenic purpura

TURP	Transurethral resection of prostate
TXA_2	Thromboxane A_2
U	Unit
U & E	Urea and electrolytes
V	Volt
VAC	Vacuum-assisted closure
VC	Vital capacity
VCO_2	Carbon dioxide production
V_D	Dead space
Vd/Vt	Dead space: tidal volume ratio
VDRL	Venereal diseases reference laboratory
VF	Ventricular fibrillation
VHF	Viral haemorrhagic fever
VILI	Ventilation-induced lung injury
VO_2	Oxygen consumption
V/Q	Ventilation/perfusion
VRE	Vancomycin-resistant *Enterococcus*
VSD	Ventricular septal defect
VSV	Volume support ventilation
V_T	Tidal volume
VT	Ventricular tachycardia
W	Watt
WBC	White blood cell
WHO	World Health Organization
wk	Week
y	Year

Detailed contents

Critical care organisation and management

Critical Care Unit layout

The Critical Care Unit should be easily accessible by departments from which patients are admitted and close to departments which share engineering services. In a new hospital, all critical care facilities should ideally be proximal to operating theatres, emergency department, laboratories, and imaging suites.

It is desirable that critically ill patients are separated from those in the recovery phase or needing coronary care where a quieter environment is needed. Providing intensive care and high dependency care in the same Critical Care Unit allows flexibility of staffing, although the differing requirements of these patients may limit such flexibility.

Size of unit

Requirements depend on the activity of the hospital with additional beds required for regional specialties such as cardiothoracic surgery or neurosurgery. Very small (<6 beds) or very large (>14 beds) units may be difficult to manage, although larger units may be divided operationally and allow better concentration of resources.

Patient areas

- Patient areas must provide unobstructed passage around the bed with a floor space of 26m^2 per bed and bed centres of at least 4.6m. Curtains or screens are required for privacy.
- Floors and ceilings must be constructed to support heavy equipment (some may weigh >1000kg).
- Doors must allow for passage of bulky equipment as well as wide beds.
- A wash hand basin with elbow-operated or proximity-operated mixer taps, soap, and antiseptic dispensers should be close to every bedspace.
- The specification should include 50% of beds as isolation cubicles. Air pressure control in cubicles should ensure effective patient isolation.
- Services must include adequate electricity supply (at least 28 sockets per bed) with an uninterruptable power supply for essential equipment. Oxygen (4), medical air (2), and high (2) and low (2) pressure suction outlets must be available for every bed.
- The bed areas should have natural daylight and patients and staff should ideally have an outside view.
- Communications systems include an adequate number of telephones, intercom systems to allow bed-to-bed communication, and a system to control entry to the department.
- Computer networks should enable communication with central hospital administration, laboratory and radiology systems, and the internet.

Other areas required

Other areas include adequate storage space, separate clean-treatment and dirty utility/sluice areas, offices, laboratory, seminar room, cleaners' room, staff rest room, staff change and locker room, toilets and shower facilities, relatives' area including a quiet area for grieving family, and an interview room.

See also:

Infection control—general principles, p544.

Critical Care Unit staffing (medical)

Critical care has evolved from its early success in simple mechanical ventilation of the lungs of polio victims to the present day where patients usually have, or are at risk of developing, failure or dysfunction of one or more organ systems requiring mechanical and pharmacological support and monitoring. The unit should have dedicated consultant sessions allocated for direct patient care with additional sessions for management, teaching, and audit activities. These sessions should be divided between several critical care-trained specialists who should be supported by trainee doctors providing round-the-clock cover on a rota which provides adequate rest.

Required skills of critical care medical staff

Management
Senior medical staff, assisted by senior nursing and pharmacy colleagues, command the primary responsibility for the structural and financial management of the unit. It is through their actions that treatment of the critically ill is initiated and perpetuated; they are ultimately responsible for the activity of the unit and patient outcome.

Decision-making
In the Critical Care Unit, most decisions are made by team consensus. Clinical decisions fall under three categories: (i) decisions relating to common or routine problems for which a unit policy exists; (ii) decisions relating to uncommon problems requiring discussion with all currently involved staff, and (iii) decisions of an urgent nature taken by critical care staff without delay.

Practical skills
Expertise in the management of complex equipment, monitoring procedures and performance of invasive procedures are required.

Clinical experience
Medical staff require experience in the recognition, prevention and management of critical illness, infection control, anaesthesia, analgesia, and organ support.

Technical knowledge
The critical care specialist has an important role in the choice of equipment used in the unit. Advice should be sought from non-medical colleagues.

Pharmacological knowledge
Drug therapy regimens are clearly open to the problems of drug interactions, while pharmacokinetics are often severely altered by the effects of major organ system dysfunction, particularly involving the liver and kidneys. Adverse reactions are common.

Teaching and training
The modern critical care specialist has acquired skills that cannot be gained outside the Critical Care Unit. Therefore, it is necessary to impart this knowledge to doctors training in the specialty.

Critical Care Unit staffing (nursing)

Critically ill patients require close nursing supervision. Many will require high-intensity nursing throughout a 24h period while others are of a lower dependency and can share nurses. In addition to the bedside nurses, the department needs additional staff to manage the day-to-day running of the unit, to assist in lifting and handLing of patients, to relieve bedside nurses for rest periods, and to collect drugs and equipment. These additional nurses (or nurse assistants) can be termed the 'fixed nursing establishment' and the nature of their duties is such that they will usually include the higher grade nurses. The bedside nurses are a 'variable establishment' and their numbers are dependent on activity such that more patients require higher numbers. Most departments fix part of their variable establishment by assuming an average activity.

Fixed establishment

Providing one nurse per shift requires a rota of 5.5 nurses. In addition, staff handover, annual leave, study leave, and sickness are usually calculated at 22% such that one additional nurse is required. Thus, the provision of one nurse in charge of each shift and one nurse to support the bedside nurses requires 11 nurses in those two roles alone. In larger units, there may be a need for additional nurses supporting the nurse in charge.

Variable establishment

The same principles apply for the provision of bedside nurses. Thus, to provide 1:1 nursing for a bed requires 5.5 nurses and to provide 1:2 nursing requires 2.75 nurses. The total number required depends on the occupancy and the nurse-to-patient ratio for each occupied bed. One of the difficulties in staffing a Critical Care Unit relates to the variable dependency and occupancy. An average dependency weighted occupancy (average occupancy × average nurse-to-patient ratio) should be used to set the establishment of bedside nurses with additional nurses being drafted in from a bank or agency to cover peak demands.

Skill mix

Nursing skill mix is the subject of much controversy as the need for economy is balanced against the need for quality. As stated above, the fixed nursing will usually be of higher grade since the role incorporates the administration of the unit and supervisory nursing. The bedside nurses will be made up of those who have received post-qualification training in critical care and those who have not. The ratio of trained to untrained critical care nurses should be of the order of 3:1 to facilitate in-service teaching.

Outreach support

Critical care outreach aims to augment the effectiveness of Critical Care Units by utilising their expertise at all stages in the evolution of critical illness. Outreach teams typically support patient care outside the Critical Care Unit to prevent admission or readmission. However, the outreach team will also expedite timely admission to a Critical Care Unit for those that need it. Outreach teams work in collaboration with staff in general ward areas and should be utilised following the identification of a deterioration in the patient's condition to provide advice, support, education, and a link to the critical care facility. Many outreach teams in the UK are developed around critical care nurses, but they also depend on support from critical care medical staff and other m embers of the multidisciplinary critical care team such as physiotherapists. In other countries such as Australia, the model of a medical emergency team, staffed by intensivists or trainees, is more commonplace.

The outreach team should support and facilitate the ability of ward staff to:

• Identify patients who are at risk of developing life-threatening acute illness. Patients suffering cardiorespiratory arrest in hospital usually show gradual deterioration over several hours (especially in conscious level and respiratory rate) rather than an abrupt collapse.
• Initiate immediate resuscitation.
• Make appropriate referral, documentation, and communication.
• Provide psychological support and physiological surveillance to patients after discharge from the Critical Care Unit.
• Educate and train general ward staff in the identification of deteriorating vital signs, the use of appropriate early warning scoring systems, and the institution of appropriate management.
• Though no study has specifically shown mortality reduction through the use of outreach or medical emergency team, ward staff and patients greatly value their support. The outreach teams can prompt decisions regarding resuscitation status and this has led to a reduction in inappropriate cardiac arrest calls.

Outreach team calling criteria

These are usually defined locally based on breaching limits of vital signs.

Early warning scoring systems

Simple risk assessment tools are available to aid the identification of patients at risk of deterioration. These are based on weighted scores given to routinely available vital sign data.

Typical outreach calling criteria

- Respiratory rate >25 or <8/min.
- Oxygen saturation <90% on FIO_2 >0.35.
- Heart rate >125 or <50 beats/min.
- Systolic blood pressure <90 or >200mmHg, or a sustained fall of >40mmHg from the patient's normal value.
- Sustained alteration in conscious level.
- Patient looks unwell or you are worried about their condition.

Early warning scoring system

	3	2	1	0	1	2	3
HR		<40	41–50	51–100	101–110	111–129	≥130
BP	<70	71–80	81–100	101–199		>200	
RR		≤8	9–14		15–20	21–29	≥30
Temp		<35.0		35.0–38.4		≥38.5	
CNS				A	V	P	U

A = alert; V = responds to voice; P = responds to pain; U = unconscious.

Key paper

Morgan RJM, Williams F, Wright MM (1997). An early warning scoring system for detecting developing critical illness. *Clin Intensive Care* **8**: 100.

See also:

Survivor follow-up, p12; Communication, p18.

Critical Care Unit admission criteria

The Critical Care Unit should be seen as the hub of critical care provision throughout the hospital. In the UK, critical illness is now defined according to patient dependency levels (see table opposite), ranging from those suitable for ward care through to true intensive care requirement. Thus, admission to the Critical Care Unit is not necessary for all of those with a critical illness, particularly where a well-functioning outreach team can support care in the general ward environment. While dependency levels do not necessarily define the need for admission to a Critical Care Unit, it is generally those requiring level 2 or 3 care who are considered for admission.

Admission criteria may be set on a priority basis related to patient dependency levels, their specific diagnosis, physiological or biochemical abnormalities, or investigational findings.

Local policies for critical care admission should:
- Identify who has day-to-day responsibility to make admission decisions.
- Include a mechanism for reviewing difficult cases and difficult ethical decisions.
- Identify those who are too well or too sick to benefit from critical care admission (in the context of other facilities available locally).
- Identify priorities for admission during times of high utilisation of beds, e.g. level 3 patients admitted as a higher priority than level 2.
- Identify when, who, and how to transfer patients to other units.
- Identify categories of patients who should or should not be admitted to Critical Care Units, including conditions where admission is mandatory.
- Identify any age criteria below which admission is precluded.
- Clarify the links with local incident management policies, contingency plans, and triggers for the implementation of these plans.

A critical care consultant should consider the nature and severity of the patient's illness, the potential reversibility of their condition, the long- and short-term probability of survival, and the wishes of the patient when deciding on Critical Care Unit admission.

Although patients with 'do not attempt resuscitation' orders or terminal illness for palliative care may fit the criteria for level 2 or 3 care, a clear assessment needs to be made on how they would benefit from admission. Admission may be justified if there is benefit to the patient in terms of avoiding cardiac arrest or better provision of palliation. However, many such patients will clearly not benefit from admission to the Critical Care Unit or from continuation of treatment once admitted. Management of such patients can be difficult. Local guidance needs to ensure decisions are reviewed regularly. Mechanisms to share decision-making between several senior members of the team (sometimes with senior staff uninvolved with the patient's care) should be in place given the potential of legal challenge of clinical decisions.

Critical care levels of dependency

Level 0

Patients are appropriately cared for in ordinary hospital wards such as are available in all acute hospitals and all general departments of surgery and medicine. Patients may need administration of medication, patient-controlled analgesia, intravenous maintenance fluids, blood transfusion, and other simple treatments. Observations would usually be required less frequently than every four hours.

Level 1

Patients are at risk of their condition deteriorating, e.g. recently relocated from higher levels of care, requiring additional monitoring or input from staff with specific expertise. In addition to level 0 requirements, patients may need administration of intravenous fluids at rates in excess of 3,000mL/d, and regular but infrequent tracheal suction via a tracheostomy. Observations would be required at least every four hours.

Level 2

Patients require single-organ monitoring and support, e.g. inotropic support for the cardiovascular system, renal replacement therapy or non-invasive ventilatory support, patients with major uncorrected physiological abnormalities, patients classified as American Society of Anaesthesiologists' 3 or 4 following minor or major surgery, patients requiring preoperative optimisation but not requiring post-operative ventilation. In addition to level 1 requirements, patients may need frequent tracheal suction via a tracheostomy tube or rapid blood transfusion (perhaps up to six units in 24h).

Level 3

Patients require advanced respiratory monitoring or support, or monitoring and support for two or more organ systems (or one organ system with chronic impairment of at least one other).

Survivor follow-up

Recovery from a critical illness continues for a prolonged period after discharge from hospital, particularly after a severe critical illness involving a long stay. Mortality after hospital discharge is up to three times higher than that of the general population for two to three years after hospital discharge. Patients often experience a variety of physical and psychological symptoms after prolonged critical illness (see table opposite). If not recognised as a sequel to critical illness, this can lead to unnecessary treatment and investigation, contributing further to their morbidity.

Many hospitals are now running critical care follow-up clinics to provide multidisciplinary support to patients after critical illness. These clinics allow patients to gain an understanding of their illness. There are usually gaps in the patient's recollection of events. They may suffer hallucinations or delusions, or misinterpret events they have patchy knowledge of. This can lead to frustration and anger. Explanations to complete their knowledge are very helpful in helping patients come to terms with what happened to them and this is usually reassuring. Provision of information that helps the patient understand a realistic timeframe for their recovery overcomes any unrealistic expectations they may harbor.

The whole family dynamic often changes as a result of a critical illness. Close family members experience anxiety and depression during the critical illness. This changes to a state of overprotection after the illness which can often be frustrating for the patient.

A follow-up clinic also gives an opportunity for patients and relatives to provide feedback on areas of care that could be improved to the benefit of subsequent patients.

Typical problems post-critical care discharge

Weakness	Stress
Weight loss	Irritability
Fatigue	Depression
Poor appetite and taste changes	Anxiety
Voice changes	Amenorrhoea
Insomnia	Lack of confidence
Skin and nail changes	Guilt
Itching	Poor concentration
Hair loss	Poor memory
Painful joints	Social isolation
Peripheral neuropathy	Sexual problems (Impotence/libido)

See also:
Outreach support, p8.

Patient safety

The nature of critical illness makes patients particularly vulnerable. They often cannot communicate or react normally to protect themselves. Normal defence mechanisms are breached by various tubes and catheters, increasing the risk of infection. Complex drug treatment regimens increase the risk of adverse reactions. Immobility increases the risk of muscle wasting or thromboembolism. It can be unclear whether deterioration in a patient's condition is a result of the disease or the treatment.

Protection in a complex environment

The critical care team must deal with an increasing array of data on multiple organ systems, support devices, monitors, treatment, and evidence on which to make decisions. Without some decision support aids, it is easy to miss some issues, with patient harm as a possible consequence. Decision support in its simplest form includes aide memoires to remind the team of what they should be doing. The Fast Hug mnemonic described in the table opposite is one such tool to ensure some of the basics of critical care are not forgotten. Other aides include communication sheets and structured record systems.

One of the most common causes of treatment error relates to drug prescription and administration. Electronic prescribing from templates will reduce errors associated with poor handwriting but these are not foolproof.

Learning from mistakes

Learning from mistakes is fundamental to the improvement of patient safety. Incident reporting systems are now widespread amongst Critical Care Units to:

- Ensure action is taken to prevent similar incidents in the future.
- Fulfill legal duties to report certain kinds of accident, violent incidents, dangerous occurrences, and occupational ill health.
- Ensure accurate information is collected to identify trends and take steps to prevent similar incidents from re-occurring.
- Provide evidence in pursuance of litigation claims, both for and against the hospital.
- Record incidents of particular interest for quality assurance, including the ability to demonstrate accident reductions, as part of a risk management strategy.

It is essential that confidentiality is maintained and disciplinary action avoided, except where acts or omissions are malicious, criminal, or constitute gross or repeated misconduct.

Deliberate harm

Because critically ill patients are vulnerable, the possibility of deliberate harm should be borne in mind. In order to protect patients, staff must undergo pre-employment health and criminal records' checks. Staff must be vigilant to ensure visitors are left with no opportunity to harm the patients. There must be clear record keeping and review by all members of the multidisciplinary critical care team to ensure unexpected changes in condition are recognised. Because deliberate harm is uncommon, recognition requires a high index of suspicion.

Fast Hug

Feeding	Oral or enteral preferred to parenteral
Analgesia	The minimum amount to avoid pain
Sedation	The minimum amount to achieve a calm patient
Thromboprohylaxis	Low molecular weight heparin
Head of bed elevated	30° head up if not contraindicated
Ulcer prophylaxis	In patients in whom evidence of benefit
Glucose control	Tight glycaemic control protocol

Key paper

Vincent JL. Give your patient a fast hug (at least) once a day (2005). *Crit Care Med* **33**: 1225–9.

See also:

Fire safety, p16; Clinical goverence, p22; Infection control—general principles, p544; Infection control—dangerous pathogens, p548.

Fire safety

Fires affecting the Critical Care Unit are rare but are particularly difficult in that patients are not easily evacuated; yet their lives depend on services which fire may disrupt. Smoke, while dangerous to staff and the less sick patient who may be breathing spontaneously, is less of a problem to those receiving mechanical ventilation since their fresh gas supply is from outside the affected environment. Therefore, it follows that in the event of fire, the priority is to ensure safety and means of escape for the staff first.

Control of smoke

Smoke and toxic gases are a common association with fire and may, in themselves, be flammable, particularly in association with high concentrations of oxygen. The main techniques for control of smoke include containment (e.g. fire-resisting walls, doors, and seals) and dispersal (e.g. positive pressure air supply), the latter being used in patient areas. The possibility of flammable or toxic fumes should be considered when equipping and furnishing the Critical Care Unit.

Escape from fire

- Escape routes should be well marked and unobstructed.
- The nature of critical illness is such that not all patients can be evacuated.
- The staff should escape first by proceeding to the nearest exit away from the fire.
- Patients should be evacuated in the order of the least sick first.
- Evacuation of patients should be managed by someone trained in the use of breathing apparatus; in most cases, this will be the fire brigade.
- If patients are to be evacuated, they should be moved to a place of safety on the same floor as the Critical Care Unit. Patients should not be moved downstairs (or lifts used) unless first approved by a Fire Officer.
- In the majority of fires, containment will reduce the need for full evacuation.

Preventing fire

- Automatic smoke or heat alarms should be provided in all areas.
- Cooking areas and laboratory areas must be separated from patient areas by fire doors.
- Fire doors are provided to protect staff and patients, and should not be wedged open.
- If a closed door would compromise the care given to patients but is essential to separate fire compartments, then an electro-mechanical device should hold the door open and be disabled by the fire alarm.
- Fire extinguishers and blankets of the appropriate types should be readily available and staff should be properly trained in their use.

Communication

Good communication is essential to the smooth running of the Critical Care Unit. This includes communication between staff, patient, visiting professionals, and relatives.

Patient communication

Critically ill patients may still be able to hear bedside conversations despite sedation or apparent unconsciousness. All procedures should be explained to the patient in simple terms before starting, even if they appear to be unconscious. The patient who is not competent to consent to treatment may still appreciate verbal discussion or explanation.

Multidisciplinary team communication

The multidisciplinary approach to critical care involves medical and non-medical staff in decision-making. Ward rounds are a forum for such interdisciplinary communication, and the specialist leading the round should ensure all present are both truly involved and understand the day's plan. The plan for the day is more likely to succeed if those effecting the plan are involved in setting it. All changes from the plan, whether due to unforeseen emergencies or failure of the patient to respond, should be fully discussed and documented.

Communication with visiting teams

The critical care staff should be responsible for the day-to-day care of critically ill patients, including coordinating the input from various non-Critical Care Unit professionals. The admitting team should be involved in major strategy decisions and should be accompanied to the bedside or relatives' area by a member of the critical care medical staff. They should be encouraged to write a clear note of their thoughts and proposed management plans in the patient records.

Communication with relatives

Relatives are often overwhelmed by the environment of a Critical Care Unit, are worried about the patient, and are easily confused by the information given. Most communication should be face to face, avoiding lengthy discussions on the telephone. Where several people are imparting information, differences in emphasis or content serve to confuse.

- All communication with relatives should be fully documented.
- It is essential the bedside nurse is present when relatives are spoken to since there are often questions and concerns which crop up later that may be directed to that nurse. Relatives have greater contact with the nurses and often build up a relationship with them.
- Where admitting teams need to communicate with relatives about a specific aspect of the illness, the bedside nurse and, ideally, a member of the Critical Care Unit medical staff, should be present.
- Most interviews with relatives should be away from the bedside although it is often helpful to impart simple information at the bedside, particularly to demonstrate particular issues. Again, it must be remembered that the patient may hear the conversation.
- While it is preferable to interview all relatives together, this is not always practical. Information changes when delivered second-hand so it may be better to communicate directly with various relatives separately in these circumstances.

Key paper

Pronovost P, Berenholtz S, Dorman T, et al. (2003) Improving communication in the ICU using daily goals. *J Crit Care* **18**: 71–5.

Medicolegal aspects

The Critical Care Unit is a source of many medicolegal problems. Patients are often not competent to consent to treatment. They may be admitted following trauma, violence, or poisoning, all of which may involve a legal process. Admission may also follow complications of treatment or medical mishaps occurring elsewhere in the hospital. The nature of critical illness is such that complications are common and litigation may follow.

Consent and agreement

Many procedures in critical care are invasive or involve significant risk. The patient is often not competent to consent for such treatment and, in many countries, surrogate consent or assent cannot be legally given by the next of kin. Nevertheless, it is, important that the risks and benefits of any major or risky procedure are explained to the next of kin and that this discussion is documented in the case records. For major decisions, particularly those involving withdrawal or withholding of life-prolonging treatments, the patient should ideally be involved in discussions. If not feasible, relatives should be asked to give their view of what the patient would want in this situation although their views should not necessarily dictate decisions, responsibility for which lies with medical staff.

Research presents consent problems in the critically ill and requires close ethical committee supervision.

Note-keeping

It is impossible to record everything that happens in critical care in the patients' notes. The 24h observation chart provides the most detailed record of what has happened but summary notes are essential. Such notes must be factual without unsubstantiated opinions about the patient or about previous treatment. All entries must be timed and signed. Records of ward rounds must include the name of the consultant leading the round. These notes may be used later in legal proceedings; they may be used against you but, if well kept, will usually form the best defence.

Errors and mishaps

In the event of an error or mishap, the episode should be clearly documented after witnessed explanation to the patient and/or relatives. An apology is not an admission of liability but is usually much appreciated, as is explanation in an open and transparent manner.

Dealing with the police

Most police enquiries relate to patients who are admitted after suspicious circumstances. While there is a duty to maintain patient confidentiality, it may be in the patient's interests to impart information about them. This may be with the consent of the patient or the next of kin. Written statements or verbal information may be requested. Any information given should be strictly factual, avoiding opinion.

Dealing with the Coroner

The Coroner must be informed of any death where a death certificate cannot be issued. Death certificates can be issued where the death is due to a natural cause and the patient has been seen professionally by the doctor within 14 days prior to death. The table opposite documents the conditions requiring the Coroner to be informed. Where there is any doubt, the Coroner should be consulted.

Deaths which must be notified to HM Coroner in the UK

No doctor attending within prior 14 days
Death without recovery from anaesthesia
Suicide
Sudden or unexplained death
Medical mishap
Industrial accident or disease or related to employment
Violence, accident, or misadventure
Suspicious circumstances
Alcoholism
Poisoning
Death in custody or shortly after detention

Clinical governance

Clinical governance is a framework through which health care organisations are accountable for continuously improving the quality of their services and safeguarding high standards of care by creating an environment in which excellence in clinical care will flourish. For critical care, clinical governance requires the culture, systems, and support mechanisms to achieve good clinical performance and ensure quality improvement is embedded into the unit's routine. This includes action to ensure risks are managed, adverse effects are rapidly detected, openly investigated, and lessons learned, that good practice is rapidly disseminated and that systems are in place to ensure continuous improvements in clinical care. There must be systems to ensure all clinicians have the right education, training, skills, and competencies to deliver the care needed by patients. There must also be systems in place to recognise and act on poor performance.

The Critical Care Unit interfaces with most of the rest of the hospital and its clinical governance arrangements must contribute to patient care throughout the hospital. Some aspects of critical illness are managed outside the Critical Care Unit, yet the critical care team retains responsibility for ensuring quality and safety of this care.

Essential components of clinical governance

Clear management arrangements
Everyone must know who they are accountable to, the limits of their decision-making, and who must be informed in the decision-making process.

Quality improvement
Through the process of clinical audit, the standard of practice is monitored and changes effected to improve quality.

Clinical effectiveness
Evidence-based practice is essential where sound evidence exists to support clinical decisions. Protocols and guidelines standardise practice.

Risk assessment and management
A register of clinical risks should be kept, to which new risks are appended as they are assessed. An action plan should be developed for managing each risk and its implementation monitored.

Staff and organisational development
Including continued professional education, clinical supervision, and professional regulation.

Patient input
Complaints monitoring should be used to learn lessons and improve practice within Intensive Care Unit (ICU). Patients' and relatives' suggestions and surveys can be used to adapt quality initiatives to the needs of patients.

See also:
Audit, p24.

Audit

Audit has become an essential part of medical practice. The main purpose is to improve quality of care. In the Critical Care Unit, this should involve all members of the multidisciplinary team. Change in practice in one discipline will inevitably have a knock-on effect in others. Audit may involve a review of activity, performance against pre-determined indicators or cost-effectiveness. Audit may focus on specific topics or may encompass the performance of several Critical Care Units. A successful audit requires commitment from senior staff to ensure practice is defined, data are collected, and change is effected where necessary. Where change is suggested by audit, a further review is required to ensure that such change has occurred.

Data collection

Ideally, a basic dataset should be common to all Critical Care Units nationally to allow meaningful comparisons to be made. This requires a dataset detailed enough to answer questions posed, but not so detailed that collection becomes unsustainable. Resources must be provided in terms of computer databases and staff to collect and analyse data. This is a skilled task that should not be delegated to junior team members. The data collector should be familiar with the fundamentals of critical care medicine, and be provided with regular summary reviews to ensure enthusiasm continues and quality control is maintained. Methods of data entry should consider the time involved and that most of those collecting data are not keyboard experts. Typographical mistakes destroy the value of collected data so error trapping and data validation must form part of the housekeeping in any database used. Some audit topics require data collection outside the basic dataset. Collecting appropriate data requires clarity in setting the question to be answered and care in choosing data items that will truly answer the question.

Audit meetings

Regular audit meetings should follow a pre-defined timetable. This helps to ensure maximum staff attendance and also sets target dates for data collection and analysis. Audit meetings should be chaired and have defined aims. Discussion of the topic being audited must lead to recommended changes in practice and these must be followed through after the meeting. It is clear that all staff cannot attend all meetings. Dissemination of information prior to implementing proposed changes is necessary to stand some chance of carrying them through.

See also:
Clinical governance, p22.

Critical care scoring systems

Various critical care scoring systems have evolved to provide:
- An index of disease severity, e.g. APACHE, SAPS.
- An index of workload and consumption of resources, e.g. TISS.
- A means of comparison for:
  - auditing performance—either in the same unit or between units.
  - research, e.g. evaluating new products or treatment regimens.
  - patient management objectives, e.g. sedation, pressure area care.

The Glasgow coma scale apart, no scoring system is practised universally. APACHE is the predominant severity score used in the USA and UK while SAPS is more popular in mainland Europe. Inter-user interpretation of the same scoring system can be highly variable.

TISS (Therapeutic intervention scoring system)

- A score is given to procedures and techniques performed on an individual patient (e.g. use and number of vasoactive drug infusions, renal replacement therapy, administering enteral nutrition).
- Some units use TISS to cost individual patients by attaching a monetary value to each TISS point scored.
- It can be used as an index of workload activity.
- A discharge TISS score can be used to estimate the amount of nursing interventions required for a patient in step-down facilities or in the general ward.
- TISS does not accurately measure nursing workload activity as it fails to cater for tasks and duties such as coping with the irritable or confused patient, dealing with grieving relatives, etc.

SoPRA (System of patient-related activities)

The SoPRA score is intended to indicate the scope of care (medical, nursing, and other) provided to critically ill patients to assess the intensity of the impact that each patient makes on the daily workload of the Critical Care Unit.

Glasgow coma scale

First described in 1974, it utilises eye opening, best motor response, and best verbal response to categorise neurological status (see table opposite). It is the only system used universally in Critical Care Units though limitations exist in mechanically ventilated, sedated patients. It can be used for prognostication and is often used for therapeutic decision-making, e.g. elective ventilation in patients presenting with a GCS <8.

Sedation

A variety of systems gauges and records the level of sedation in a mechanically ventilated patient. They assist staff to titrate the dose of sedatives to avoid either over- or under-sedation. The forerunner, developed in 1974, was the Ramsay Sedation Score. This is a 6-point scoring system separated into three awake and three asleep levels where the patient responds to a tap or loud auditory stimulus with either brisk, sluggish, or no response at all. The main problem lies in achieving reproducibility of the tap or loud auditory stimulus. We currently use an 8-point system developed in-house (UCLH sedation scale) (see table opposite).

Glasgow coma scale

Score	Eyes open	Best motor response	Best verbal response
6	–	Obeys commands	–
5	–	Localises pain	Orientated
4	Spontaneously	Flexion withdrawal	Confused
3	To speech	Decerebrate flexion	Inappropriate words
2	To pain	Decerebrate extension	Incomprehensible sounds
1	Never	No response	Silent

Key paper
Teasdale G, Jennet B (1974). Assessment of coma and impared consciousness: a practical scale. *Lancet* **2**: 81–4.

UCLH sedation scale

3	Agitated and restless
2	Awake and uncomfortable
1	Aware but calm
0	Roused by voice, remains calm
–1	Roused by movement
–2	Roused by noxious or painful stimuli
–3	Unrousable
A	Natural sleep

APACHE scoring

- The APACHE (Acute physiology and chronic health evaluation) score utilises a point score derived from the degree of abnormality of readily obtainable physiological and laboratory variables in the first 24h of ICU admission, plus extra points for age and chronic ill health.
- The summated score provides a measure of severity while the percentage risk of subsequent death can be computed from specific coefficients applied to a wide range of admission disorders (excluding burns and cardiac surgery).
- APACHE I, first described in 1981, utilised 34 physiological and biochemical variables.
- A simplified version (APACHE II) utilising just 12 variables was published in 1985 and extensively validated in different countries.

A further refinement published in 1990, APACHE III, claims to improve upon the statistical predictive power by adding five new physiological variables (albumin, bilirubin, glucose, urea, urine output), changing thresholds and weighting of existing variables, comparing both admission and 24h scores, incorporating the admission source (e.g. ward, operating theatre), and reassessing effects of age, chronic health, and specific disease category. Wide acceptance of APACHE III may be limited as its risk stratification system is proprietary and has to be purchased.

Key paper

Knaus WA, Draper EA, Wagner DP, et al. (1985) APACHE II: a severity of disease classification system. *Crit Care Med* **13**: 818–29.

Acute physiology score

+4	+3	+2	+1	0	+1	+2	+3	+4
Core temperature (°C)								
≥41	39–40.9		38.2–38.9	36–38.4	34–35.9	32–33.9	30–31.9	≤29.9
Mean BP (mmHg)								
≥160	130–159	110–129		70–109		50–69		≤49
Heart rate (bpm)								
≥180	140–179	110–139		70–109		55–69	40–54	≤39
Respiratory rate (/min)								
≥50	35–49		25–34	12–24	10–11	6–9		≤5
If FIO2≥0.5: A–aDO2 (mmHg)								
≥500	350–499	200–349		<200				
If FIO2<0.5: PaO2 (mmHg)								
				>70	61–70		55–60	≤55
Arterial pH								
≥7.7	7.6–7.69		7.5–7.59	7.33–7.49		7.25–7.32	7.15–7.24	≤7.15
Serum Na+ (mmol/L)								
≥180	160–179	155–159	150–154	130–149		120–129	111–119	≤110
Serum K+ (mmol/l)								
≥7	6–6.9		5.5–5.9	3.5–5.4	3–3.4	2.5–2.9		<2.5
Serum creatinine (µmol/L) (NB. double points score if acute renal failure)								
≥300	171–299	121–170		50–120		<50		
Haematocrit (%)								
≥60		50–59.9	46–49.9	30–45.9		20–29.9		<20
Leukocytes (/mm3)								
≥40		20–39.9	15–19.9	3–14.9		1–2.9		<1
Neurological points = 15 (Glasgow coma score)								

Age points

Years	≤44	45–54	55–64	65–74	≥75
Points	0	2	3	5	6

Chronic health points

Two points for elective post-operative admission or five points if emergency operation or non-operative admission, if patient has either:
- Biopsy-proven cirrhosis, portal hypertension, or previous hepatic failure.
- Chronic heart failure (NYHA Grade 4).
- Chronic hypoxia, hypercapnia, severe exercise limitation, 2° polycythaemia, or pulmonary hypertension.
- Dialysis-dependent renal disease.
- Immunosuppression by disease or drugs.

SAPS score

- Has a similar role to APACHE II, but more widely utilised in mainland Europe; the Simplified Acute Physiology Score (SAPS) was devised by LeGall *et al.* in 1984 (SAPS I) and modified by the same group in 1993 (SAPS II).
- As for APACHE II, burns and cardiac surgical patients are excluded from analysis.
- The original version used 14 readily measured clinical and biochemical variables while the updated version, SAPS II, comprises 12 physiology variables, age, type of admission (medical, scheduled, or unscheduled surgical), and three underlying disease variables (see table opposite).
- A point score is based on the degree and prognostic importance of derangement of these variables in the first 24h following ICU admission. The point scoring was assigned following logistic regression modelling of data obtained from 8,369 patients in 137 adult ICUs in both Europe and North America and validated in a further 4,628 patients.
- The claimed advantage of this system is that it estimates the risk of death without having to specify a primary diagnosis.

Key paper

Le Gall JR, Lemeshow S, Saulnier F. (1993) A new Simplified Acute Physiology Score (SAPS II) based on a European/North American multicentre study. *JAMA* **270**: 2957–63.

SAPS II score

Age	<40 (0); 40–59 (7); 60–69 (12); 70–74 (15); 75–79 (16); ≥80 (18)
Heart rate (bpm)	<40 (11); 40–69 (2); 70–119 (0); 120–159 (4); ≥160 (7)
Systolic BP (mmHg)	<70 (13); 70–99 (5); 100–199 (0); ≥200 (2)
Body temp (°C)	<39 (0); ≥39 (3)
PaO_2/FIO_2 (kPa) if ventilated/CPAP	<13.3 (11); 13.3–26.5 (9); ≥26.6 (6)
Urine output (L/d)	<0.5 (11); 0.5–0.999 (4); ≥1 (0)
Serum urea (mmol/L)	<10 (0); 10–29.9 (6); ≥30 (10)
White cell count (/mm³)	<1 (12); 1–19.9 (0); ≥20 (3)
Serum K^+ (mmol/L)	<3 (3); 3–4.9 (0); ≥5 (3)
Serum Na^+ (mmol/L)	<125 (5); 125–144 (0); ≥145 (1)
Serum HCO_3^- (mmol/L)	<15 (6); 15–19 (3); ≥20 (0)
Serum bilirubin (μmol/L)	<68.4 (0); 68.4–102.5 (4); ≥102.6 (9)
Glasgow coma score	<6 (26); 6–8 (13); 9–10 (7); 11–13 (5); 14–15 (0)
Chronic disease	Metastatic cancer (9); haematological malignancy (10); AIDS (17)
Type of admission	Scheduled surgical (0); medical (6); unscheduled surgical (8)

Point score in brackets

SOFA score

A limitation of the APACHE and SAPS scoring systems is that they were designed and validated on data obtained during the first 24h of intensive care admission. Various systems have been developed to enable daily scoring (e.g. Sequential Organ Failure Assessment (SOFA), Riyadh Intensive Care Program (RIP) score, Multiple Organ Dysfunction Score (MODS), etc.) to allow a better assessment of change in the patient's condition.

As the physiological and biochemical status of the patient is determined in part by the disease severity, but also by the degree of medical intervention, these sequential scoring systems incorporate the use of various therapies and procedures.

The SOFA system was initially designed to improve patient characterisation for multicentre drug trials in sepsis (SOFA initially stood for 'Sepsis organ failure assessment'), but has subsequently been applied to intensive care patients in general, with 'Sequential' being substituted for 'Sepsis'.

Although it has not been validated in the sense that a point score denoting severity of dysfunction in one organ system does not translate directly to an equivalent severity in another organ, it has been used successfully to prognosticate and to follow changes in patient status throughout their intensive care stay (see table opposite).

Key paper

Moreno R, Vincent JL, Matos R, et al. (1999) The use of maximum SOFA score to quantify organ dysfunction/failure in intensive care. Results of a prospective, multicentre study. Working Group on Sepsis related Problems of the ESICM. *Intensive Care Med* **25**: 686–96.

SOFA score

	0	1	2	3	4
Respiratory $PaO_2:FIO_2$ ratio (mmHg)	>400	>400	≤300	≤200[*]	<100[*]
Renal Creatinine (mg/dL) or urine output (mL/d)	<1.2	1.2–1.9	2.0–3.4	3.5–4.9 or <500mL/d	≤5.0 or <200mL/d
Hepatic Bilirubin (mg/dL)	<1.2	1.2–1.9	2.0–5.9	6.0–11.9	12.0
Cardiovascular Mean arterial pressure (mmHg)	No hypotension	MAP >70	Dopamine ≤5 or dobutamine (any dose)[†]	Dopamine >5 or epinephrine ≤0.1 epinephrine ≤0.1[†]	Dopamine >15 or epinephrine >0.1 epinephrine >0.1[†]
Haematological Platelet count ($\times10^3/mm^3$)	>150	<150	≤100	≤50	≤20
Neurological Glasgow coma score	15	13–14	10–12	6–9	<6

[*] With ventilatory support; [†] Adrenergic agents administered for at least 1h (doses in mcg/kg/min).

Conversion factors

- $PaO_2:FIO_2$ to kPa: divide by 7.5.
- Creatinine to μmol/L: multiply by 88.
- Bilirubin to μmol/L: multiply by 17.1.

Trauma score

Scoring systems have been developed in trauma for:
- Rapid field triage to direct the patient to appropriate levels of care.
- Quality assurance.
- Developing and improving trauma care systems by categorising patients and identifying problems within the systems.
- Making comparisons between groups from different hospitals, in the same hospital over time, and/or undergoing different treatments.

The Injury severity score (ISS) is a severity scoring for patients based on the anatomical injuries sustained. The Revised trauma score (RTS) utilises measures of physiological abnormality to predict survival (see table opposite). A combination of ISS and RTS—TRISS—was developed to overcome the shortcomings of anatomical or physiological scoring alone. The TRISS methodology uses ISS, RTS, patient age, and whether the injury was blunt or penetrating to provide a measure of the probability of survival.

Injury severity score

Use AIS90 (Abbreviated Injury Score 1990) dictionary to score injury. Identify highest abbreviated injury scale score for each of the following:
- Head and neck.
- Abdomen and pelvic contents.
- Bony pelvis and limbs.
- Face.
- Chest.
- Body surface.

Add together the squares of the three highest area scores.

Revised trauma score

	Measure	Coded value	x Weighting	= Score
Respiratory rate (breaths/min)	10–29	4		
	>29	3		
	6–9	2	0.2908	
	1–5	1		
	0	0		
Systolic BP (mmHg)	>89	4		
	76–89	3		
	50–75	2	0.7326	
	1–49	1		
	0	0		
Glasgow coma scale	13–15	4		
	9–12	3		
	6–8	2	0.9368	
	4–5	1		
	3	0		
		Total = revised trauma score		

See also:
Multiple trauma (1), p582; Multiple trauma (2), p584.

Respiratory therapy techniques

Oxygen therapy

All critically ill patients should receive additional inspired O_2 on a 'more not less is best' philosophy.

Principles

- High flow, high concentration O_2 should be given to any acutely dyspnoeic or hypoxaemic patient until accurate titration can be performed using arterial blood gas analysis.
- In general, maintain SaO_2 between 92–98%. Compromises may need to be made during acute on chronic hypoxaemic respiratory failure, or prolonged severe ARDS, when lower values may suffice provided tissue O_2 delivery is maintained.
- When starting mechanical ventilation use a high FIO_2 until accurate titration is performed using arterial blood gas analysis.
- Apart from patients being treated for carbon monoxide poisoning or hyperbaric therapy, e.g. diving accidents, there is no need to maintain supranormal levels of PaO_2. Indeed this may cause harm.

Type II respiratory failure

Patients in chronic type II (hypoxaemic, hypercapnic) respiratory failure may develop apnoea if their central hypoxic drive is removed by supplemental O_2. This is seldom (if ever) abrupt; a period of deterioration and increasing drowsiness will prompt consideration of either (i) FIO_2 reduction if overall condition allows; (ii) non-invasive or invasive mechanical ventilation if fatiguing; or (iii) use of respiratory stimulants such as doxepram. Close supervision and monitoring is necessary.

Oxygen toxicity

This is well described in animal models. Normal volunteers become symptomatic (chest pain, dyspnoea) after several hours of breathing pure O_2. Washout of nitrogen can cause microatelectasis. O_2 may induce direct oxidant damage to proteins, lipids, and DNA, and is a potent vasoconstrictor; high levels of PaO_2 may paradoxically compromise regional O_2 delivery. The relative importance of O_2 toxicity to the lung compared to other forms of ventilator trauma in critically ill patients remains unclear. Efforts should be made to minimise FIO_2 whenever possible. Debate continues as to whether FIO_2 or other ventilator settings (e.g. PEEP, V_T, inspiratory pressures) should be reduced first. The authors' present view is to minimise the risks of ventilator trauma and accept progressively lower values of SaO_2/PaO_2 rather than continue with a high FIO_2.

Monitoring

- A normal pulse oximetry reading may obscure deteriorating gas exchange and progressive hypercapnia.
- An O_2 analyser in the inspiratory limb of the ventilator or CPAP/BiPAP circuit confirms the patient is receiving a known FIO_2. Some ventilators have built-in calibration devices.
- Adequacy and any changes in arterial O_2 saturation can be monitored continuously by pulse oximetry and intermittently with laboratory blood gas analysis.

Oxygen masks

- Hudson-type masks or nasal 'spectacles' give an imprecise FIO_2 and should only be used when hypoxaemia is not a major concern. Hudson-type masks do allow delivery of humidified gas (e.g. via an 'Aquapak'). Valves fitted to the Aquapak system do not deliver an accurate FIO_2 unless gas flow is at the recommended level.
- Masks fitted with a Venturi valve deliver a reasonably accurate FIO_2 (0.24 at 2L/min, 0.28 at 4L/min, 0.35 at 8L/min, 0.40 at 10L/min, 0.60 at 15L/min) except in patients with very high inspiratory flow rates. Pure O_2 is delivered via a fixed jet drawing in air from around the jet to give a known dilution of O_2 to the desired concentration. These masks do not allow delivery of humidified gas but are preferable in the short term for dyspnoeic patients as they enable more precise monitoring of PaO_2 /FIO_2 ratios.
- A tight-fitting anaesthetic mask and reservoir bag allows 100% O_2 to be delivered.

Airway maintenance

The airway may become occluded by secretions, vomitus, blood, or foreign body. Reduced muscle tone in the obtunded patient may result in occlusion by the tongue and surrounding structures.

Opening the airway

- Clear secretions, vomitus, debris, or blood with a Yankauer sucker and/or Magill's forceps.
- In the absence of neck injury, and with the patient supine, tilt the head back with one hand on the forehead, and lift the chin with the fingers of the other hand.
- If there is a suspected neck injury or an inadequate airway with the head tilt and chin lift, perform a jaw thrust. With the patient supine, place the fingers behind the angle of the mandible on both sides and lift the mandible forward and upward until the lower teeth (or gum) are in front of the upper teeth (or gum).

Maintaining the airway

If the patient can be turned and is breathing adequately, it may suffice to adopt a lateral recovery position. If manual ventilation is required or the patient must remain supine, an oropharyngeal or nasopharyngeal airway may be used.

Oropharyngeal (Guedel) airway

- This is a hard plastic tube shaped to keep the tongue forward.
- It should only be used in obtunded patients.
- The correct size should be selected by comparing the airway to the distance between the teeth and the angle of the jaw.
- Open the patient's mouth and remove any obstruction by suction.
- Insert the airway into the mouth with the curve pointing toward the skull.
- Rotate the airway through 180° once the soft palate is reached.
- The curve of the airway will retain its position in the oropharynx once fully inserted.

Nasopharyngeal airway

- This soft shaped plastic tube fits the passage from nares to pharynx.
- It is better tolerated in the semi-conscious patient, but should be avoided where there is a suspected/known basal skull fracture.
- Assess the correct size by approximating the diameter of the airway to the diameter of the patient's fifth finger.
- Insert a safety pin through the flange of the airway to prevent accidental inhalation after insertion.
- Pass the lubricated airway into the patent nostril with a slight twisting motion.

See also:
Endotracheal intubation, p42; Basic resuscitation, p338; Airway obstruction, p348.

Endotracheal intubation

Indications

An artificial airway is necessary in the following circumstances:
- Apnoea: provision of mechanical ventilation, e.g. unconsciousness, severe respiratory muscle weakness, self-poisoning.
- Respiratory failure: provision of mechanical ventilation, e.g. ARDS, pneumonia.
- Airway protection: GCS <8, trauma, aspiration risk, poisoning.
- Airway obstruction: maintain airway patency, e.g. trauma, laryngeal oedema, tumour, burns.
- Haemodynamic instability: facilitate mechanical ventilation, e.g. shock, cardiac arrest.

Choice of endotracheal tube

Most adults require a standard high volume, low pressure, cuffed endotracheal tube. Average sized adults require a size 8.0–9.0mm id tube (size 7.5–8.0mm id for females), cut to a length of 23cm (21cm for females). Particular problems with the upper airway, e.g. trauma, oedema, may require a smaller tube. In specific situations, non-standard tubes may be used, e.g. armoured tubes to avoid external compression or double lumen tubes to isolate the right or left lung.

Route of intubation

The usual routes are orotracheal and nasotracheal. Orotracheal intubation is generally preferred. The nasotracheal route has the advantages of increased patient comfort, easier blind placement, and easier to secure the tube. However, there are several disadvantages. The tube is usually smaller, there is a risk of sinusitis and otitis media, and is generally contraindicated in coagulopathy, CSF leak, and nasal/base-of-skull fractures.

Difficult intubation

If predicted, this should not be attempted by an inexperienced, unaccompanied operator except in life-threatening situations. Difficulty may be predicted in patients with a small mouth, high arched palate, large upper incisors, hypognathia, large tongue, anterior larynx, short neck, immobile temporomandibular joints, immobile cervical joints, or morbid obesity. If a difficult intubation presents unexpectedly, the use of a stylet, a straight bladed laryngoscope, a laryngeal mask airway, or a fibreoptic laryngoscope may help. It is important not to persist for too long; revert to bag-and-mask ventilation to ensure adequate oxygenation.

Complications of intubation

Early complications
- Trauma, e.g. haemorrhage, mediastinal perforation.
- Haemodynamic collapse, e.g. positive pressure ventilation, vasodilatation, arrhythmias, or rapid correction of hypercapnia.
- Tube malposition, e.g. failed intubation or endobronchial intubation.

Later complications
- Infection, including maxillary sinusitis if nasally intubated.
- Cuff pressure trauma (avoid by maintaining cuff pressure <25cmH$_2$O).
- Mouth/lip or pharyngeal trauma.

Equipment required

- Suction (Yankauer tip).
- O$_2$ supply, rebreathing bag, and mask.
- Laryngoscope (two curved blades and straight blade).
- Stylet/bougie.
- Endotracheal tubes (preferred size and smaller).
- Water-based gel to lubricate tube.
- Magill forceps.
- Drugs (Induction agent, muscle relaxant, sedative).
- Syringe for cuff inflation.
- Tape to secure tube.
- Capnograph.

See also:

Airway maintenance, p40; Ventilatory support—indications, p44; Airway obstruction, p348; Respiratory failure, p350; Coma, p438; Acute weakness, p440; Poisoning—general principles, p520.

Ventilatory support—indications

Oxygenation failure (Type I respiratory failure)

Hypoxaemia is defined by PaO_2 <11kPa on $FIO_2 \geq 0.4$. May be due to:

- Ventilation/perfusion mismatch (reduced ventilation in, or preferential perfusion of, some lung areas), e.g. pneumonia, pulmonary oedema, pulmonary vascular disease, very high cardiac output.
- Shunt (normal perfusion but absent ventilation in some lung zones), e.g. pneumonia, pulmonary oedema.
- Diffusion limitation (reduced alveolar surface area with normal ventilation), e.g. emphysema, or reduced inspired O_2 tension, e.g. altitude, suffocation.
- Acute ventilatory insufficiency (as above).

Acute ventilatory insufficiency (Type II respiratory failure)

Defined by an acute rise in $PaCO_2$ and significant respiratory acidosis. $PaCO_2$ is directly proportional to the body's CO_2 production and inversely proportional to alveolar ventilation (minute ventilation minus dead space ventilation). Causes include:

- Respiratory centre depression, e.g. drugs or intracranial pathology.
- Peripheral neuromuscular disease, e.g. Guillain-Barré syndrome, myasthenia gravis, or spinal cord pathology.
- Therapeutic muscle paralysis, e.g. as part of balanced anaesthesia, for management of tetanus or status epilepticus.
- Loss of chest wall integrity, e.g. chest trauma, diaphragm rupture.
- High CO_2 production, e.g. burns, sepsis or severe agitation.
- Reduced alveolar ventilation, e.g. airways obstruction (asthma, acute bronchitis, foreign body), atelectasis, pneumonia, pulmonary oedema (ARDS, cardiac failure), pleural pathology, fibrotic lung disease, obesity.
- Pulmonary vascular disease (e.g. pulmonary embolus, ARDS).

To reduce intracranial pressure

Reduction of $PaCO_2$ to approximately 4kPa causes cerebral vasoconstriction, and therefore, reduces intracranial pressure after brain injury. Studies suggest this effect is transient and may impair an already critical cerebral blood flow.

To reduce work of breathing

Assisted ventilation ± sedation and muscle relaxation reduces respiratory muscle activity and the work of breathing. In cardiac failure or non-cardiogenic pulmonary oedema, the resulting reduction in myocardial O_2 demand is more easily matched to the supply of O_2.

Indications for ventilatory support

Consider ventilatory support (invasive or non-invasive) if:
- Respiratory rate >30/min.
- Vital capacity <10–15mL/kg.
- PaO_2 <11kPa on $FIO_2 \geq 0.4$.
- $PaCO_2$ high with significant respiratory acidosis (e.g. pH <7.2).
- V_d/V_T >60%.
- Q_s/Q_t >15–20%.
- Exhaustion.
- Confusion.
- Severe shock.
- Severe LVF.
- Raised ICP.

See also:
Respiratory failure, p350; Acute weakness, p440.

IPPV—description of ventilators

Classification of mechanical ventilators

Modern ventilators deliver a gas flow with a cycling mechanism to cut flow during expiration. They may be classified by the method of cycling from inspiration to expiration, i.e. when a preset time has elapsed (time-cycled), a preset pressure is reached (pressure-cycled), or a preset volume delivered (volume-cycled). The ventilator breath may be volume-controlled (a pre-determined tidal volume (V_T) is delivered), pressure-controlled (gas flow is at a pre-determined pressure), or volume controlled with a limited pressure (the ventilator delivers a preset V_T within a pressure limit unless the lungs are non-compliant or airway resistance is high). The latter is useful to avoid high airway pressures. Various 'mixed' modes are available. In volume-cycled mode with a time limit, the inspiratory flow is reduced; the ventilator delivers the preset V_T unless impossible at the set respiratory rate (limiting airway pressure). In time-cycled mode with pressure control, preset pressure is delivered throughout inspiration with cycling determined by time. V_T is dependent on respiratory compliance and airway resistance.

Setting up the mechanical ventilator

Tidal volume

Values of 6–7mL/kg ideal body weight are related to better outcomes in severe acute respiratory failure, by reducing ventilator-associated trauma and distant inflammatory effects. In severe airflow limitation (e.g. asthma, acute bronchitis), smaller V_T and minute volume may be needed to allow prolonged expiration.

Respiratory rate

Usually set in accordance with V_T to provide minute ventilation of 85–100mL/kg/min. In time-cycled or time-limited modes, the set respiratory rate determines the timing of the ventilator cycles.

Inspiratory flow

Usually set between 40–80L/min. Higher flow rates are more comfortable for alert patients. This allows for longer expiration in patients with severe airflow limitation, but may result in higher peak airway pressures. The flow pattern may be adjusted on most ventilators. A square waveform is often used, but decelerating flow may reduce peak airway pressure.

I:E ratio

A function of respiratory rate, V_T, inspiratory flow, and inspiratory time. Prolonged expiration is useful in severe airflow limitation while a prolonged inspiratory time is used in ARDS to allow slow-reacting alveoli time to fill. Alert patients are more comfortable with shorter inspiratory times and high inspiratory flow rates.

FIO_2

Set according to arterial blood gases. Usual to start at $FIO_2 = 0.6$–1, then adjust according to arterial blood gases and pulse oximetry.

Airway pressure

In pressure-controlled or -limited modes, a peak airway pressure (circuit rather than alveolar pressure) can be set (ideally ≤30cmH$_2$O). PEEP is often increased to maintain FRC when compliance is low.

Initial ventilator set-up

- Check for leaks.
- Check O_2 is flowing.
- FIO_2 0.6–1.
- V_T 5–10mL/kg.
- Rate   10–15/min.
- I:E ratio   1:2.
- Peak pressure   ≤35cmH₂O.
- PEEP   3–5cmH₂O.

Key paper

Acute Respiratory Distress Syndrome Network. (2000) Ventilation with lower tidal volumes compared with traditional tidal volumes for acute lung injury and the acute respiratory distress syndrome. *N Engl J Med* **342**: 1301–8.

See also:

IPPV—modes of ventilation, p48; High frequency jet ventilation, p62; High frequency oscillatory ventilation, p64; Continuous positive airway pressure, p70; Non-invasive respiratory support, p76.

IPPV—modes of ventilation

Controlled mechanical ventilation (CMV)

A preset number of breaths are delivered to supply all the patient's ventilatory requirements. Breaths may be at a preset V_T (volume-controlled) or at a preset inspiratory pressure (pressure-controlled).

Assist-control mechanical ventilation (ACMV)

Patients can breathe, triggering the ventilator to determine the respiratory rate. However, a preset number of breaths are delivered if the spontaneous respiratory rate falls below the preset level.

Intermittent mandatory ventilation (IMV)

A number of breaths are preset, but patients are free to breathe spontaneously in between. Mandatory breaths may be synchronised with spontaneous efforts (synchronised IMV) to avoid mandatory breaths occurring on top of spontaneous breaths ('stacking'). This may lead to excessive V_T, high airway pressure, incomplete exhalation, and air trapping. Positive pressure support may be added to spontaneous breaths to reduce the work of breathing.

Pressure support ventilation (PSV)

A preset positive inspiratory pressure is added to the ventilator circuit during inspiration in spontaneously breathing patients. Preset pressures should be adjusted to an adequate (but not excessive) V_T.

Volume support ventilation (VSV)

A target V_T is set and pressure support is adjusted to achieve the target volume.

Choosing the appropriate mode

Pressure-controlled ventilation avoids the dangers associated with high airway pressure, although it may result in marked changes in V_T if respiratory compliance alters. Allowing the patient to make some spontaneous respiratory effort may reduce sedation requirements, retrain respiratory muscles, and reduce mean airway pressure.

Apnoeic patient

Use of IMV or ACMV in totally apnoeic patients provides total minute volume requirement if the preset rate is high enough (effectively CMV), but allows spontaneous respiratory effort on recovery.

Patient taking limited spontaneous breaths

A guaranteed minimum minute volume is assured with both ACMV and IMV, depending on the preset rate. The work of spontaneous breathing is reduced by supplying the preset V_T for spontaneously triggered breaths with ACMV or by adding pressure support to spontaneous breaths with IMV. With ACMV, the spontaneous tidal volume is guaranteed, whereas with IMV and pressure support, spontaneous tidal volume depends on lung compliance and may be less than preset tidal volume. The advantage of IMV and pressure support is that gradual reduction of preset rate, as spontaneous effort increases, allows a smooth transition to pressure support ventilation. Subsequent weaning is by reduction of pressure support level.

IPPV—adjusting the ventilator

See also:
IPPV—description of ventilators, p46; High frequency jet ventilation, p62; High frequency oscillatory ventilation, p64; Continuous positvie airway pressure, p70; Non-invasive respiratory support, p76.

IPPV—adjusting the ventilator

Adjustments are usually made in response to blood gases, pulse oximetry or capnography, patient agitation or discomfort, or during weaning. 'Migration' of the endotracheal tube, either distally to the carina or beyond, or proximally such that the cuff is at vocal cord level, may result in agitation, excess coughing, and a deterioration in blood gases. Tube migration or obstruction should be considered and rectified before changing ventilator settings or sedative dosing.

The choice of ventilator mode depends upon conscious level, the number of spontaneous breaths being taken, and blood gas values. Many spontaneously breathing patients can cope adequately with pressure support ventilation alone. However, a few intermittent mandatory breaths (SIMV) may be needed to assist gas exchange or slow an excessive spontaneous rate. The paralysed/heavily sedated patient will require either volume- or pressure-controlled mandatory breaths.

The order of change will be dictated by the severity of respiratory failure and individual operator preference. Earlier use of increased PEEP is advocated to recruit collapsed alveoli and thus improve oxygenation in severe respiratory failure.

Low PaO_2 considerations
- Increase FIO_2.
- Increase PEEP (may raise peak airway pressure or reduce cardiac output).
- Increase I:E ratio.
- Consider tolerating low PaO_2 ('permissive hypoxaemia').
- Consider increasing pressure support/pressure control or V_T.
- In CMV, consider increasing sedation ± muscle relaxants.
- Prone ventilation, inhaled nitric oxide.

High PaO_2 considerations
- Decrease FIO_2.
- Decrease I:E ratio.
- Decrease PEEP.
- Decrease level of pressure control/pressure support if V_T adequate.

High $PaCO_2$ considerations
- Consider tolerating high level ('permissive hypercapnia').
- Increase V_T (if low and peak airway pressure allows).
- Increase respiratory rate.
- Reduce rate if too high (to reduce intrinsic PEEP).
- Reduce dead space.
- In CMV, increase sedation ± muscle relaxants.

Low $PaCO_2$ considerations
- Decrease respiratory rate.
- Decrease V_T.

See also:
IPPV—modes of ventilation, p48; IPPV—failure to tolerate ventilation, p52; IPPV—failure to deliver ventilation, p54; IPPV—complications of ventilation, p56; IPPV—weaning techniques, p58; IPPV—assessment of weaning, p60.

IPPV—failure to tolerate ventilation

Agitation or 'fighting the ventilator' may occur at any time. If paralysed or heavily sedated, poor ventilator tolerance may be indicated by hypoxaemia, hypercapnia, ventilator alarms, or cardiovascular instability. The first priority is to assess the patient.

- Is the patient cyanosed?
- Is the chest moving?
- Are breath sounds present and equal?
- Are there abnormal breath sounds?
- Has the SpO_2 changed?

Basic clinical assessment is necessary to judge how serious the problem is and whether immediate resuscitative steps are required. If the problem is serious, the first response must be to disconnect the ventilator and manually ventilate.

Manual ventilation with 100% O_2 and a non-rebreathing bag allows assessment of how difficult it is to inflate the lungs, how long exhalation takes, and whether the problem with ventilation relates to patient (problem persists) or ventilator (problem resolved) factors.

Poor initial tolerance

- Increase FIO_2 to 1.0 and start manual ventilation.
- Check endotracheal tube is correctly positioned and both lungs are being inflated. Consider tube replacement, intra-tracheal obstruction, pneumothorax, or bronchospasm.
- Check ventilator circuit is both intact and patent, and ventilator is functioning correctly. Check ventilator settings, including FIO_2, PEEP, I:E ratio, set tidal volume, respiratory rate, and/or pressure control. Check 'pressure limit' settings as these may be set too low causing ventilator to cycle to expiration prematurely.

Poor tolerance after previous good tolerance

If agitation occurs in a patient who has previously tolerated mechanical ventilation, either the patient's condition has deteriorated, or there is a problem in the ventilator circuit (including artificial airway) or the ventilator itself.

- The patient should be removed from the ventilator and placed on manual ventilation with 100% O_2 while the problem is resolved. Resorting to increased sedation ± muscle relaxation in this circumstance is dangerous until the cause is understood.
- Check patency of the endotracheal tube (e.g. with a suction catheter) and re-intubate if in doubt.
- Consider chest X-ray to identify endotracheal tube malposition (e.g. cuff above vocal cords, tip at carina, tube in main bronchus).
- Seek and treat changes in the patient's condition, e.g. bronchospasm, tension pneumothorax, sputum plug, pain, raised intra-abdominal pressure, pulmonary oedema.
- Where patients are making spontaneous respiratory effort, consider increasing pressure support or adding mandatory breaths.
- If patients fail to synchronise with IMV by stacking spontaneous and mandatory breaths, increasing pressure support and reducing mandatory rate may help. Use of pressure support ventilation may also be appropriate.

See also:

IPPV—modes of ventilation, p48; IPPV—adjusting the ventilator, p50; IPPV—failure to deliver ventilation, p54; IPPV—complications of ventilation, p56; IPPV—weaning techniques, p58; IPPV—assessment of weaning, p60.

IPPV—failure to deliver ventilation

Failure to ventilate despite apparently appropriate ventilator settings and exclusion of patient factors requires assessment of which ventilator settings are not being delivered.

Poor gas exchange

- Increase FIO_2 to 1.0 and start manual ventilation.
- Exclude patient factors.
- Check endotracheal tube is correctly positioned, patent, and both lungs are being inflated. Consider tube replacement.
- Check ventilator circuit is both intact and patent, and ventilator is functioning correctly. Check ventilator settings, including FIO_2, PEEP, I:E ratio, set V_T, respiratory rate and/or pressure control.

Low V_T or low pressure alarm

Expired V_T will be lower than inspired V_T with bronchopleural fistula. In other situations where expired V_T is suddenly significantly lower than inspired V_T, or maintenance of circuit pressure is not possible, there is a leak in the ventilator circuit. The patient should be manually ventilated while the leak is identified and corrected. If the leak persists with manual ventilation, repositioning or replacement of the endotracheal tube is required.

High pressure alarm

A sudden increase in airway pressure indicates a change in resistance to gas flow. After patient factors have been excluded:

- Check patency of the endotracheal tube (e.g. with a suction catheter); re-intubate if in doubt.
- Check patency of ventilator circuit and catheter mount. Look for excessive trapped water partially occluding the catheter mount.
- Check for sputum obstructing the HME.
- Consider a chest X-ray to identify endotracheal tube malposition (e.g. cuff above vocal cords, tip at carina, tube in main bronchus).

See also:

IPPV—modes of ventilation, p48; IPPV—adjusting the ventilator, p50; IPPV—failure to tolerate ventilation, p52; IPPV—complications of ventilation, p56; IPPV—weaning techniques, p58; IPPV—assessment of weaning, p60; Fibreoptic bronchoscopy, p88; Chest physiotherapy, p90; Bronchodilators, p254; Positive end expiratory pressure (1), p66; Positive end expiratory pressure (2), p68.

IPPV—complications of ventilation

Haemodynamic complications

Venous return depends on passive flow from central veins to right atrium. An increase in intrathoracic pressure is transmitted across compliant lungs to increase right atrial pressure and reduce venous return. This is less of a problem with stiff lungs (e.g. ARDS), but will be exacerbated by inverse I:E ratio and high PEEP. As lung volume is increased by IPPV, the pulmonary vasculature is constricted. Pulmonary vascular resistance and diastolic volume of the right ventricle rise and, by septal shift, left ventricular filling is impeded. These effects all contribute to a reduced stroke volume. This can be minimised by reducing airway pressure, avoiding prolonged inspiratory time, and maintaining blood volume.

Ventilator trauma

Barotrauma relates to gas escape into cavities and interstitial tissues during IPPV. Distending volume and high shear stress are probably responsible rather than high pressures. It is most likely to occur with high V_T. It occurs in IPPV and conditions associated with lung overinflation (e.g. asthma). Tension pneumothorax is life-threatening and should be suspected in any patient on IPPV who becomes suddenly agitated, tachycardic, hypotensive, or exhibits sudden deterioration in their blood gases. An immediate chest drainage tube should be inserted if tension pneumothorax develops. Prevention of ventilator trauma relies on avoidance of high V_T and high airway pressures.

Nosocomial infection

Endotracheal intubation bypasses normal defence mechanisms. Ciliary activity and cellular morphology in the tracheobronchial tree are altered. The requirement for endotracheal suction further increases susceptibility to infection. In addition, the normal heat and moisture exchanging mechanisms are bypassed, requiring artificial humidification of inspired gases. Failure to provide adequate humidification increases the risk of sputum retention and infection. Maintaining ventilated patients at 30° upright, head tilt reduces the incidence of nosocomial pneumonia.

Acid–base disturbance

Over-ventilating patients with chronic respiratory failure may, by rapid correction of hypercapnia, cause respiratory alkalosis. This reduces pulmonary blood flow and may contribute to hypoxaemia. Respiratory acidosis due to hypercapnia may be due to inappropriate ventilator settings or may be desired to avoid high V_T and ventilator trauma.

Water retention

Vasopressin released from the anterior pituitary is increased due to a reduction in intrathoracic blood volume and psychological stress. Reduced urine flow thus contributes to water retention. In addition, the use of PEEP reduces lymphatic flow with consequent peripheral oedema, especially affecting the upper body. High airway pressure reduces venous return, again contributing to oedema.

Respiratory muscle wasting

Prolonged ventilation may lead to disuse atrophy of the respiratory muscles with subsequent weaning difficulty.

IPPV—weaning techniques

See also:

IPPV—modes of ventilation, p48; IPPV—adjusting the ventilator, p50; IPPV—failure to tolerate ventilation, p52; IPPV—failure to deliver ventilaion, p54; High frequency jet ventilation, p62; Positive end expiratory pressure (1), p66; Positive end expiratory pressure (2), p68.

IPPV—weaning techniques

Patients may require all or part of their respiratory support to be provided by a mechanical ventilator. Weaning from mechanical ventilation may follow several patterns. In patients ventilated for short periods (no more than a few days), it is common to allow 20–30min breathing on a 'T' piece before removing the endotracheal tube. For patients who have received longer term ventilation, it is unlikely that mechanical support can be withdrawn suddenly; several methods are commonly used to wean these patients from mechanical ventilation. There is no strong evidence that any technique is superior in terms of weaning success.

Intermittent 'T' piece or continuous positive airway pressure (CPAP)

Spontaneous breathing is allowed for increasingly prolonged periods with a rest on mechanical ventilation in between. The use of a 'T' piece for longer than 30min may lead to basal atelectasis since the endotracheal tube bypasses the physiological PEEP effect of the larynx. Therefore, it is common to use 5cmH$_2$O CPAP as spontaneous breathing periods get longer. In the early stages of weaning, mechanical ventilation is often continued at night to encourage sleep, avoid fatigue, and rest respiratory muscles.

Intermittent mandatory ventilation (IMV)

The set mandatory rate is gradually reduced as the spontaneous rate increases. Spontaneous breaths are usually pressure-supported to overcome circuit and ventilator valve resistance. With this technique, it is important that the patient's required minute ventilation is provided by the combination of mandatory breaths and spontaneous breaths without an excessive spontaneous rate. The reduction in mandatory rate should be slow enough to maintain adequate minute ventilation. It is also important that the patient can synchronise his own respiratory efforts with mandatory ventilator breaths; many cannot, particularly where there are frequent spontaneous breaths, some of which may 'stack' with mandatory breaths causing hyperinflation.

Pressure support ventilation

All respiratory efforts are spontaneous but positive pressure is added to each breath, the level being chosen to maintain an appropriate tidal volume. Weaning is performed by a gradual reduction of the pressure support level while the respiratory rate is <30/min. The patient is extubated or allowed to breathe with 5cmH$_2$O CPAP when pressure support is minimal (<10–15cmH$_2$O with modern ventilators).

Choice of ventilator

Modern ventilators have enhancements to aid weaning; however, weaning most patients from ventilation is possible with a basic ventilator and the intermittent 'T' piece technique, provided an adequate fresh gas flow is provided. If IMV and/or pressure support are used, the ventilator should provide the features listed in the table opposite.

Key features in the choice of ventilator

- Ventilator must allow patient triggering (i.e. not a minute volume divider).
- Fresh gas flow must be greater than spontaneous peak inspiratory flow.
- Minimum circuit resistance (short, wide bore, and smooth internal lumen).
- Low resistance ventilator valves.
- Sensitive pressure or flow trigger (ideally monitored close to the ET tube).
- Synchronised IMV (avoids 'stacking' mandatory on spontaneous breaths).

See also:

IPPV—modes of ventilation, p48; IPPV—assessment of weaning, p60; Continuous positive airway pressure, p70; Non-invasive respiratory support, p76.

IPPV—assessment of weaning

Prior to weaning, it is important that the cause of respiratory failure and any complications arising have been corrected.

- Sepsis should be eradicated as should factors that increase O_2 demand.
- Attention is required to nutrition, fluid and electrolyte balance.
- The diaphragm should be allowed to contract unhindered by choosing the optimum position for breathing (sitting up unless the diaphragm is paralysed) and ensuring that intra-abdominal pressure is not high. Adequate analgesia must be provided.
- Sedatives are often withdrawn by this point, but may still be needed in specific situations, e.g. residual agitation, raised intracranial pressure.

Weaning should start after adequate explanation has been given to the patient. Factors predicting weaning success are detailed in the table opposite. Spontaneous (pressure-supported) breathing should generally start as soon as possible to allow a reduction in sedation levels and to maintain respiratory muscle function. Weaning with the intention of removing mechanical support is unlikely to be successful while FIO_2 >0.4.

Continuous pulse oximetry and regular clinical review are essential during weaning. Arterial blood gases should be taken after 20–30min of spontaneous breathing. After short-term ventilation, extubate if arterial gases and respiratory pattern remain satisfactory, the cough reflex is adequate, and the patient can clear sputum. Patients being weaned from longer-term ventilation (>1wk) should generally be allowed to breathe spontaneously for at least 24h before extubation.

Indications for re-ventilation

If spontaneous respiration is discoordinate or the patient is exhausted, agitated, or clammy, the ventilator should be reconnected. Successful weaning is more easily accomplished if excessive fatigue is not allowed to set in. Tachypnoea (>30/min), tachycardia (>110/min), respiratory acidosis (pH <7.2), rising $PaCO_2$, and hypoxaemia (SaO_2 <90%) should all prompt reconnection of the ventilator.

Factors associated with weaning failure

Failure to wean is associated with:

- Increased O_2 cost of breathing.
- Muscle fatigue (malnutrition, peripheral neuropathy or myopathy, drugs, (e.g. muscle relaxants, aminoglycosides), and electrolyte abnormalities (e.g. low Mg^{2+}, K^+, and perhaps phosphate).
- Inadequate respiratory drive (alkalosis, opiates, sedatives, malnutrition, cerebrovascular accident, coma).
- Inadequate cardiac reserve and heart failure.

In the latter case, monitor cardiac function during spontaneous breathing periods. Any deterioration in cardiac function should be treated aggressively (e.g. optimal fluid therapy, vasodilators, inotropes). Early muscle fatigue due to prolonged disuse requires regular and controlled exercise after correction of nutritional deficit. Weaning should be stopped during periods when exercise is provided. Patients who are building up muscle on an exercise programme may also benefit from rest periods at night so that the time free of mechanical ventilator support is gradually increased.

Factors predicting weaning success

- PaO_2 >11kPa on FIO_2 = 0.4 (PaO_2/FIO_2 ratio >27.5kPa).
- Minute volume <12L/min.
- Vital capacity >10mL/kg.
- Maximum inspiratory force (PImax) >20cmH$_2$O.
- Respiratory rate/tidal volume <100.
- Q_s/Q_t <15%.
- Dead space/tidal volume <60%.
- Haemodynamic stability.
- A ratio of respiratory rate to tidal volume (f/V$_T$, shallow breathing index) ≤105 has a 78% positive predictive value for successful weaning.

Key paper

Yang KL, Tobin MJ. (1991) A prospective study of indexes predicting the outcome of trials of weaning from mechanical ventilation. *N Engl J Med* **324**: 1445–50.

See also:

IPPV—weaning techniques, p58; Pluse oximetry, p144; CO$_2$ monitoring, p146; Pulmonary function tests, p148; Blood gas analysis, p154.

High frequency jet ventilation

- High frequency jet ventilation (HFJV) involves a high pressure jet of gas entraining further fresh gas which is directed by the jet towards the lungs.
- Respiratory rates of 100–300/min ensure minute ventilation of about 20L/min although tidal volume may be lower than dead space. CO_2 elimination is usually more efficient than conventional IPPV.
- The method of gas exchange is not fully elucidated, but includes turbulent gas mixing and convection.
- Oxygenation is dependent on mean airway pressure. Peak airway pressures are lower than with conventional mechanical ventilation, but auto-PEEP and mean airway pressures are maintained.
- SaO_2 often falls when starting HFJV, but usually improves with time.
- The high gas flow rates employed require additional humidification (30–100mL/h); this is usually nebulised with the jet.

Indications

Bronchopleural fistula is the only proven ICU indication for HFJV. It may assist weaning from mechanical ventilation as the open circuit allows spontaneous breaths without the drawbacks of demand valves. HFJV also ensures adequate ventilation if the patient fails to breathe adequately. Reducing the driving pressure and increasing the respiratory rate may facilitate weaning further. In ARDS, conventional ventilation can lead to ventilator trauma if a high V_T is used. HFJV avoids problems associated with high V_T, but is often unable to provide adequate ventilation in isolation for patients with severe ARDS.

Setting up HFJV

- A jet must be provided via a modified endotracheal tube or catheter mount. Entrainment gas is provided via a T-piece.
- V_T cannot be set directly, but is altered by adjusting jet size, I:E ratio, driving pressure, and respiratory rate from inbuilt algorithms.
- Respiratory rate is usually set between 100–200/min. As the rate increases at a constant driving pressure, $PaCO_2$ may increase (increasing PEEPi increases effective physiological dead space).
- The I:E ratio is usually set between 1:3 and 1:2. V_T is determined by airway pressure and I:E ratio.
- Driving pressure is usually set between 1–2bar. These pressures are much higher than the 60–100cmH$_2$O used in conventional ventilation. PEEPi is related to the driving pressure, I:E ratio, and respiratory rate.
- External PEEP may be added to increase mean airway pressure should this be necessary to improve oxygenation.

Combined HFJV and conventional CMV

May be useful in conditions of poor lung compliance where HFJV alone cannot provide adequate gas exchange. Low frequency pressure limited ventilation with PEEP provides an adequate mean airway pressure to ensure oxygenation while CO_2 clearance is effected by HFJV. Care must be taken to avoid excessive peak airway pressure when HFJV and CMV breaths stack.

Adjusting HFJV according to blood gases

Increasing PaO$_2$
- Increase FIO$_2$.
- Increase I:E ratio.
- Increase driving pressure.
- Add external PEEP.
- Consider reducing respiratory rate.

Decreasing PaCO$_2$
- Increase driving pressure.
- Decrease respiratory rate.

See also:

IPPV—description of ventilators, p46; IPPV—modes of ventilation, p48; High frequency oscillatory ventilation, p64; Positive end expiratory pressure (1), p66; Positive end expiratory pressure (2) p68; Acute respiratory distress syndrome (1), p360; Acute respiratory disress syndrome (2), p362; Pneumothorax, p368.

High frequency oscillatory ventilation

High frequency oscillation (HFO) is an extreme form of standard ventilation with high rates, sub-deadspace tidal volumes (1–3mL/kg), and significantly higher levels of PEEP (equal to the continuous distending pressure or mean airway pressure during HFO). It may thus be viewed as a CPAP device that allows generation of pressure oscillations around a continuous distending pressure eliminating CO_2 by accelerating molecular diffusion processes. Precise mechanisms of action on gas exchange are uncertain. Whereas bulk convection and diffusion predominate, during standard ventilation, HFO may provide:

- Inter-regional gas mixing between respiratory units with different time constants (Pendelluft ventilation).
- Convective transport from asymmetric inspiratory and expiratory velocity profiles.
- Longitudinal dispersion via interaction between the axial velocity profile and the radial concentration gradient.

During HFO, high frequencies (180–360bpm = 3–6Hz) generally maintain normal $PaCO_2$ levels. At lower frequencies (3Hz), CO_2 clearance usually improves because of the larger V_T generated. CO_2 clearance can also be enhanced by higher proximal driving pressures (range 60–90cmH$_2$O) and longer inspiratory times (range 30–50%)—both have a similar effect on V_T.

Indications

This technique is used as a rescue therapy for refractory hypoxaemia or ventilatory failure in ARDS. It is now being considered as an early strategy in patients with milder forms of acute lung injury to prevent further deterioration. However, there are no controlled data showing superiority over conventional techniques. Theoretically, low V_T and high PEEP in HFO reduce the risk of cyclical alveolar collapse and over-distension, both important factors in ventilator-induced lung injury (VILI). The higher mean airway pressure, but lower cycling and plateau pressures, will also improve oxygenation and allow reduction in the FIO_2.

Lung recruitment can often be achieved by temporarily increasing lung volumes by a stepwise increase in continuous distending pressure to an oxygenation or chest X-ray target.

The incidence of pneumothorax is thought to be similar to conventional ventilation in adults. HFO may reduce the size of an air leak and promote healing by reducing high peak airway pressures and the alveolar–pleural pressure gradient. Reducing the diameter of the leak increases resistance to gas flow and this facilitates lung healing. Changes in mean airway pressure will result in the greatest percentage change in the size of the air leak.

Potential problems with HFO

- Inability to maintain spontaneous breathing such that the patient often requires heavy sedation ± paralysis. Novel technical developments incorporating a flow-demand system to enable flow compensation may reduce the imposed work of breathing, increase patient comfort, and allow continued spontaneous breathing.
- Haemodynamic compromise that usually responds to volume loading. This is more common during recruitment manoeuvres.

See also:

IPPV—description of ventilators, p46; IPPV—modes of ventilation, p48; High frequency jet ventilation, p62; Positive end expiratory pressure (1), p66; Positive end expiratory pressure (2), p68; Acute respiratory distress syndrome (1), p360; Acute respiratory distress syndrome (2), p362; Pneumothorax, p368.

Positive end expiratory pressure (1)

Positive end expiratory pressure (PEEP) is a modality used in positive pressure ventilation to prevent the alveoli returning to atmospheric pressure during expiration. It is routinely set between 3–5cmH$_2$O; however, in severe respiratory failure, it will often need to exceed 10cmH$_2$O to be above the lower inflexion point of the pressure–volume curve. This has been suggested as beneficial in patients with severe ARDS. It rarely needs to exceed 20cmH$_2$O to avoid cardiorespiratory complications and alveolar over-distension (see below). It neither prevents nor attenuates ARDS, reduce capillary leak, or lung water.

Respiratory effects

PEEP improves oxygenation by recruiting collapsed alveoli, re-distributing lung water, decreasing A–V mismatch, and increasing functional residual capacity (FRC).

Haemodynamics

PEEP usually lowers both left and right ventricular preload, and increases RV afterload. Though PEEP may increase cardiac output in left heart failure and fluid overload states by preload reduction, in most other cases, cardiac output falls, even at relatively low PEEP levels. PEEP may also compromise a poorly functioning right ventricle. Improved PaO$_2$ resulting from decreased venous admixture may sometimes arise solely from reductions in cardiac output.

Physiological PEEP

A small degree of PEEP (2–3cmH$_2$O) is usually provided physiologically by a closed larynx. It is lost when the patient is intubated or tracheostomised and breathing spontaneously on a T-piece with no CPAP valve (see CPAP).

Intrinsic PEEP (auto-PEEP, air trapping, PEEPi)

Increased level of PEEP due to insufficient time for expiration, leading to 'air trapping', CO$_2$ retention, increased airway pressures, and increased FRC. Seen in pathological conditions of increased airflow resistance (e.g. asthma, emphysema) and when insufficient expiratory time is set on the ventilator. Used clinically in inverse ratio ventilation to increase oxygenation and decrease peak airway pressures. However, high levels of PEEPi can slow weaning by an increased work of breathing; use of extrinsic PEEP may overcome this. PEEPi can be measured by temporarily occluding the expiratory outlet of ventilator at end-expiration for a few seconds to allow equilibration of pressure between upper and lower airway, and then reading the ventilator pressure gauge (or print-out).

'Best' PEEP

Initially described as the level of PEEP producing the lowest shunt value. Now generally considered to be the lowest level of PEEP that achieves SaO$_2$ ≥90% allowing, wherever possible, lowering of FIO$_2$ (ideally ≤0.6), though not at the expense of peak airway pressures >35–40cmH$_2$O or significant reductions in DO$_2$.

See also:
IPPV—description of ventilators, p46; IPPV—modes of ventilation, p48; IPPV—adjusting the
ventilator, p50; IPPV—complications of ventilation, p56; Positive end expiratory pressure (2),
p68; Continuous positive airway pressure, p70; Lung recruitment, p72; Atelectasis and pulmonary
collapse, p352.

Positive end expiratory pressure (2)

Adjusting PEEP

1. Measure blood gases and monitor haemodynamic variables.
2. If indicated, alter level of PEEP by 3–5cmH$_2$O increments.
3. Re-measure gases and haemodynamic variables after 15–20min.
4. Consider further changes as necessary (including additional changes in PEEP, fluid challenge, or vasoactive drugs)

A number of clinical trials have adjusted PEEP levels according to FIO$_2$ requirements (see table below). Although unlikely to constitute 'optimal PEEP' for an individual patient, this provides a useful approximation and starting point for further titration of therapy.

FIO$_2$	0.3	0.4	0.4	0.5	0.5	0.6	0.7	0.7	0.7	0.8	0.9	0.9	0.9	1.0
PEEP (cmH$_2$O)	5	5	8	8	10	10	10	12	14	14	14	16	18	≥18

Indications

- Hypoxaemia requiring high FIO$_2$.
- Optimising the pressure–volume curve in severe respiratory failure.
- Hypoxaemia secondary to left heart failure.
- Improvement of cardiac output in left heart failure.
- Reduced work of breathing while weaning patients with high PEEPi.
- Neurogenic pulmonary oedema (i.e. non-cardiogenic pulmonary oedema following relief of upper airway obstruction).

Complications

- Reduced cardiac output. May need additional fluid loading or even inotropes. This should generally be avoided unless higher PEEP is necessary to maintain adequate arterial oxygenation. Caution should be exercised in patients with myocardial ischaemia.
- Increased airway pressure (and potential risk of ventilator trauma).
- Overinflation leading to air trapping and raised PaCO$_2$. Use with caution in patients with chronic airflow limitation or asthma. In pressure-controlled ventilation, over-distension is suggested when an increase in PEEP produces a significant fall in tidal volume.
- High levels will decrease venous return, raise intracranial pressure, and increase hepatic congestion.
- PEEP may change the area of lung in which a pulmonary artery catheter tip is positioned from West zone III to non-zone III. This is suggested by a rise in wedge pressure of at least half the increase in PEEP and requires re-siting of the catheter.

See also:

IPPV—description of ventilators, p46; IPPV—modes of ventilation, p48; IPPV—adjusting the ventilator, p50; IPPV—complications of ventilation, p56; Positive end expiratory pressure (1), p66; Continuous positive airway pressure, p70; Lung recruitment, p72; Atelectasis and pulmonary collapse, p352.

Continuous positive airway pressure

Continuous positive airway pressure (CPAP) is the addition of positive pressure to the expiratory side of the breathing circuit of a spontaneously ventilating patient who may or may not be intubated. This sets the baseline upper airway pressure above atmospheric pressure, prevents alveolar collapse, and may recruit already collapsed alveoli. It is usually administered in $2.5cmH_2O$ increments to a maximum of $10cmH_2O$. It is applied either via a tight-fitting face mask (face CPAP), nasal mask (nasal CPAP), a whole head helmet, or the expiratory limb of a T-piece breathing circuit. A high-flow (i.e. above peak inspiratory flow) inspired air–oxygen supply or a large reservoir bag in the inspiratory circuit is necessary to keep the valve open. CPAP improves oxygenation and may reduce the work of breathing by reducing the alveolar-to-mouth pressure gradient in patients with high levels of intrinsic PEEP. Transient periods of high CPAP (e.g. $40cmH_2O$ for 40s) may be a useful manoeuvre for recruiting collapsed alveoli and improving oxygenation in ARDS.

Indications
- Hypoxaemia requiring high respiratory rate, effort, and FIO_2.
- Left heart failure to improve hypoxaemia and cardiac output.
- Weaning modality.
- Reduces work of breathing in patients with high PEEPi (e.g. asthma, chronic airflow limitation). NB. Use with caution, monitor closely.

Management
1. Measure blood gases, monitor haemodynamic variables and respiratory rate.
2. Prepare T-piece circuit with a $5cmH_2O$ CPAP valve on the expiratory limb. Connect inspiratory limb to flow generator/large volume reservoir bag. Adjust air–oxygen mix to obtain desired FIO_2 (measured by O_2 analyser in circuit). Use a heat-moisture exchanger to humidify the inhaled gas. If not intubated, consider nasal, face, or helmet CPAP. Attach mask to the patient's face by an appropriate harness, attach a T-piece to the mask, and ensure no air leak is present. If using a nasal mask, encourage patient to keep their mouth closed.
3. Repeat measurements after 15–20min.
4. Consider further changes in CPAP (by $2.5cmH_2O$ increments).
5. Consider: (i) fluid challenge (or vasoactive drugs) if circulatory compromise, and (ii) nasogastric tube if gastric atony present.

Complications
- With mask CPAP, the risk of aspiration increases as gastric dilatation may occur from swallowed air. Insert a nasogastric tube, especially if consciousness is impaired or gastric motility is reduced.
- Reduced cardiac output due to reduced venous return (raised intrathoracic pressure). May need additional fluid or even inotropes.
- Overinflation leading to air trapping and high $PaCO_2$. Caution is urged in patients with chronic airflow limitation or asthma.
- May reduce venous return and increase intracranial pressure.
- Occasional poor patient compliance with tight-fitting face mask due to feelings of claustrophobia and discomfort on bridge of nose.
- Inspissated secretions due to high flow, dry gas.

Lung recruitment

There has been considerable interest in recent years in the concept of lung recruitment. The rationale is that re-opening of collapsed alveoli results in improved gas exchange, with resulting reductions in airway pressures and FIO_2. Timing is crucial as collapsed alveoli are more likely to be recruitable in the early stages of respiratory failure.

It appears that benefit is more likely in extra-pulmonary causes of ARDS rather than in cases of direct pulmonary pathology such as pneumonia. Some animal studies suggest that recruitment procedures may even be potentially injurious in the latter situation.

Consideration should be given to lung recruitment soon after intubation of patients with severe respiratory failure, and procedures causing de-recruitment, e.g. endotracheal suction, airway disconnection.

Recruitment techniques

- Several techniques are used to recruit collapsed alveoli, e.g. applying 40cmH$_2$O PEEP for 40s with no ventilator breaths; delivering a few large-volume, ventilator-delivered breaths; or by using a combination of varying levels of PEEP and increasing pressure-delivered breaths to obtain optimal gas exchange.
- Although anecdotal successes are reported, with occasionally dramatic improvements in lung compliance and gas exchange, no comparative trials have been performed and outcomes have not been assessed prospectively. Haemodynamic compromise may occur during the procedure though this usually recovers on cessation.

Key paper

Brower RG, Morris A, MacIntyre N, et al. for the ARDS Clinical Trials Network.(2003) Effects of recruitment manoeuvres in patients with acute lung injury and acute respiratory distress syndrome ventilated with high positive end-expiratory pressure. *Crit Care Med* **31**: 2592–7.

See also:

IPPV—modes of ventilation, p48; IPPV—failure to deliver ventilation, p54; High frequency oscillatory ventilation, p64; Positive end expiratory pressure (1), p66; Positive end expiratory pressure (2), p68; Continuous positive airway pressure, p70; Chest physiotherapy, p90; Atelectasis and pulmonary collapse, p352.

Prone positioning

Prone positioning is used to treat patients with ARDS to improve gas exchange. Various theories have been proposed to explain improvement, including: reduction in compression atelectasis of dependent lung regions (temporary), reduction in chest wall compliance, increasing intrathoracic pressure and alveolar recruitment, better regional diaphragmatic movement, better V/Q matching, improved secretion clearance, and less alveolar distension leading to better oxygenation.

Indications

Prone positioning may be considered when: PaO_2 <8.5, FIO_2 0.6, PEEP >10cmH$_2$O despite optimisation of other ventilatory support.

Technique

Positioning the patient takes time and preparation. Four members of staff are required to turn a patient and one person to secure the head and ET tube. The turn itself is a two-stage procedure via the lateral position. The arm on which the patient is to be rolled is tucked under the hip with the other arm laid across the chest. Pillows are placed under the abdomen and chest prior to rotation to the lateral position. If stable, the turn may be completed to prone. Pillows are placed under shoulders and pelvis. The head of bed is raised and one arm is extended at the patient's side while the other is flexed with head facing opposite way.

Frequency of turns

The response to prone ventilation is difficult to predict. Some patients may have no improvement in gas exchange; others may have a temporary benefit, requiring frequent turns; and others may have difficulty returning to a supine position. For compression atelectasis, it is likely that benefit will last up to 2h before resumption of supine position is required. For other conditions, up to 18h prone position may be required. The head and arms should be repositioned 2-hourly.

Complications

There are problems associated with positioning the patient prone, including; facial oedema, incorrect positioning of limbs leading to nerve palsy, and accidental removal of drains and catheters, pressure necrosis, myositis ossificans. These problems are preventable so long as awareness of their potential is understood.

Contraindications

There are two absolute contraindications to prone position: severe head, spinal, or abdominal injury; and severe haemodynamic instability. Relative contraindications include:
- Recent abdominal surgery.
- Large abdomen.
- Pregnancy.
- Spinal instability (though special beds are available for turning affected patients).
- Frequent seizures.
- Multiple trauma.
- Raised intracranial pressure.

Key paper

Gattinoni L, Tognoni G, Pesenti A. et al. for the Prone-Supine Study Group. (2001) Effect of prone positioning on the survival of patients with acute respiratory failure. *N Engl J Med* **345**: 568–73.

See also:

Acute respiratory distress syndrome (1), p360; Acute respiratory distress syndrome (2), p362.

Non-invasive respiratory support

Devices of varying sophistication are available to augment spontaneous breathing in the compliant patient by either assisting inspiration (inspiratory support) and/or providing CPAP. Non-invasive support is usually delivered by tight-fitting face or nasal mask, or via a helmet. Inspiratory support can also be delivered via a mouthpiece. Some devices allow connection to an endotracheal tube for the intubated but spontaneously breathing patient.

Indications

- Hypoxaemia requiring high respiratory rate, effort, and FIO_2.
- Hypercapnia in a fatiguing patient.
- Weaning modality.
- To avoid endotracheal intubation where desirable (e.g. severe chronic airflow limitation, immunosuppressed patients).
- Reduces work of breathing in patients with high PEEPi (e.g. asthma, chronic airflow limitation). Use with caution and monitor closely.
- Physiotherapy technique for improving FRC.
- Sleep apnoea.

Inspiratory support (IS)

A preset inspiratory pressure is given when triggered by the patient's breath. The trigger can be adjusted according to the degree of patient effort. Some devices deliver breaths automatically at adjustable rates. The I:E ratio may also be adjustable. The V_T delivered for a given level of inspiratory support varies according to the patient's respiratory compliance. An example of an IS device is the Bird ventilator, commonly used by physiotherapists to improve FRC and expand lung bases.

BiPAP (Bilevel positive airways pressure)

This device delivers adjustable levels of pressure support and PEEP. Delivered breaths can be either patient-triggered and/or mandatory. Some BiPAP devices are driven by air; to increase the FIO_2, supplemental O_2 can be given via a circuit connection or through a portal in the mask.

Management

1. Select type and delivery mode of ventilatory support.
2. Connect patient as per device instructions.
3. Use an appropriate-sized mask that is comfortable and leak-free.
4. A delivered pressure (IPAP) of 10–15cmH_2O is a usual starting point which can be adjusted according to patient response (respiratory rate, degree of fatigue, comfort, blood gases, etc.).
5. Expiratory pressure support (EPAP) is usually in the 5–12cmH_2O range.
6. Patients in respiratory distress may have initial difficulty in coping. Constant attention and encouragement will help to accustom them to the device and/or mask while different levels of support, I:E ratios, etc. are tested to find optimal settings. Cautious administration of low dose opiate injections (e.g. diamorphine 2.5mg SC) may help to calm the patient without depressing respiratory drive. The tight-fitting mask may become increasingly claustrophobic after a few days' use. Pre-empt if possible by allowing the patient regular breaks. Protect pressure areas such as the bridge of the nose.

Key papers

Brochard L, Mancebo J, Wysocki M, et al. (1995) Non-invasive ventilation for acute exacerbations of chronic obstructive pulmonary disease. *N Engl J Med* **333**: 817–22.

Antonelli M, Conti G, Rocco M, et al. (1998) A comparison of non-invasive positive-pressure ventilation and conventional mechanical ventilation in patients with acute respiratory failure. *N Engl J Med* **339**: 429–35.

See also:

Ventilatory support—indications, p44; IPPV—description of ventilators, p46; IPPV—modes of ventilation, p48; IPPV—failure to tolerate ventilation, p52; IPPV—weaning techniques, p58; IPPV—assessment of weaning, p60; Continuous positive airway pressure, p70.

Extracorporeal respiratory support

These techniques have declined in popularity over recent years after several trials failed to demonstrate clear outcome benefit in adults with very severe respiratory failure. Survival rates of 50–60% are reported, but clear superiority over conventional ventilation has not yet been demonstrated in controlled studies. A large, prospective, randomised study (the 'CESAR' trial) has recently been completed, but failed to show benefit from extracorporeal support.

Extracorporeal CO_2 removal ($ECCO_2R$)

An extracorporeal veno-venous circulation allows CO_2 clearance via a gas exchange membrane. Blood flows of 25–33% cardiac output are typically used, allowing only partial oxygenation support. Low frequency (4–5/min) positive pressure ventilation is usually used with $ECCO_2R$, with continuous oxygenation throughout inspiration and expiration. The lungs are 'held open' with high PEEP (20–25cmH$_2$O), limited peak airway pressures (35–40cmH$_2$O), and a continuous fresh gas supply. Thus, oxygenation is provided with lung rest to aid recovery. Anticoagulation of the extracorporeal circuit can be reduced by using heparin-bonded tubing and membranes.

Extracorporeal membrane oxygenation (ECMO)

An extracorporeal veno-arterial circulation with high blood flows (approaching cardiac output) through a gas exchange membrane enables most if not all of the body's gas exchange requirements to be met. Main disadvantages compared to $ECCO_2R$ are the need for large bore arterial puncture with its consequent risks and high extracorporeal blood flows with the potential for cell damage.

Indications

Failure of maximum intensive therapy and ventilatory support to sustain adequate gas exchange as evidenced by the criteria opposite.

Contraindications

- Chronic systemic disease involving any major organ system (e.g. irreversible chronic CNS disease, chronic lung disease with FEV_1 <1L, FEV_1/FVC <0.3 of predicted, chronic $PaCO_2$ >6.0kPa, emphysema or previous admission for chronic respiratory insufficiency, incurable or rapidly fatal malignancy, chronic failure of heart, kidney or liver, HIV-related disease).
- Lung failure for >7d (although treatment with extracorporeal respiratory support may persist for longer than 14d).
- Burns (>40% of body surface).
- More than three organ failures in addition to lung failure.

Criteria for ECCO$_2$R/ECMO

- Rapid failure of ventilatory support: immediate use of these techniques should be considered in those meeting the following criteria for a period >2h despite maximum intensive care:
  - PaO$_2$ <6.7kPa.
  - FIO$_2$ 1.0.
  - PEEP >5–10cmH$_2$O.
- Slow failure of ventilatory support: consider use after 48h maximum intensive care for those meeting the following gas exchange and mechanical pulmonary function criteria for a period >12h:
  - PaO$_2$ <6.7kPa.
  - PEEP >5–10cmH$_2$O.
  - Q$_s$/Q$_t$ >30% on FIO$_2$ of 1.0.
  - PaO$_2$/FIO$_2$ <11.2kPa.
  - TSLC <30mL/cmH$_2$O at 10mL/kg inflation.

See also:

Anticoagulants, p318; Prostaglandins, p330; Acute respiratory distress syndrome (1), p360; Acute respiratory distress syndrome (2), p362.

Tracheotomy

The technique of creating a hole (the tracheostomy) in the trachea.

Indications

To provide an artificial airway in place of orotracheal or nasotracheal intubation. This may be to provide better patient comfort, avoid vocal cord, mouth or nasal trauma or, in an emergency, bypass acute upper airway obstruction. The optimal time to perform a tracheotomy in an intubated patient is not known; a prospective randomised study (the 'TracMan' trial) is underway in the UK. Reduced need for sedation, the potential to eat, drink and speak, and facilitation of mouth care are all advantages.

Percutaneous tracheotomy

Percutaneous tracheotomy can be performed in the ICU. Coagulopathy should be excluded or treated first. Subcutaneous tissues are infiltrated with 1% lidocaine and epinephrine (adrenaline). After a 1–1.5cm midline skin crease incision, the subcutaneous tissue is blunt-dissected to the anterior tracheal wall. The ET tube tip is withdrawn to the level of the vocal cords. The trachea is then punctured in the midline with a 14G needle between the 1st and 2nd tracheal cartilages (or lower), allowing guide wire insertion. The stoma is created by dilatation to 32–36Fr (Ciaglia technique) or by a guided forceps dilating tool (Schachner–Ovill technique). In the former case, the tracheostomy tube is introduced over an appropriate-sized dilator, and in the latter, through the open dilating tool. End-tidal CO_2 monitoring confirms adequate ventilation during the procedure. Fibreoptic bronchoscopy may be used to confirm correct tracheal placement and no trauma to the posterior tracheal wall.

Complications

The main early complication is haemorrhage from vessels anterior to the trachea. This is usually controlled with direct pressure or, occasionally, sutures. Bleeding into the trachea may result in clot obstruction of the airway; endotracheal suction is usually effective. Paratracheal placement should be rare, but promptly recognised by the inability to ventilate the lungs. Later complications include tracheostomy tube displacement, stomal infection, and tracheal stenosis. Stenosis is often related to low-grade infection and is claimed to be more common with open tracheotomy. Rare complications include tracheo-oesophageal fistula due to trauma or pressure necrosis of the posterior tracheal wall, or erosion through the lateral tracheal wall into a blood vessel.

Maintenance of a tracheostomy

Since the upper air passages have been bypassed, artificial humidification is required. Cough is less effective without a functioning larynx so regular tracheal suction will be necessary. Natural laryngeal PEEP is lost with a tracheostomy. The risk of basal atelectasis can be overcome with CPAP or attention to respiratory exercises that promote deep breathing. After 3–5d, the tracheostomy tube can be safely replaced.

Tracheostomy tube removal

Before removing the tube, ensure the upper airway is patent, either by allowing the patient to exhale passed an occluded tube or by visualisation.

Tracheotomy tubes

Standard high volume, low pressure cuff

Fenestrated, with or without cuff

Useful where airway protection is not a primary concern. May be closed during normal breathing while providing intermittent suction access.

Fenestrated, with inner tube

As above, but with an inner tube to facilitate closure of the fenestration during intermittent mechanical ventilation.

Fenestrated, with speaking valve

Inspiration allowed through the tracheostomy to reduce dead space and inspiratory resistance. Expiration through the larynx via the fenestration, allowing speech and the advantages of laryngeal PEEP.

Adjustable flange

Accommodates extreme variations in skin to trachea depth while ensuring the cuff remains central in the trachea.

Pitt speaking tube

A non-fenestrated, cuffed tube for continuous mechanical ventilation and airway protection with a port to direct airflow above the cuff to the larynx. When airflow is directed through the larynx, some patients are able to vocalise.

Passy–Muir speaking valve

This expiratory occlusive valve is placed onto the tracheostomy tube to permit inspiration through the tracheostomy and expiration through the glottis. The tracheostomy tube cuff must be first deflated. The valve allows phonation, facilitates swallowing, and may reduce aspiration. Small studies have suggested that it may reduce the work of breathing. The potential tidal volume drop through cuff deflation makes this valve only suitable in those patients requiring no (or relatively low level) invasive ventilatory support.

Silver tube

An uncuffed tube used occasionally in ENT practice to maintain a tracheostomy fistula.

See also:
Endrotracheal intubation, p42; Ventilatory support-indications, p44; Minitracheotomy, p82; Airway obstruction, p348; Respiratory failure, p350.

Mini-tracheotomy

The technique of placing a small diameter, uncuffed plastic tube through the cricothyroid membrane under local anaesthetic.

Indications
- Removal of retained secretions, usually if patient's cough is weak.
- Emergency access to lower airway if upper airway obstructed.

Contraindications/cautions
- Coagulopathy.
- Non-compliant, agitated patient (unless sedated).

Technique
Some commercial kits rely on blind insertion of a blunt introducer; others use a Seldinger technique where a guidewire is inserted via the crico-thyroid membrane into the trachea. An introducer passed over the wire dilates the track, allowing easy passage of the tube.

1. Use an aseptic technique. Cleanse site with antiseptic. Locate cricothyroid membrane (midline, 'spongy' area between cricoid and thyroid cartilages).
2. Infiltrate local skin and subcutaneous tissues with 1% lidocaine ± epinephrine (adrenaline). Advance needle into deeper tissues, aspirating to confirm absence of blood, then infiltrate with lidocaine until cricothyroid membrane is pierced and air is easily aspirated.
3. If using Seldinger technique, insert the guidewire through the membrane into the trachea. Tether thyroid cartilage with one hand, incise skin and tissues vertically in midline (alongside wire) using a short-bladed guarded scalpel provided with pack. Insert scalpel to blade guard level to make adequate hole through cricothyroid membrane. Remove scalpel.
4. Insert introducer through incision site into trachea (or over guidewire). Angle caudally. Relatively light resistance is felt during correct passage; do not force introducer if resistance is excessive.
5. Lubricate plastic tube and slide it over introducer into trachea.
6. Remove introducer (+ wire), leaving plastic tube *in situ*.
7. Confirm correct position by placing own hand over tube and feeling airflow during breathing. Suction down tube to aspirate intratracheal contents (check pH if in doubt). Cap opening of tube. Suture to skin.
8. Perform CXR (unless very smooth insertion and no change in cardiorespiratory variables).
9. O_2 can be entrained through the tube, or a catheter mount placed to allow bagging, the use of intermittent positive pressure breathing and/ or short-term assisted ventilation.

Complications
- Puncture of blood vessel at cricothyroid membrane may cause significant intratracheal or external bleeding. Apply local pressure if this occurs after blade incision. If bleeding continues, insert mini-tracheotomy tube for a tamponading effect. If bleeding persists, insert deep sutures either side of mini-tracheotomy; if this fails, contact surgeon for assistance.
- Perforation of oesophagus.
- Mediastinitis (rare).
- Pneumothorax.

See also:
Tracheotomy, p80; Chest physiotherapy, p90; Atelectasis and pulmonary collapse, p352.

Chest drain insertion

Indications include drainage of air (pneumothorax), fluid (effusion), blood (haemothorax), or pus (empyema) from the pleural space.

Insertion technique

1. Use 28Fr drain (or larger) for haemothorax or empyema; 20Fr will suffice for a pure pneumothorax. Seldinger-type drains with an integral guidewire are now available. The drain is usually inserted through the 5th intercostal space in the mid-axillary line, first anaesthetising skin and pleura with 1% lidocaine. Ensure that air/fluid is aspirated.
2. Make a 1–1.5cm skin crease incision, create a track with gloved finger (or forceps) to separate muscle fibres and open pleura.
3. Insert drain through open pleura without trochar.
4. Angle and insert drain to correct position (toward lung apex for pneumothorax and lung base for haemothorax/effusion). CT scan or ultrasound is useful for directing placement for small collections.
5. Connect to the underwater seal and keep bottle below level of heart.
6. Secure drain to chest wall by properly placed sutures.
7. Perform chest X-ray to ensure correct siting and lung reinflation.
8. Place on 5–10cmH$_2$O (0.5–1.3kPa) negative pressure (low pressure wall suction) if lung has not fully expanded.

Subsequent management

- Do not clamp drains prior to removal or during transport of patient.
- Drains may be removed when lung has re-expanded and no air leak is present (no respiratory swing in fluid level nor air leak on coughing).
- Unless long-term ventilation is necessary, a drain inserted for a pneumothorax should usually be left in situ during IPPV.
- Remove drain at end-expiration. Cover hole with thick gauze and Elastoplast®; a purse-string suture is not usually necessary. Repeat chest X-ray if indicated by deteriorating clinical signs or blood gas analysis.

Complications

- Morbidity associated with chest drainage may be up to 10%.
- Puncture of an intercostal vessel may cause significant bleeding. Consider: (i) correcting any coagulopathy, (ii) placing deep tension sutures around drain, or (iii) removing drain, inserting a Foley catheter, inflating the balloon, and applying traction to tamponade bleeding vessel. If these measures fail, contact (thoracic) surgeon.
- Puncture of lung tissue may cause a bronchopleural fistula. Consider suction (up to 15–20cmH$_2$O), pleurodesis, high frequency ventilation, a double-lumen endobronchial tube or surgery. Extubate if feasible.
- Perforation of major vessel (often fatal); clamp but do not remove drain, resuscitate, contact surgeon, consider double-lumen ET tube.
- Infection: take cultures; antibiotics (staphylococcal ± anaerobic cover); consider removing/resiting drain.
- Local discomfort/pain from pleural irritation may impair cough. Consider simple analgesia, subcutaneous lidocaine, instilling local anaesthetic, local or regional anaesthesia, etc.
- Drain dislodgement; if needed, replace/resite new drain, depending on cleanliness of site. Don't advance old drain (infection risk).
- Lung entrapment/infarction: avoid milking drain in pneumothorax.

See also:
Pleurla aspiration, p86; Basic resuscitation, p338; Pneumothorax, p368; Haemothorax, p370.

Pleural aspiration

Drainage of fluid from the pleural space using needle, cannula, or flexible small-bore drain. Increasingly being performed under ultrasound guidance. Blood/pus often requires large-bore drain insertion.

Indications
- Improvement of blood gases.
- Symptomatic improvement of dyspnoea.
- Diagnostic 'tap'.

Contraindications/cautions
- Coagulopathy.

Technique
1. Confirm presence of effusion by CXR or ultrasound.
2. Select drainage site either by maximum area of stony dullness under percussion or under ultrasound guidance.
3. Use aseptic technique. Clean area with antiseptic and infiltrate local skin and subcutaneous tissues with 1% lidocaine. Advance into deeper tissues, aspirating to confirm absence of blood, then infiltrate with local anaesthetic until pleura is pierced and fluid can be aspirated.
4. Advance drainage needle/cannula/drain slowly through chest wall and intercostal space (above upper border of rib to avoid neurovascular bundle). Apply gentle suction until fluid is aspirated.
5. Withdraw 50mL for microbiological (M, C & S, TB stain, etc.), biochemical (protein, glucose, etc.) and histological/cytological (pneumocystis, malignant cells, etc.) analysis, as indicated.
6. Either leave drain *in situ* connected to a drainage bag or connect needle/cannula by a three-way tap to a drainage apparatus.
7. Continue aspiration/drainage until no further fluid can be withdrawn or if patient becomes symptomatic (pain/dyspnoea). Dyspnoea or haemodynamic changes may occur due to removal of large volumes of fluid (>1–2L) and subsequent fluid shifts; if this is considered to be a possibility, remove no more than 1L at a time, either by clamping/declamping drain or repeating needle aspiration after an equilibration interval (e.g. 4–6h).
8. Remove needle/drain. Cover puncture site with firmly applied gauze dressing.

Complications
- Puncture of lung or subdiaphragmatic viscera.
- Bleeding.

Fluid protein level
- Protein >30g/L (NB. This should be viewed in the context of the plasma protein level) is an exudates; caused by: inflammatory, e.g. pneumonia, pulmonary embolus, neoplasm, collagen vascular diseases.
- Protein <30g/L is a transudate caused by: (i) raised venous pressure (e.g. heart failure, fluid overload), (ii) decreased colloid osmotic pressure (e.g. critical illness leading to reduced [plasma protein] from capillary leak and hepatic dysfunction, hepatic failure, nephrotic syndrome).

See also:
Chest drain insertion, p84; Basic resuscitation, p338; Pneumothorax, p368; Haemothorax, p370.

Fibreoptic bronchoscopy

Indications

Diagnostic

- Collection of microbiological ± cytological specimens (by bronchoalveolar lavage, protected brush specimen, biopsy).
- Cause of bronchial obstruction (e.g. clot, foreign body, neoplasm).
- Extent of inhalation injury.
- Diagnosis of ruptured trachea/bronchus.

Therapeutic

- Clearance of secretions, inhaled vomitus, etc.
- Removal of obstructing matter (e.g. mucus plug, blood clot, food, tooth). Proximal obstruction rather than consolidation is suggested by the X-ray appearance of a collapsed lung/lobe and no air bronchogram.
- Cleansing/removing soot or other toxic materials, irrigation with saline.
- Directed physiotherapy ± saline to loosen secretions.
- Directed placement of balloon catheter to arrest pulmonary bleeding.
- To aid difficult endotracheal intubation.

Contraindications/cautions

- Coagulopathy.
- Severe hypoxaemia.

Procedure

It is difficult to perform bronchoscopy in a nasally intubated patient. A narrow lumen scope can be used but suction is limited.

1. Pre-oxygenate with FIO_2 1.0. Monitor with pulse oximetry.
2. Increase pressure alarm limit on ventilator.
3. Lubricate scope with lubricant gel/saline.
4. If unintubated, apply lidocaine gel to nares ± spray to pharynx.
5. Consider short-term IV sedation ± paralysis.
6. Insert scope nasally in a non-intubated patient or via the catheter mount port if intubated. An assistant should support the ET tube during the procedure to minimise trauma to trachea and/or scope.
7. Inject 2% lidocaine into trachea to prevent coughing and haemodynamic effects from tracheal/carinal stimulation.
8. Perform thorough inspection and any necessary procedures. If SpO_2 ≤85% or haemodynamic disturbance occurs, remove scope and allow re-oxygenation before continuing.
9. Bronchoalveolar lavage is performed by instillation of at least 60mL of (preferably warm) isotonic saline into affected lung area without suction, followed by aspiration into a sterile catheter trap. All bronchoscopic samples should be sent promptly to the lab.
10. After procedure, reset ventilator as appropriate.

Complications

- Hypoxaemia: from suction, loss of PEEP, partial obstruction of endotracheal tube, and non-delivery of tidal volume.
- Haemodynamic disturbance, including hypertension and tachycardia (related to hypoxaemia, agitation, tracheal stimulation, etc.).
- Bleeding.
- Perforation (unusual though more common if biopsy taken).

See also:
Endotracheal intubtion, p42; Chest physiotherapy, p90; Atelectasis and pulmonary collapse, p352;
Haemoptysis, p372; Inhalation injury, p374.

Chest physiotherapy

The aim is to expand collapsed alveoli, mobilise chest secretions, or re-inflate collapsed lung segments. Though anecdotal experience suggests benefit, no scientific validation of effectiveness has been reported. The current view is routine 'prophylactic' suctioning/bagging should be avoided in the critically ill.

Indications
- Mobilisation of secretions.
- Re-expansion of collapsed lung/lobes.
- Prophylaxis against alveolar collapse and secondary infection.

Contraindications/cautions
- Aggressive hyperinflation in already hyperinflated lungs, e.g. asthma, emphysema—though can be very useful in removing mucus plugs.
- Undrained pneumothorax.
- Raised intracranial pressure.

Techniques
Hyperinflation
Hyperinflating to 50% above ventilator-delivered V_T, aiming to expand collapsed alveoli and mobilise secretions. V_T is rarely measured, so either excessive or inadequate hyperinflations may be given, depending on lung compliance and operator technique. Pressure-limiting devices ('blow-off valves') or manometers can avoid excessive airway pressures. A recommended technique is slow inspiration, a 1–2s plateau phase, and then rapid release of the bag to simulate a 'huff' and mobilise secretions. Preoxygenation may be needed as PEEP may be lost and the delivered V_T may be inadequate. Cardiac output often falls with variable blood pressure and heart rate responses. Sedation may blunt haemodynamic response. Full deflation avoids air trapping.

Suction
Removing secretions from trachea and main bronchi (usually right). A cough reflex may be stimulated to mobilise secretions further. Tenacious secretions may be loosened by instillation of 2–5mL 0.9% saline. Falls in SaO_2 and cardiovascular disturbance may be avoided by pre-oxygenation.

Percussion and vibration
Drumming and shaking actions over chest wall to mobilise secretions.

Inspiratory pressure support (Bird ventilator)
The aim is to increase FRC and expand collapsed alveoli.

Postural drainage
Patient positioning to assist drainage—depends on affected lung area(s).

Complications of chest physiotherapy
- Hypoxaemia: from suction, loss of PEEP, etc.
- Haemodynamic disturbance affecting cardiac output, heart rate, and blood pressure (may be related to high V_T, airway pressure, hypoxaemia, agitation, tracheal stimulation, etc.).
- Direct trauma from suctioning.
- Barotrauma/volutrauma, including pneumothorax.

General care to avoid need for urgent physiotherapy

- Adequate humidification avoids tenacious sputum and mucus plugs.
- Pain relief is important to encourage good chest expansion and cough.
- Position semi-recumbent to optimise use of respiratory muscles.
- Ensure nutrition is adequate to maintain muscle strength.
- Mobilisation and encouraging deep breathing may avoid infection.

Requesting urgent physiotherapy

Request	Don't request
Collapsed lung/lobe with no air bronchogram visible, i.e. suggesting proximal obstruction rather than consolidation.	Clinical signs of chest infection with no secretions being produced.
Mucus plugging causing subsegmental collapse, e.g. asthma.	Radiological consolidation with air bronchogram but no secretions present.

See also:

Minitracheotomy, p80; Fibreoptic bronchoscopy, p88; Atelectasisa and pulmonary collapse, p352.

Cardiovascular therapy techniques

Electrical cardioversion

Electrical conversion is used to convert a tachyarrhythmia to normal sinus rhythm. This may be:
- Emergency—when the circulation is absent or severely compromised.
- Semi-elective—when the circulation is compromised to a lesser degree.
- Elective—when synchronised cardioversion is performed to restore sinus rhythm for a non-compromising supraventricular tachycardia.

Synchronisation requires initial connection of ECG leads from the patient to the defibrillator so that the shock is delivered on the R wave to minimise the risk of ventricular fibrillation. Newer, biphasic defibrillators require approximately half the energy setting of monophasic defibrillators.

Indications
- Cardiac arrest, e.g. VF.
- Compromised circulation, e.g. VT.
- Restoration of sinus rhythm and more effective cardiac output.
- Lessens risk of cardiac thrombus formation.

Contraindications/cautions
- Aware patient.
- Severe coagulopathy.
- Caution with recent thrombolysis.
- Digoxin levels in toxic range.

Complications
- Surface burn.
- Pericardial tamponade.
- Electrocution of bystanders.

Technique
(See algorithm opposite, figure 3.1).
- The chances of maintaining sinus rhythm are increased in elective cardioversion if K^+ >4.5mmol/L and plasma Mg^{2+} levels are normal.
- Prior to defibrillation, ensure self and onlookers are not in contact with patient, things attached to the patient, or the bed frame.
- To reduce the risk of superficial burns, replace gel/gelled pads after every three shocks.
- Consider resiting paddle position (e.g. anteroposterior) if defibrillation fails.
- The risk of intractable VF following defibrillation in a patient receiving digoxin is small unless the plasma digoxin levels are in the toxic range or the patient is hypovolaemic.

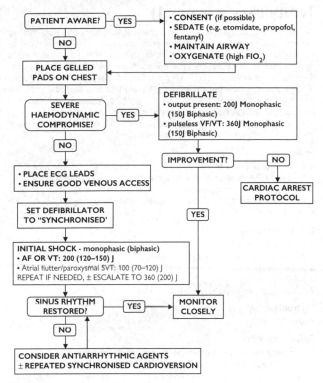

Fig. 3.1 Algorithm for use of electrical cardioversion.

Key paper
Deakin CD, Nolan JP. European Resuscitation Council Guidelines for Resuscitation 2005. Section 3. (2005) Electrical therapies: Automated external defibrillators, defibrillation, cardioversion and pacing. *Resuscitation* **67**(Suppl 1), S25–37.

See also:
Chronotropes, p274; Cardiac arrest, p340; Tachyarrhythmias, p384.

Temporary pacing (1)

When the heart's intrinsic pacemaking ability fails, temporary internal or external pacing can be instituted. Internal electrodes can be endocardial (inserted via a central vein) or epicardial (placed on the external surface of the heart at thoracotomy). The endocardial wire may be placed under fluoroscopic control or 'blind' using a balloon flotation catheter. External pacing can be rapidly performed by placement of two electrodes on the front and rear chest wall when asystole or third degree heart block has produced acute haemodynamic compromise. It is often used as a bridge to temporary internal pacing. It can also be used as a prophylactic measure, e.g. for Mobitz type II second degree heart block.

Indications
- Third degree heart block.
- Mobitz type II second degree heart block when the circulation is compromised or an operation is planned.
- Overpacing (rarely; more successful with internal pacing).
- Asystole.

Complications
Internal pacing
- As for central venous catheter insertion.
- Arrhythmias.
- Infection (including endocarditis).
- Myocardial perforation (rare).

External pacing
- Discomfort.

Failure to pace
1. No pacemaker spikes seen: check connections, check battery.
2. No capture (pacing spikes but no QRS complex following): poor positioning/dislodgement of wire. Temporarily increase output as this may regain capture. Reposition/replace internal pacing wire.

General
1. Check threshold daily as it will rise slowly over 48–96h, probably due to fibrosis occurring around the electrodes.
2. Overpacing may be used for a tachycardia unresponsive to anti-arrhythmic therapy or cardioversion. For SVT, pacing is usually attempted with the wire sited in the right atrium. Pace at rate 20–30bpm above patient's heart rate for 10–15s, then either decrease rate immediately to 80bpm or slowly by 20bpm every 5–10s.
3. If overpacing fails, underpacing may be attempted with the wire situated in either atrium (for SVT) or usually ventricle (for either SVT or VT). A paced rate of 80–100bpm may produce a refractory period sufficient to suppress the intrinsic tachycardia.
4. Epicardial pacing done during cardiac surgery uses either two epicardial electrodes or one epicardial and one skin electrode (usually a hypodermic needle). The pacing threshold of epicardial wires rises quickly and may become ineffective after 1–2d.
5. In asystole, paced rhythm does not guarantee cardiac output.

See also:
Temporary pacing (2), p98; Chronotropes, p274; Cardiac arrest, p340; Bradyarrhythmias, p386.

Temporary pacing (2)

Technique (for endocardial electrode placement)

1. If using fluoroscopy, move patient to X-ray suite or place lead shields around bed area. Place patient on 'screening table'. Staff should wear lead aprons.
2. Use aseptic technique throughout. Insert 6Fr sheath in internal jugular or subclavian vein. Suture in position.
3. Connect pacing wire electrodes to pacing box (black = negative polarity = distal, red = positive polarity = proximal). Set pacemaker to demand. Check box is working and battery charge adequate. Turn pacing rate to 30bpm above patient's intrinsic rhythm. Set voltage to 4V.
4. Insert pacing wire through sheath into central vein. If using balloon catheter, insert to 15–20cm depth, then inflate balloon. Advance catheter, viewing ECG monitor for change in ECG morphology and capture of pacing rate. If using screening, direct wire toward the apex of the right ventricle. Approximate insertion depth from a neck vein is 35–40cm.
5. If pacing impulses not captured, (deflate balloon), withdraw wire to 15cm insertion depth, then repeat step 4.
6. Once pacing captured, decrease voltage by decrements to determine threshold at which pacing is no longer captured. Ideal position determined by a threshold ≤0.6V. If not achieved, re-position wire.
7. If possible, ask patient to cough to check that wire does not dislodge.
8. Set voltage at three times threshold and desired heart rate on 'demand' mode. Tape wire securely to patient to prevent dislodgement.

Technique (for external pacing)

1. Connect pacing wire gelled electrodes to pacemaker. Place black (= negative polarity) electrode on the anterior chest wall to the left of the lower sternum and red (= positive polarity) electrode to the corresponding position on the posterior hemithorax.
2. Connect ECG electrodes from ECG monitor to external pacemaker and another set of electrodes from pacemaker to patient
3. Set pacemaker to demand. Turn pacing rate to 30bpm above patient's intrinsic rhythm. Set current to 70mA.
4. Start pacing. Increase current (by 5mA increments) until pacing rate captured on monitor.
5. If pacing rate not captured at current of 120–130mA, resite electrodes and repeat steps 3–4.
6. Once pacing captured, set current at 5–10mA above threshold.

See also:
Temporary pacing (1), p96; Chronotropes, p274; Cardiac arrest, p340; Bradyarrhythmias, p386.

Therapeutic hypothermia

Induced (therapeutic) hypothermia is being increasingly used as a tool to achieve neuroprotection and/or cardioprotection. Clear benefit in terms of neurological outcome exists for victims of cardiac arrest following VT or VF, and following asphyxia in neonates. Ongoing work is examining its efficacy in ischaemic stroke, traumatic head injury, subarachnoid haemorrhage, hepatic encephalopathy, and haemorrhagic shock. Study results are either conflicting or too preliminary to make firm recommendations.

Timing and duration

The optimal period following neurological injury for which outcomes may be positively influenced by hypothermia is uncertain. Human studies show benefit from treatment durations ranging from 12–72h. From animal experiments, optimal effects are achieved when hypothermia is induced as rapidly as possible—'time is brain'. Studies show benefits can be realised even after delays of 8h before commencement. Ideally, target temperature (currently 32–34°C) should be maintained as closely as possible, and rewarming should be slow and controlled to minimise reperfusion injury.

Various cooling systems are currently available, each with specific advantages and disadvantages.

Cooling techniques

These can be subdivided into non-invasive and invasive.

Non-invasive

- Air- or water-circulating cooling blankets or pads.
- Ice packs in groins and axillae.
- Covering body in wet sheets or spraying with alcohol.
- Exposing head.
- Fans to increase air circulation.
- Immersion of body in cold water.

Invasive

- Infusion of cold fluids.
- Irrigating (or instilling and draining at regular intervals) bladder and/or stomach and/or peritoneum with iced water.
- Specialised endovascular catheters placed in a central vein, with iced sterile saline pumped through integral cooling balloons.
- Extracorporeal circulation.

Infusion of cold fluid can be used in the induction phase of hypothermia maintained by non-invasive methods.

Potential side effects

- Infection.
- Pressure sores.
- Electrolyte disorders.
- Hyperglycaemia.
- Arrhythmias (low risk if core temperature kept >30°C).
- Increased bleeding tendency.
- Alterations in drug metabolism.
- Bradycardia.
- Thrombocytopaenia, leucopaenia.

Key papers

The Hypothermia after Cardiac Arrest Study Group. (2002) Mild therapeutic hypothermia to improve the neurologic outcome after cardiac arrest. *N Engl J Med* **346**: 549–56.

Polderman KH. (2004) Keeping a cool head: How to induce and maintain hypothermia. *Crit Care Med* **32**: 2558–60.

See also:

Cardiac arrest, p340; Coma, p438; Head injury (1), p586 Head injury (2), p588; Hypothermia, p600.

Intra-aortic balloon counterpulsation

Principle
A 30–40mL balloon is placed in the descending aorta. The balloon is inflated with helium during diastole, increasing diastolic blood pressure above the balloon which thus improves coronary and cerebral perfusion. The balloon is deflated during systole, decreasing peripheral resistance and increasing stroke volume. No drug therapy exists which can increase coronary blood flow while reducing peripheral resistance. Intra-aortic balloon counterpulsation may improve cardiac performance in situations where drugs are ineffective (see figure 3.2).

Indications
It can be used to support the circulation where a structural cardiac defect is to be repaired surgically. It may also be used for acute circulatory failure where resolution of the cause of the cardiac dysfunction is expected. In acute MI, resolution of peri-infarct oedema may allow spontaneous improvement in myocardial function; the use of balloon counterpulsation may provide temporary circulatory support and promote healing by improving myocardial blood flow. Other indications include acute myocarditis and poisoning with myocardial depressants. It should not be used in aortic regurgitation as the rise in diastolic blood pressure would increase regurgitant flow.

Insertion of the balloon
The usual route is via a femoral artery. Percutaneous Seldinger catheterisation (± an introducer sheath) provides a rapid, safe technique with minimal arterial trauma and bleeding. Open surgical catheterisation may be needed in elderly patients with atheromatous disease. Check the balloon position on a chest X-ray to ensure that the radio-opaque tip is at the level of the 2nd intercostal space.

Anticoagulation
The presence of a large foreign body in the aorta requires systemic anticoagulation to prevent thrombosis. The balloon should not be left deflated for longer than a minute while in situ, otherwise thrombosis may develop despite anticoagulation.

Control of balloon inflation and deflation
Helium is used to inflate the balloon, its low density facilitating rapid transfer from pump to balloon. Deflation is commonly timed to the 'R' wave of the ECG, although timing may be taken from an arterial pressure waveform. Minor adjustment may be made to the timing to ensure that inflation occurs immediately after closure of the aortic valve (after the dicrotic notch of the arterial pressure waveform) and deflation occurs at the end of diastole. The filling volume of the balloon can be varied up to the maximum balloon volume. The greater the filling volume, the greater the circulatory augmentation. The rate at which balloon inflation occurs may coincide with every cardiac beat or every 2nd or 3rd cardiac beat. Slower rates are necessary in tachyarrhythmias. Weaning of intra-aortic balloon counterpulsation may be achieved by reducing augmentation or the rate of inflation.

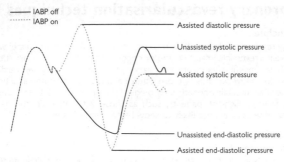

Fig. 3.2 Arterial waveform with and without intra-aortic counterpulsation.

See also:
Inotropes, p264; Vasopressors, p268; Anticoagulants, p318; Heart failure—assessment, p392; Heart failure—management, p394.

Coronary revascularisation techniques

Principle

Early restoration of blood flow through an obstructed coronary vessel will prevent irreversible infarction and/or ongoing ischaemia. Revascularisation leads to benefit after acute coronary syndromes, including myocardial infarction. However, this is more often confined to symptom reduction rather than mortality benefit over medical therapy with efforts to reduce risk factors. High-risk patients, such as those with left main coronary artery disease, are more likely to show better survival rates.

Techniques

Pharmacological

Thrombolytic agents remain in common usage, though contraindicated in 15–20%. Older drugs such as streptokinase are being replaced by recombinant tissue plasminogen activators (rtPA) such as alteplase, reteplase, and tenecteplase—these are easier to administer and appear more effective. However, the rate of recanalisation at 90min is only 55–60% and there is a 5–15% risk of early or late reocclusion. There is also a 1–2% risk of intracranial haemorrhage (with 40% mortality) and an increased risk of bleeding elsewhere (e.g. gastrointestinal tract, cannula sites). Other anticoagulant agents are administered alongside rtPA or PCI (see below), including heparin, warfarin, and antiplatelet agents—aspirin, clopidogrel, and the glycoprotein IIb/IIIa inhibitors (e.g. abciximab, eptifibatide, and tirofiban).

Percutaneous

Percutaneous coronary intervention (PCI) has evolved since the 1980s, when stenotic lesions were simply dilated by transluminal coronary angioplasty (PTCA), to now include stenting of these dilated areas using baremetal and, more recently, drug-eluting stents. Though drug-eluting stents reduce the risk of restenosis and the need for repeat PCI, they carry an increased risk of 'very late stent thrombosis' plus undesired effects related to the stent polymer and the stent itself. Next-generation stents using new drugs, polymers, and drug delivery systems are in development to improve on current devices.

Surgical

Coronary artery bypass grafting (CABG), though declining in recent years due to the increasing use of preventive health measures and PCI techniques, still has an important role to play in bypassing stenotic lesions not amenable or suitable for PCI. While PCI is targeted at the 'culprit' lesion(s), CABG is directed at the epicardial vessel, including the 'culprit' lesion(s) and possible future culprits.

Patients with single-vessel disease are more likely to have PCI, while those with triple-vessel disease are more likely to undergo CABG. Despite the increased morbidity and recovery time of CABG, mortality is similar to PCI.

The advantages of CABG over PCI are better relief of angina and a lower likelihood of subsequent reocclusion. The magnitude of the latter benefit may decrease with drug-eluting stents. However, the increase in the rate of stroke with CABG offsets these advantages.

Critical care issues

- Increased bleeding risk with the use of anticoagulant agents. The prolonged action of aspirin and clopidogrel on platelet function (lasting 3–7d after discontinuation) will heighten the risk of bleeding, both peri-operatively and during critical illness. Fresh platelet transfusions may be needed to restore platelet functionality. Similarly, warfarin has a prolonged duration of action that can be reversed with fresh frozen plasma, prothrombin complex concentrates (e.g. Octaplex®), or recombinant factor VIIa. A balance has to be sought between bleeding risk (or severity of an existing haemorrhage) and stent thrombosis from discontinuation of the drug(s).
- Arrhythmias—commonly related to reperfusion and may occasionally be life-threatening.
- Mishaps related to PCI, including coronary artery rupture plus restenosis and acute occlusion of the stent.
- Complications related to CABG, including stroke, bleeding, and transient myocardial depression.

See also:

Anticoagulants, p318; Thrombolytics, p320; Acute coronary syndrome (1), p388; Acute coronary syndrome (2), p390.

Renal therapy techniques

Haemo(dia)filtration (1)

Conventional haemodialysis requires a pressurised, purified water supply, and a greater risk of haemodynamic instability due to rapid fluid and osmotic shifts. Haemo(dia)filtration can be arterio-venous, using the patient's BP to drive blood through the haemofilter, or pumped veno-venous. The latter is preferable as it does not depend on the patient's BP, and the pump system incorporates alarms and safety features. Continuous veno-venous haemo(dia)filtration (CVVH or CVVHD) is increasingly the technique of choice. Blood is usually drawn and returned via a 10–12Fr double-lumen, central venous catheter (see figure 4.1).

Indications

- Azotaemia (uraemia).
- Hyperkalaemia.
- Anuria/oliguria; to make space for nutrition.
- Severe metabolic acidosis of non-tissue hypoperfusion origin.
- Fluid overload.
- Drug removal.
- Hypothermia/hyperthermia.

Techniques

CVVH relies on convection (bulk transfer of solute and water) to clear solute. In CVVHD, dialysate flows countercurrent to the blood, allowing small molecules to diffuse according to their concentration gradients.

Membranes are usually hollow fibre polyacrylonitrile, polyamide, or polysulphone with a surface area of 0.6–1m^2.

Both CVVH and CVVHD are effective for small molecule clearance (e.g. urea). CVVH is better at larger molecule clearance and can remove substances up to the membrane pore size cut-off (usually 30–35kD). Filtrate is usually removed at 20–35mL/kg/h; fluid balance is adjusted by varying the rate of fluid replacement. High volume haemofiltration involves much higher ultrafiltration rates (e.g. 50–100mL/kg/h, usually for short periods, e.g. 4h) in an effort to remove inflammatory mediators. Variable outcomes are reported in studies.

Creatinine and K$^+$ clearances are higher with CVVHD, but filtration alone is usually sufficient if ultrafiltrate volume is adequate. (1000mL/h approximates to a creatinine clearance of 16mL/min). CVVHD is preferred for pharmacologically-resistant hyperkalaemia.

Replacement fluid

A balanced electrolyte solution buffers acidaemia and is titrated to desired fluid and electrolyte balance. Buffers include lactate (liver metabolised to bicarbonate) and bicarbonate. Acetate (metabolised by muscle) causes most haemodynamic instability and is now rarely used. Bicarbonate may be more efficient than lactate at reversing severe acidosis, but no outcome benefit has been shown. Care is needed when giving Ca^{2+} since calcium bicarbonate may crystallise. In hypoperfused liver, lactate may be inadequately metabolised.

Increasing metabolic alkalosis may be due to excessive buffer so use low buffer (30mmol/L lactate) replacement fluid. K$^+$ can be added to maintain normokalaemia. 20mmol KCl in a 4.5L bag provides a concentration of 4.44mmol/L. K$^+$ clearance is increased by reducing the concentration within replacement fluid or dialysate.

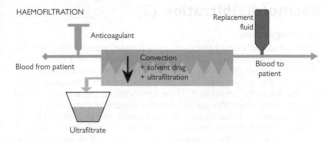

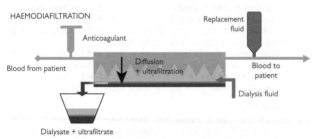

Fig. 4.1 Circuit arrangement for haemo(dia)filtration.

Key papers

Ronco C, Bellomo R, Homel P, et al. (2000) Effects of different doses in continuous veno-venous haemofiltration on outcomes of acute renal failure: a prospective randomised trial. *Lancet* **356**: 26–30.

Bouman CS, Oudermans-Van Straaten HM, et al. (2002) Effects of early high-volume continuous venovenous haemofiltration on survival and recovery of renal function in intensive care patients with acute renal failure: a prospective, randomized trial. *Crit Care Med* **30**: 2205–11.

The VA/NIH Acute Renal Failure Trial Network. (2008) Intensity of renal support in critically ill patients with acute kidney injury. *N Engl J Med* **359**: 7–20.

See also:

Haemo(dia)filtration (2), p110; Oliguria, p398; Acute renal failure—diagnosis, p400; Acute renal failure—management, p402.

Haemo(dia)filtration (2)

Anticoagulation

The circuit can be anticoagulated with unfractionated heparin (200–2000IU/h), a prostanoid (prostacyclin or PGE_1) at 2–10ng/kg/min, or a combination of the two. Other alternatives include regional citrate anticoagulation, the low molecular weight heparinoid danaparoid, or direct thrombin inhibitors (e.g. lepirudin, argatroban). These agents are, as yet, under-evaluated for renal replacement therapy and they risk important complications such as hypocalcaemia (with citrate) and prolonged bleeding with the long half-lives of the thrombin inhibitors. Bivalirudin is a new agent related to hirudin and lepirudin but is reversible with a short half-life of only 25min. No anticoagulant may be needed if the patient is auto-anticoagulated.

Premature clotting may be due to mechanical kinking/obstruction of the circuit, insufficient anticoagulation, inadequate blood flow rates, or lack of endogenous anticoagulants such as antithrombin III.

Usual filter lifespan should be at least two days, but is often decreased in septic patients due to decreased endogenous anticoagulant levels. In this situation, consider use of fresh frozen plasma, a synthetic protease inhibitor such as aprotinin, or antithrombin III replacement (costly).

Filter blood flow

Flow through the filter is usually 100–200mL/min. Too slow a flow rate promotes clotting. Too high a flow rate will increase transmembrane pressures and decrease filter lifespan without significant improvement in clearance of 'middle molecules' (e.g. urea).

Complications

- Disconnection leading to haemorrhage.
- Infection risk (sterile technique must be employed).
- Electrolyte, acid-base or fluid imbalance (due to excess input or removal).
- Haemorrhage (vascular access sites, peptic ulcers) related to anticoagulation therapy or consumption coagulopathy. Heparin-induced thrombocytopaenia may rarely occur.

Cautions

- Haemodynamic instability related to hypovolaemia (especially at start).
- Vasoactive drug removal by the filter (e.g. catecholamines).
- Membrane biocompatibility problems (especially with cuprophane).
- Drug dosages may need to be revised (consult pharmacist).
- Amino acid losses through the filter.
- Heat loss leading to hypothermia.
- Masking of pyrexia.

See also:
Haemo(dia)filtration (1), p108; Coagulation monitoring, p222; Anticoagulants, p318.

Peritoneal dialysis

A slow form of dialysis, utilising the peritoneum as the dialysis membrane. It is now rarely used in UK Critical Care Units, having been largely superseded by continuous haemofiltration. The technique does not require complex equipment although continuous flow techniques do require continuous generation of dialysate. Treatment is labour-intensive and there is considerable risk of peritoneal infection.

Peritoneal access

For acute peritoneal dialysis, a trochar and cannula are inserted through a small skin incision under local anaesthetic. The skin is prepared and draped as for any sterile procedure. The commonest approach is through a small midline incision 1cm below the umbilicus. The subcutaneous tissues and peritoneum are punctured by the trocar which is withdrawn slightly before the cannula is advanced towards the pouch of Douglas. In order to avoid damage to intra-abdominal structures, 1–2L warmed peritoneal dialysate may be infused into the peritoneum by a standard, short intravascular cannula prior to placement of the trochar and cannula system. If the midline access site is not available, an alternative is to use a lateral approach, lateral to a line joining the umbilicus and the anterior superior iliac spine (avoiding the inferior epigastric vessels).

Dialysis technique

Warmed peritoneal dialysate is infused into the peritoneum in a volume of 1–2L at a time. During the acute phase, fluid is flushed in and drained continuously (i.e. with no dwell time). Once biochemical control is achieved, it is usual to leave fluid in the peritoneal cavity for 4–6h before draining. Heparin (500IU/L) may be added to the first six cycles to prevent fibrin catheter blockage. Thereafter, it is only necessary if there is blood or cloudiness in the drainage fluid.

Peritoneal dialysate

The dialysate is a sterile balanced electrolyte solution with glucose at 75mmol/L for a standard fluid or 311mmol/L for a hypertonic fluid (used for greater fluid removal). The fluid is usually potassium-free since potassium exchanges slowly in peritoneal dialysis although potassium may be added if necessary.

Complications

- Fluid leak
  - Poor drainage
  - Corticosteroid therapy
  - Obese or elderly patient
- Catheter blockage
  - Bleeding
  - Omental encasement
- Infection — White cells >50/mL, cloudy drainage fluid
- Hyperglycaemia — Absorption of hyperosmotic glucose
- Diaphragm splinting

Treatment of infection

It is possible to sterilise the peritoneum and catheter by adding appropriate antibiotics to the dialysate. Suitable regimens include:

- Cefuroxime 500mg/L for two cycles, then 200mg/L for 10d.
- Gentamicin 8mg/L for one cycle daily.

See also:
Oliguria, p398; Acute renal failure—diagnosis, p400; Acute renal failure—management, p402.

Plasma exchange

Indications

Plasma exchange may be used to remove circulating toxins or to replace missing plasma factors. It may be used in sepsis (e.g. meningococcaemia). In patients with immune mediated disease (e.g. Guillain–Barré syndrome, thrombotic thrombocytopaenic purpura), plasma exchange is usually a temporary measure while systemic immunosuppression takes effect. Most diseases require a daily 3–4L plasma exchange repeated for at least four further occasions over 5–10 days.

Techniques

Cell separation by centrifugation

Blood is separated into components in a centrifuge. Plasma (or other specific blood components) is discarded and a plasma replacement fluid is infused in equal volume. Centrifugation may be continuous (where blood is withdrawn and returned by separate needles) or intermittent (where blood is withdrawn and separated, then returned via the same needle).

Membrane filtration

Plasma is continuously filtered through a large pore filter (molecular weight cut-off typically 1,000,000D). Plasma is discarded and replaced by infusion of an equal volume of replacement fluid. The technique is similar to haemofiltration and uses the same equipment.

Replacement fluid

Most patients will tolerate replacement with a plasma substitute. Some fresh frozen plasma will be necessary after the exchange to replace coagulation factors. The only indication to replace plasma loss with all fresh frozen plasma is where plasma exchange is being performed to replace missing plasma factors.

Complications

- Circulatory instability   Intravascular volume changes

  Removal of circulating catecholamines

  Hypocalcaemia
- Reduced intravascular COP   If replacement with crystalloid
- Infection   Reduced plasma opsonisation
- Bleeding   Removal of coagulation factors

Indications

Autoimmune disease	Goodpasture's syndrome
	Guillain–Barré syndrome
	Myasthenia gravis
	Pemphigus
	Rapidly progressive glomerulonephritis
	Systemic lupus erythematosus
	Thrombotic thrombocytopaenic purpura
Immunoproliferative disease	Cryoglobulinaemia
	Multiple myeloma
	Waldenstrom's macroglobulinaemia
Poisoning	Paraquat
Others	Meningococcaemia (possible benefit)
	Sepsis (possible benefit)
	Reye's syndrome

See also:
Guillain Barré syndrome, p456; Myasthenia gravis, p458; Platelet disorders, p478; Vasculitides, p574.

Gastrointestinal therapy techniques

Sengstaken-type tube

Used to manage oesophageal variceal haemorrhage that continues despite pharmacological ± per-endoscopic therapy. The device (Sengstaken–Blakemore or similar) is a large-bore rubber tube, usually containing two balloons (oesophageal and gastric) and two further lumens (oesophageal and gastric) that open above and below the balloons. This device works usually by the gastric balloon alone compressing the varices at the cardia. Inflation of the oesophageal balloon is rarely necessary.

Insertion technique

The tubes are usually kept in the fridge to provide added stiffness for easier insertion.

1. The patient often requires judicious sedation or mechanical ventilation (as warranted by conscious state/level of agitation) prior to insertion.
2. Check balloons inflate properly beforehand. Lubricate end of tube.
3. Insert via mouth. Place to depth of 55–60cm, i.e. to ensure gastric balloon is in stomach prior to inflation.
4. Inflate gastric balloon with water to volume instructed by manufacturer (usually 200mL). A small amount of radio-opaque contrast may be added. Negligible resistance to inflation should be felt. Clamp gastric balloon lumen.
5. Pull tube back until resistance is felt, i.e. gastric balloon is at cardia. Fix tube in place by applying countertraction at the mouth. Old-fashioned methods, such as attaching the tube to a free-hanging litre bag of saline, have been superseded by more manageable techniques. For example, two wooden tongue depressors, 'thickened' by having Elastoplast® wound around them, are placed on either side of the tube at the mouth and then attached to each other at both ends by more Elastoplast®. The tube remains gripped at the mouth/cheek by the attached tongue depressors, but can be retracted until adequate but not excessive traction is being applied.
6. Perform X-ray to check satisfactory position of gastric balloon.
7. If bleeding continues (continued large aspirates from gastric or oesophageal lumens), inflate oesophageal balloon (approximately 50mL).

Subsequent management

1. The gastric balloon is usually kept inflated for 12–24h and deflated prior to endoscopy ± sclerotherapy. The traction on the tube should be tested hourly by the nursing staff. The oesophageal lumen should be placed on continuous drainage while enteral nutrition and administration of drugs can be given via the gastric lumen.
2. If the oesophageal balloon is used, deflate for 5–10min every 1–2h to reduce the risk of oesophageal pressure necrosis. Do not leave oesophageal balloon inflated for >12h after sclerotherapy.
3. The tube may need to stay *in situ* for 2–3d though periods of deflation should then be allowed.

Complications

- Aspiration.
- Perforation.
- Ulceration.
- Oesophageal necrosis.

See also:
Upper gastrointestinal haemorrhage, p412; Bleeding varices, p414.

Upper gastrointestinal endoscopy

Oesophago-gastro-duodenoscopy is performed identically in ventilated and non-ventilated patients. Additional sedation may be needed, especially if the patient is awake and/or agitated. A protected airway facilitates the procedure and also offers additional safety if the patient's conscious level if obtunded, and there is a high risk of aspiration of gastric contents (blood or food/liquid if ileus or obstruction is present).

Indications

- Investigation of upper GI signs/symptoms. e.g. bleeding, pain, mass, obstruction.
- Therapeutic, e.g. sclerotherapy and/or banding for varices, local epinephrine (adrenaline) injection or heat probe (thermocoagulation) for discrete bleeding points, e.g. in peptic ulcer base.
- Placement of nasojejunal tube (when gastric atony prevents enteral feeding) or percutaneous gastrostomy (PEG).
- ERCP—relatively unusual in the ICU patient but may be needed for bile duct/pancreatic duct obstruction.

Complications

- Local trauma causing haemorrhage or perforation.
- Abdominal distension with gas, compromising respiratory function.
- Aspiration of gastric contents.

Contraindications/cautions

- Severe coagulopathy should ideally be corrected.
- Caution with upper GI tract pathology as risk of perforation.

Procedure

Upper GI endoscopy should be performed by an experienced operator to minimise the duration and trauma of the procedure, and to minimise gaseous distension of the gut.

1. The patient is usually placed in a lateral position.
2. Increase FIO$_2$ and ventilator pressure alarm settings. Consider increasing sedation and adjusting ventilator mode.
3. Monitor ECG, SpO$_2$, airway pressures, and haemodynamic variables throughout. If patient is on pressure support or pressure control ventilatory modes, also monitor tidal volumes. The operator should cease the procedure, at least temporarily, if the patient becomes compromised.
4. At the end of the procedure, the operator should aspirate as much air as possible out of the GI tract to decompress the abdomen, and resite a nasogastric tube which often becomes displaced.

See also:
Upper gastrointestinal haemorrhage, p412; Bleeding varices, p414.

Enteral feeding and drainage tubes

Types of tube

Nasogastric

Enteral tube routinely placed in critical care patients to provide nutrition and oral medication, or to drain/decompress the stomach.

- Never use excessive force during insertion if tube does not pass smoothly. Due to external compression from the endotracheal tube, cuff, McGill forceps, or similar may aid passage through the pharynx in intubated patients (under laryngoscopic guidance).
- Before food, liquid, or drug administration, correct positioning of tip should be verified by two of: aspiration of acidic fluid (pH <5), positive auscultation over gastric area when air is injected, and radiological confirmation. Auscultation is the least specific technique and should not be relied upon alone.
- The tube should be tethered securely to the nose. In agitated patients, this may require a sling or suture, especially if repeatedly removed.
- Tube insertion depth should be recorded and regularly checked to ensure non-migration proximally.

A nasogastric tube is contraindicated if there is:

- Any nasopharyngeal or upper GI pathology that obstructs lumen or increases risk of perforation/bleeding, unless expert advice is first obtained (e.g. ENT, GI specialist).
- Bleeding oesophageal varices (non-bleeding varices are not an absolute contraindication).
- Base of skull fracture.
- Severe coagulopathy.

Orogastric

- Sited if contraindication to nasal route, e.g. basal skull fracture.
- Otherwise, similar rules as above apply to NG tube though it is difficult to securely tether and is less well tolerated by patient.

Nasoduodenal/nasojejunal

- Used for gastric outlet obstruction or prolonged gastric ileus.
- Sited radiologically under endoscopic guidance or blind (a weighted tube migrates distally from the stomach over time).

Percutaneous enterogastrotomy (PEG)/jejunostomy (PEJ)

Feeding tube inserted percutaneously under radiological or endoscopic guidance or by direct surgical placement.

- Mainly used for long-term nutrition in patients who cannot maintain adequate oral intake, such as head and neck pathology (e.g. cancer), swallowing difficulties (e.g. stroke, severe head injury). The risk of aspiration pneumonia is reduced.
- Avoid in patients with severe coughing.
- Correct coagulopathy before insertion (platelets >50x10^9/L and INR <1.5).
- Usually retained with an intraluminal balloon ± attachment to skin.
- Follow local guidelines (antibiotic prophylaxis, period of delay before use, initial introduction of water pre-feeding, site care, etc.).
- Such tubes carry a 3–8% morbidity rate and mortality <1% from infection, perforation, internal leakage, peritonitis, bleeding.

See also:
Enteral nutrition, p128; Vomiting/gastric stasis, p406.

Nutrition and metabolic therapy

Nutrition—use and indications

Malnutrition leads to an increased risk of infection due to immune compromise (related to decreased intake of trace elements, amino acids and vitamins, plus decreased production of leptin), increased fatigability and inability to wean/mobilise due to loss of muscle bulk, and poor wound healing. Gut mucosal atrophy occurs within days of non-feeding and may compromise the ability to feed enterally.

Adequate nutritional support should, in general, be provided early during critical illness. Improved outcomes from early nutritional support exist for patients with trauma and burns. Enteral feed is also a gastric protectant. However, the patient should be resuscitated and stabilised before enteral feeding is contemplated as gut hypoperfusion will compromise the ability to absorb, and feeding may render the gut more ischaemic. Increasing abdominal distension, pain/discomfort, large gastric aspirates, and diarrhoea suggest the need for a period of bowel rest rather than persisting with feeding and addition of prokinetics.

Enteral nutrition is indicated when swallowing is inadequate or impossible but GI function is otherwise intact. Parenteral nutrition is indicated when the GI tract cannot be used to provide adequate nutritional support, e.g. obstruction, ileus, high small bowel fistula, or malabsorption. Parenteral nutrition may be used to supplement enteral nutrition.

Calorie requirements

As with nitrogen requirements below, this is inexact and optimal day-to-day intake is not known for individual patients. Various formulae can calculate basal metabolic rate but are misleading in critical illness. Metabolic rate can be measured by indirect calorimetry, but most patients are assumed to require 2000–2700Cal/d or less if starved or underweight. Burn-injured patients generally receive more feed.

Nitrogen requirements

Nitrogen excretion can be calculated in the absence of renal failure according to the 24h urea excretion.

$$\text{Nitrogen (g/24h)} = 2 + \text{urinary urea (mmol/24h)} \times 0.028$$

However, as with most formulae, this method lacks accuracy. Most patients require 7–14g/d.

Other requirements

The normal requirements of substrates, vitamins, and trace elements are tabled opposite. Most long-term, critically ill patients require folic acid and vitamin supplementation during nutritional support. Trace elements are usually supplemented in parenteral formulae but should not be required during enteral nutrition.

Consequences of malnutrition

Underfeeding	Overfeeding
Loss of muscle mass	Increased VO_2
Reduced respiratory function	Increased VCO_2
Reduced immune function	Hyperglycaemia
Poor wound healing	Fatty infiltration of liver
Gut mucosal atrophy	
Reduced protein synthesis	

Normal daily requirements (for a 70kg adult)

Water	2100mL
Energy	2000–2700Cal
Nitrogen	7–14g
Glucose	210g
Lipid	140g
Sodium	70–140mmol
Potassium	50–120mmol
Calcium	5–10mmol
Magnesium	5–10mmol
Phosphate	10–20mmol
Vitamins	
Thiamine	16–19mg
Riboflavin	3–8mg
Niacin	33–34mg
Pyridoxine	5–10mg
Folate	0.3–0.5mg
Vitamin C	250–450mg
Vitamin A	2800–3300IU
Vitamin D	280–330IU
Vitamin E	1.4–1.7IU
Vitamin K	0.7mg
Trace elements	
Iron	1–2mg
Copper	0.5–1.0mg
Manganese	1–2mcg
Zinc	2–4mg
Iodide	70–140mcg
Fluoride	1–2mg

Additional requirements are needed to satisfy excess loss or increased metabolic activity.

See also:
Enteral nutrition, p128; Parenteral nutrition, p130.

Enteral nutrition

Routes include nasogastric, nasoduodenal/jejunal, gastrostomy, and jejunostomy. Nasal tube feeding should be via a soft, fine-bore tube to aid patient comfort and avoid ulceration of the nose or oesophagus. Prolonged enteral feeding may be accomplished via a percutaneous/per-operative gastrostomy or jejunostomy. Enteral feeding provides a more complete diet than parenteral nutrition, maintains structural integrity of the gut, improves bowel adaptation after resection, and reduces infection risk.

Feed composition

Most patients tolerate iso-osmolar, non-lactose feed. Carbohydrates are provided as sucrose or glucose polymers; protein as whole protein or oligopeptides (may be better absorbed than free amino acids in 'elemental' feeds); fats as medium chain or long chain triglycerides. Medium chain triglycerides are better absorbed. Standard feed is formulated at 1Cal/mL. Special feeds are available, e.g. high fibre, high protein-calorie, restricted salt, high fat or concentrated (1.5 or 2Cal/mL) for fluid restriction. Immune-enhanced feeds (e.g. glutamine-enriched or Impact®, a feed supplemented with nucleotides, arginine, and fish oil) may reduce nosocomial infections, but no evidence of outcome benefit has yet been shown from large prospective studies.

Management of enteral nutrition

Once a decision is made to start enteral nutrition, 30mL/h full strength standard feed may be started immediately. Starter regimens incorporating dilute feed are not necessary. After 4h at 30mL/h, the feed should be stopped for 30min prior to aspiration of the stomach. Since gastric juice production is increased by the presence of a nasogastric tube, it is reasonable to accept an aspirate of <200mL as evidence of gastric emptying, and therefore, to increase the infusion rate to 60mL/h. This process is repeated until the target feed rate is achieved. Thereafter, aspiration of the stomach can be reduced to 8-hourly. If gastric aspirate volume >200mL, the infusion rate is not increased though feed is continued. If aspirates remain at high volume, consider either prokinetics to promote gastric emptying (e.g. metoclopramide, erythromycin), bowel rest (especially if abdominal distension or discomfort increases), nasoduodenal/jejunal or parenteral feeding.

Complications

- Tube misplacement: tracheobronchial, nasopharyngeal perforation, intracranial penetration (basal skull fracture), oesophageal perforation.
- Reflux.
- Pulmonary aspiration.
- Nausea and vomiting.
- Abdominal distension is occasionally reported with features including a tender, distended abdomen, and an increasing metabolic acidosis. Laparotomy and bowel resection may be necessary in severe cases.
- Refeeding syndrome.
- Diarrhoea: large volume, bolus feeding, high osmolality, infection, lactose intolerance, antibiotic therapy, high fat content.
- Constipation.
- Metabolic: dehydration, hyperglycaemia, electrolyte imbalance.

Key paper

Atkinson S, Sieffert E, Bihari D. (1998) A prospective, randomised, double-blind, controlled clinical trial of enteral immunonutrition in the critically ill. *Crit Care Med* **26**: 1164–72.

See also:

Nutrition—use and indications, p126; Gut motility agents, p294; Vomiting/gastric stasis, p406; Diarrhoea, p408.

Parenteral nutrition

Feed composition
Carbohydrate is normally provided as concentrated glucose. 30–40% of total calories are usually given as lipid (e.g. soya bean emulsion). The nitrogen source is synthetic, crystalline L-amino acids which should contain appropriate quantities of all essential and most non-essential amino acids. Carbohydrate, lipid, and nitrogen sources are usually mixed into a large bag in a sterile pharmacy unit. Vitamins, trace elements, and appropriate electrolyte concentrations can be achieved in a single infusion, thus avoiding multiple connections. Volume, protein and calorie content of the feed should be determined on a daily basis in conjunction with the dietician.

Choice of parenteral feeding route
Central venous
A dedicated catheter (or lumen of a multi-lumen catheter) is placed under sterile conditions. For long-term feeding, a subcutaneous tunnel is often used to separate skin and vein entry sites. This probably reduces the risk of infection and clearly identifies the special purpose of the catheter. Ideally, blood samples should not be taken nor other injections or infusions given via the feeding lumen. The central venous route allows infusion of hyper-osmolar solutions, providing adequate energy intake in reduced volume.

Peripheral venous
Parenteral nutrition via the peripheral route requires a solution with osmolality <800mOsm/kg. Either the volume must be increased or the energy content (particularly from carbohydrate) reduced. Peripheral cannulae sites must be changed frequently.

Complications

Catheter-related	Misplacement
	Infection
	Thromboembolism
Fluid excess	
Hyperosmolar, hyperglycaemic state	
Electrolyte imbalance	
Hypophosphataemia	
Metabolic acidosis	Hyperchloraemia
	Metabolism of cationic amino acids
Rebound hypoglycaemia (from high endogenous insulin levels)	
Vitamin deficiency	Folate (pancytopaenia)
	Thiamine (encephalopathy, neuropathy, heart failure)
	Vitamin K (hypoprothrombinaemia)
Vitamin excess	Vitamin A (dermatitis)
	Vitamin D (hypercalcaemia)
Fatty liver	

See also:
Nutrition—use and indications, p126; Indirect calorimetry, p234; Electrolyte management, p482; Hypophosphataemia, p498; Metabolic acidosis, p502; Hyperglycaemia, p508.

Tight glycaemic control/intensive insulin therapy

Rationale

Hyperglycaemia and insulin resistance occur commonly in critically ill patients and are associated with an increased risk of mortality. This may be related to immune compromise, an increased rate of bacterial growth, and the effects of glycation and free radical production on protein, lipid and mitochondrial function and integrity.

In two landmark papers by van den Berghe et al., a combination of tight glucose control (aiming for blood glucose levels of 4.5–6.1mmol/L) plus additional glucose and insulin administration reduced mortality and morbidity in both surgical and medical critical care patients. Benefit was only seen in those receiving >3–4 days' therapy.

Controversy has since existed regarding how tight the glucose control should be, with some advocating a 5–8mmol/L target range to reduce the risk of potentially injurious hypoglycaemia, particularly as regular testing introduces a significant nurse workload. The introduction of (semi-) continuous, (semi-) automated blood glucose monitoring devices should facilitate closer maintenance of normoglycaemia.

Protocol

Several protocols and algorithms have been devised by different groups. None are perfect, but suit the particular circumstances of their units in terms of staffing levels and expertise.

Key papers

Van den Berghe G, Wouters P, Weekers F, et al. (2001) Intensive insulin therapy in critically ill patients. *N Engl J Med* **345**: 1359–67.

Van den Berghe G, Wilmer A, Hermans G, et al. (2006) Intensive insulin therapy in the medical ICU. *N Engl J Med* **354**: 449–61.

Brunkhorst FM, Engel C, Bloos F, et al. (2008) Intensive insulin therapy and pentastarch resuscitation in severe sepsis. *N Engl J Med* **358**: 125–39.

See also:

Hypoglycaemia, p506.

Wound and pressure area management

Wound management principles

Wound management attempts to promote wound healing, prevent contamination and wound breakdown, and reduce pain and discomfort.

A wound heals through the phases of haemostasis, inflammation, granulation, and maturation.

The first two processes arrest bleeding and help remove contamination.

- Granulation involves rebuilding of the tissues, angiogenesis contraction, and epithelialisation. This process normally takes about 21 days, but may be delayed by age, infection, dehydration, or poor nutrition.
- Maturation may take several years and involves remodelling of the dermis to increase the strength of the healed wound.

A wound that fails to go through these process steps may become chronic.

It is important to keep the wound warm and moist since all human cells (with the exception of the dead, keratinised, superficial skin cells) require moisture to survive, and warmth to grow and divide. An exudate provides the best environment for healing by supporting cells involved in wound repair with nutrients. Although angiogenesis is increased in a low oxygen environment (e.g. under occlusive dressings), most large, randomised trials show reduction in post-operative wound infection from administering supplemental oxygen.

Wound cleansing

Wounds should be cleaned by irrigation with isotonic saline. Soaps irritate the wound but may be useful on the surrounding skin. Both iodine and peroxide irritate the wound, are unnecessary, and best avoided.

Wound infection

The hallmarks of wound infection are:
- Pain.
- Redness.
- Increased warmth.
- Tenderness.
- Oedema.
- Purulent discharge.
- Foul odour.

Systemic or spreading signs of infection (e.g. cellulitis) may be present and mandate systemic antibiotic therapy. The wound should be swabbed prior to treatment. Otherwise, local treatments may be sufficient, e.g. silver preparations, iodine-based preparations, and topical antibiotic (e.g. silver sulfadiazine). The latter should only be used for short-term treatment in mild cases. Surgical debridement may occasionally be needed.

Pressure sores

Pressure sores occur due to compression of tissue between bone and the support surface, and due to shearing forces, friction, and maceration of tissues against the support surface. A pressure sore requires cleansing, debridement of eschar or necrotic tissue, staging (see table opposite), and packing if there is crater formation. Packing should occlude the ulcer, but should be loose to avoid adding to the pressure damage. Dressings should keep the ulcer moist.

Staging of pressure sores

Stage 1	Skin intact with persistent redness due to pressure
Stage 2	Ulcer involving the epidermis or dermis.
Stage 3	Ulcer involving subcutaneous tissue layer. May be undermined.
Stage 4	Ulcer extends through the fascia to muscle, tendon, or bone. Undermining and tunnelling may be present.
Unstageable	Ulcer bed cannot be visualised due to slough or eschar.

Modified from the National Pressure Ulcer Advisory Panel, February 2007.

See also:
Dressing techniques, p138; Special support surfaces, p140.

Dressing techniques

Wound dressings serve to reduce pain, protect the wound from further injury and infection, and reduce moisture loss. Dressings should be non-adherent, sterile, and cover the wound completely. Adherent dressings delay wound healing.

When dressings are applied to wounds, an aseptic technique must be used.

Bio-occlusive dressings
These allow air and water vapour to permeate, thus accelerating healing; they are transparent to allow wound assessment and are waterproof.

Calcium alginate
Calcium exchanges with sodium from the wound to convert exudates to a gel. This reduces moisture loss. They are not effective for dry wounds since they depend on absorption of exudates to be active.

Foam dressing
Foam dressings absorb excessive exudates while allowing air and vapour permeation to accelerate healing. They require absorption of exudates to be effective. They are thermally insulating and non-adherent.

Hydrocolloids
Hydrocolloid dressings provide slow absorption of exudates to create a soft, non-adherent gel which occludes the wound and retains moisture. They are effective when exudates are low volume. They should not be used in infected wounds as growth of anaerobes may be encouraged by their occlusive properties.

Hydrogels
Hydrogels have hydrophilic sites to enable absorption of excess exudates. They retain moisture.

Vacuum-assisted closure (VAC)
A foam dressing is placed in the ulcer absorbing excessive exudates. The ulcer is sealed with an adhesive drape and negative pressure is applied for up to 24h per day. The VAC dressing reduces oedema and improves local blood supply while removing surface debris and exudate. Intermittent treatment may be more effective than continuous. Use of VAC dressing is advantageous in perineal pressure sores because the vacuum helps keep the dressing in place.

Properties of wound dressings
- Maintain warmth.
- Maintain moisture.
- Remove exudates.
- Allow vapour and gas permeation.
- Minimise contamination.
- Non-adherent.

See also:
Wound management principles, p136.

Special support surfaces

The use of special support surfaces attempts to reduce the pressure at the contacting skin surface to a level below capillary occlusion pressure. In most cases, it is sufficient to use postural changes to minimise the time the support surface contacts with any one area of skin.

Factors suggesting need for special support surfaces

- Patients with severely restricted mobility due to external traction or cardiorespiratory instability cannot be turned frequently, if at all.
- Patients with decreased skin integrity, e.g. burns, pressure sores already present, chronic corticosteroid use, diabetes mellitus.
- Patients on vasoactive drug infusions and/or poor tissue perfusion.

Types of special support surface

Air mattress
This either replaces or is placed on top of a standard hospital bed mattress. Although providing minimum reduction in contact pressure, they should be considered as minimum support for patients with any of the above factors.

Low air loss bed
These purpose-built, pressure-relieving beds allow easier patient mobility than other support surfaces. Contact pressure may still be higher than capillary occlusion pressure so positioning is still required. Patients who are haemodynamically unstable should usually be managed on a low air loss bed, particularly if receiving vasoconstrictor drugs. The presence of pressure sores with intact skin is an indication for a low air loss bed. Rotational low air loss beds allow automated lateral rotation at variable time intervals to facilitate chest drainage. These may also be useful where manual positioning is impractical.

Air fluidised bed
This is the only support surface that consistently lowers contact pressure to below capillary occlusion pressure. Consequently, most benefit is seen in patients with severe cardiorespiratory instability who cannot be turned, and those with pressure sores and broken skin. The additional ability to control temperature of the immediate environment is advantageous in hypothermic patients and those with large surface area burns. Any exudate from the skin is adsorbed into the silicone beads on which the patient floats. This drying effect is particularly useful in major burns (although it must be taken into account for fluid replacement therapy). The air fluidised bed also has a role in pain relief.

Rotation therapy
Rotation therapy beds continuously change the pressure with the contacting surface by lateral turning to each side. This reduces shear and minimises pain and discomfort associated with manual turning.

See also:
Wound management principles, p136.

Respiratory monitoring

Pulse oximetry

Continuous, non-invasive monitoring of arterial oxygen saturation by placement of a probe emitting red and near-infrared light over a pulse on a digit, ear lobe, cheek, or bridge of the nose. It is unaffected by skin pigmentation, hyperbilirubinaemia, or anaemia (unless profound).

Physics

The colour of blood varies with oxygen saturation due to the optical properties of the haem moiety. As the haemoglobin molecule gives up O_2, it becomes less permeable to red light and takes on a blue tint. Saturation is determined spectrophotometrically by measuring the 'blueness', utilising the ability of compounds to absorb light at a specific wavelength. The use of two wavelengths (650 and 940nm) permits the relative quantities of reduced and oxyhaemoglobin to be calculated, thereby determining saturation. The arterial pulse is used to provide timepoints to allow subtraction of the constant absorption of light by tissue and venous blood. The accuracy of pulse oximetry is $\pm$ 2% at values above 70% SaO_2.

Indications

- Continuous monitoring of arterial oxygen saturation.

Cautions

- As only two wavelengths are used, pulse oximetry measures functional rather than fractional oxyhaemoglobin saturation. Erroneously high readings are given with carboxyhaemoglobin and methaemoglobin.
- With poor peripheral perfusion or intense vasoconstriction, the reading may be inaccurate ('fail soft') or, in newer models, absent ('fail hard').
- Motion artefact and high levels of ambient lighting may affect readings.
- Erroneous signals may be produced by significant venous pulsation from tricuspid regurgitation or venous congestion. Venous pulsatility accounts for differences between ear and finger SpO_2 in the same subject.
- Ensure a good LED signal indicator or a pulse waveform (if available) is seen on the monitor.
- Vital dyes, e.g. methylthioninium chloride (methylene blue) and indocyanine green, may affect SpO_2 readings as may nail varnish.

See also:

Oxygen therapy, p38; Ventilatory support—indications, p44; IPPV—adjusting the ventilator, p50; Vasopressors, p268.

CO_2 monitoring

Capnography

For capnography, respiratory gases must be sampled continuously and measured by a rapid response device attached to (sidestream sampling) or within the breathing circuit (mainstream sampling). As CO_2 has an absorption band within the infrared spectrum, CO_2 tension is usually measured by infrared absorption. Other gases can interfere, but this may be overcome by calibrating the instrument with known concentrations of CO_2 in the required measurement range, i.e. diluted with a gas mixture similar to exhaled gas.

The capnogram

The CO_2 concentration of exhaled gas consists of four phases (see figure 8.1). The presence of significant concentrations of CO_2 in phase 1 implies rebreathing of exhaled gas. Failure of an expiratory valve to open is the most likely cause of rebreathing during manual ventilation, although an inadequate flow of fresh gas into a rebreathing bag is a common cause. The slope of phase 3 is dependent on the rate of alveolar gas exchange. A steep slope may indicate ventilation-perfusion mismatch since alveoli that are poorly ventilated but well-perfused discharge late in the respiratory cycle. A steep slope is seen in patients with significant auto-PEEP.

Colorimetric devices

The underlying principle is that the change in pH produced by different CO_2 concentrations in solution will change the colour of an indicator. These are small devices that fit onto an ET tube or the ventilator circuit and respond rapidly (up to 60 breaths/min). They can be affected by excessive humidity and generally only work in the range 0–4% CO_2. They are useful to confirm tracheal intubation during patient transfer and in the cardiac arrest situation.

End-tidal PCO_2

End-tidal PCO_2 approximates $PaCO_2$ in patients with normal lung function. In ICU patients, pulmonary function is rarely normal, thus end-tidal PCO_2 is a poor approximation of $PaCO_2$. Large differences may represent an increased dead space to tidal volume ratio, poor pulmonary perfusion or intra-pulmonary shunting. A progressive rise in end-tidal PCO_2 may represent hypoventilation, airway obstruction, or increased CO_2 production due to increased metabolic rate. End-tidal PCO_2 falls with hyperventilation and in low cardiac output states. It is absent with ventilator disconnection and during cardiac arrest, but rises with effective CPR or restoration of a spontaneous circulation.

Dead space to tidal volume ratio

The arterial to end-tidal PCO_2 difference may be used to calculate the physiological dead space to tidal volume ratio via the Bohr equation:

$$\frac{V_D}{V_T} = \left(\frac{PaCO_2 - PetCO_2}{PaCO_2} \right)$$

In health, a value between 30 and 45% should be expected.

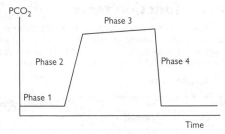

Fig. 8.1 The components of the normal capnogram.

Phase 1
During the early part of the exhaled breath, anatomical dead space and sampling device dead space gas are sampled. There is negligible CO$_2$ in phase 1.

Phase 2
As alveolar gas begins to be sampled, there is a rapid rise in CO$_2$ concentration.

Phase 3
Phase 3 is known as the alveolar plateau and represents the CO$_2$ concentration in mixed expired alveolar gas. There is normally a slight increase in PCO$_2$ during phase 3 as alveolar gas exchange continues during expiration. Airway obstruction or a high rate of CO$_2$ production will increase the slope. End-tidal PCO$_2$ will be less than the PCO$_2$ of ideal alveolar gas since the sampled exhaled gas is mixed with alveolar dead space gas.

Phase 4
As inspiration begins, there is a rapid fall in sample PCO$_2$.

See also:
Endotracheal intubation, p42; Ventilatory support-indications, p44; IPPV—adjusting the ventilator, p50; Tracheotomy, p80; Blood gas analysis, p154.

Pulmonary function tests

Few of the numerous pulmonary function tests available currently impact upon clinical management of the critically ill, particularly if the patient has to be moved to a laboratory. A number of other tests require highly specialised equipment and fulfil a predominant research role.

Clinically relevant tests

Measurement	Test	Common clinical use
PaO_2, SaO_2, $PaCO_2$	Arterial blood gases	
SpO_2	Pulse oximetry	
End-tidal PCO_2	Capnography	
Vital capacity, tidal volume (see figure 8.2)	Spirometry, electronic flowmetry	Serial measurement of borderline function (VC <10–15mL/kg) e.g. Guillain–Barré syndrome
Peak expiratory flow rate	Wright peak flow meter	(Spontaneous ventilation) asthma
FEV_1, FVC (see figure 8.2)	Spirometry, electronic flowmetry	(Spontaneous ventilation) asthma, obstructive/restrictive disease
Lung/chest wall compliance	The change in pressure litre increase in volume above FRC	Ventilator adjustments, monitoring disease progression
Flow-volume loop, pressure-volume loop	Pneumotachograph, manometry	Ventilator adjustments

Notes
- The alveolar–arterial oxygen difference ($A–aDO_2$) is <2kPa in youth and <3.3kPa in old age.
- The Bohr equation calculates physiological deadspace (V_D). The normal value is <30%.
- The shunt equation estimates the proportion of blood shunted past poorly ventilated alveoli (Q_S) compared to total lung blood flow (Q_T). The normal range is <15%.

Equations

Alveolar gas equation

$$P_AO_2 = (FIO_2 \times 94.8) - \left(\frac{PaCO_2}{RQ}\right)$$

Respiratory quotient (RQ) is often approximated to 0.8.

Alveolar–arterial oxygen difference (A–aDO₂)

$$A - aDO_2 = (FIO_2 \times 94.8) - (PaCO_2/RQ) - PaO_2$$

Dead space to tidal volume ratio (Bohr equation)

$$\frac{V_D}{V_T} = \left(\frac{PaCO_2 - PetCO_2}{PaCO_2}\right)$$

Shunt equation

$$\frac{Q_S}{Q_T} = \left(\frac{CcO_2 - CaO_2}{CcO_2 - CvO_2}\right)$$

CcO_2 = end-capillary O_2 content, a = arterial, v = mixed venous.

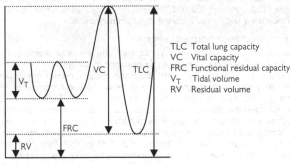

TLC   Total lung capacity
VC   Vital capacity
FRC   Functional residual capacity
V_T Tidal volume
RV   Residual volume

Fig. 8.2 Lung volumes and capacities.

See also:
Pulse oximetry, p144; CO_2 monitoring, p146.

Volume-pressure relationship

This is determined by the compliance of the lungs and chest wall. The inspiratory volume-pressure relationship contains three components: an initial increase in pressure with no significant volume change; a linear increase in volume as pressure increases (the slope of which represents respiratory system compliance); and a further period of pressure increase with no volume increase. These three phases are separated by two inflexion zones, the lower representing the opening pressure of the system after flow resistance has been overcome in smaller airways, and the upper approximating to total lung capacity. The expiratory pressure-volume relationship should normally approximate the inspiratory curve, returning to functional residual capacity. In patients with small airway collapse, separation of the inspiratory and expiratory curves occurs (hysteresis) as gas is trapped in smaller airways at the end of expiration.

Dynamic measurement

A pressure-volume loop may be viewed on most modern mechanical ventilators. A square wave inspiratory waveform (constant flow) and no inspiratory pause are necessary for waveform interpretation.

Static measurement

Small, incremental lung volumes (200mL) are delivered with a calibrated syringe. The pressure measurement after each increment is taken under zero flow conditions, allowing construction of a pressure-volume curve. A quasi-static curve can be constructed by setting incremental tidal volumes (e.g. between 100 and 1000mL) for successive ventilator breaths and measuring the pressure during an inspiratory pause.

Use of volume-pressure curves

Since respiratory muscle activity can alter intrathoracic pressure, the volume-pressure curve is more easily obtained in the relaxed, fully ventilated patient (see figure 8.3). Both static and dynamic respiratory system compliance can be determined as the slope of the linear portion of the curve, i.e. where incremental pressure inflates the lungs. Below the lower inflexion zone the small airways are closed and expiration does not reach functional residual capacity. Therefore, the lower inflexion zone represents the appropriate setting for external PEEP to avoid gas trapping. Above the upper inflexion zone, the lungs cannot inflate further. Therefore, the upper inflexion zone represents the maximum setting for peak airway pressure.

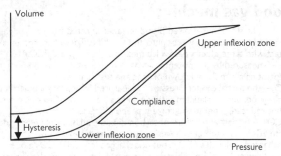

Fig. 8.3 Volume-pressure curve.

Compliance: calculations

Lung compliance (L/cmH$_2$O) = $\Delta V_L/\Delta P_L$ where L, the litre above FRC, is the slope of the linear portion of the curve.

Total respiratory system compliance is derived from the equation:

(1/total compliance) = (1/lung compliance) + (1/chest wall compliance)

Total compliance can be calculated in well-sedated, ventilated patients as: tidal volume/(end-inspiratory pause pressure — PEEP).

See also:

IPPV—adjusting the ventilator, p50; Positive end expiratory pressure (1), p66; Positive end expiratory pressure (2), p68.

Blood gas machine

A small amount of heparinised blood is either injected from a syringe or aspirated from a capillary tube into the machine. The blood comes into contact with three electrodes which measure pH, PO_2, and PCO_2.

- pH—measured by the potential across a pH-sensitive glass membrane separating a sample of known pH and the test sample.
- PO_2—the partial oxygen pressure, is measured by applying a polarising voltage between a platinum cathode and a silver anode (Clark electrode). O_2 is reduced, generating a current proportional to the PO_2.
- PCO_2—the partial pressure of carbon dioxide, utilises a pH electrode with a Teflon membrane (Severinghaus electrode) that allows through uncharged molecules (CO_2), but not charged ions (H^+). CO_2 alone thus changes the pH of a bicarbonate electrolyte solution, the change being linearly related to the PCO_2.
- Hb—estimated photometrically; this is not as accurate as co-oximetry (see below).
- Bicarbonate—calculated by the Henderson–Hasselbach equation. Actual HCO_3^- includes bicarbonate, carbonate, and carbamate.

$$pH = 6.1 + \log_{10} \frac{\text{arterial}\left[HCO_3^-\right]}{PaCO_2 \times 0.03}$$

- Actual base excess (deficit)—the difference in concentration of strong base (acid) in whole blood and that titrated to pH 7.4, at PCO_2 5.33kPa and 37°C.
- Standard base excess (deficit)—a calculated *in vivo* base excess (deficit).
- Standard bicarbonate—the plasma concentration of hydrogen carbonate equilibrated at PCO_2 5.33kPa, PO_2 13.33kPa, and temperature 37°C.

Blood gas values can be given either as 'pHstat' or 'alphastat', the former correcting for body temperature by shifting the calculated Bohr oxyhaemoglobin dissociation curve (hyperthermia to the right, hypothermia to the left). Alphastat measures true blood gas levels in the sample.

Co-oximeter

This differs from a blood gas machine in that the blood is haemolysed to calculate: (i) total Hb and fetal Hb, and (ii) oxyHb, carboxyhaemoglobin (COHb), methaemoglobin, and sulphaemoglobin by utilising absorbance at six wavelengths (535, 560, 577, 622, 636, 670nm).

Taking a good blood gas sample

Use a 1mL syringe containing preferably a dry heparin salt (if not, liquid sodium heparin 1000IU/mL solution just filling the hub). Take sample, expel air, mix sample thoroughly, and insert without delay.

Cautions

- Too much heparin causes dilution errors and is acidic.
- Nitrous oxide or halothane anaesthesia may give unreliable PO_2 values.
- Intravenous lipid administration may affect pH values.
- Abnormal (high/low) plasma protein concentrations affect base deficit.

See also:
Blood gas analysis, p154.

Blood gas analysis

A heparinised (arterial, venous, capillary) blood sample can be inserted into a blood gas machine and/or co-oximeter for measurement of gas tensions and saturations, and acid-base status.

Measurements

- Identification of arterial hypoxaemia and hyperoxia, hypercapnia and hypocapnia—enabling monitoring of disease progression and efficacy of treatment. Ventilator and FIO_2 adjustments can be made precisely.
- pH, $PaCO_2$ and base deficit (or bicarbonate) values can be reviewed in parallel for diagnosis of acidosis and alkalosis, whether it is respiratory or metabolic in origin, and whether any compensation has occurred. (see figure 8.4).
- Using a co-oximeter, accurate measurement can be made of haemoglobin oxygen saturation and also the total Hb level. The more sophisticated co-oximeters permit measurement of the fraction of metHb, COHb, deoxyHb, and fetal Hb.
- Measurement of mixed venous oxygen saturation—for calculation of oxygen consumption and monitoring of 'oxygen supply:demand balance'.

Causes of acid-base disturbances

Respiratory acidosis	pH↓, $PaCO_2$↑	Excess CO_2 production and/or inadequate excretion, e.g. hypoventilation, excess narcotic.
Respiratory alkalosis	pH↑, $PaCO_2$↓	Reduction in PCO_2 due to hyperventilation
Metabolic acidosis	pH↓, $PaCO_2$ → or ↓	Usually lactic, keto, renal, or tubular. Consider tissue hypoperfusion, ingestion of acids (e.g. aspirin), loss of alkali (e.g. diarrhoea, renal tubular acidosis), diabetic ketoacidosis, and hyperchloraemia (e.g. from excess normal saline administration).
Metabolic alkalosis	pH↑, $PaCO_2$ → or ↑	Consider excess alkali (e.g. bicarbonate or buffer infusion), loss of acid (e.g. large gastric aspirates, renal), hypokalaemia, drugs (e.g. diuretics).

Normal values

pH	7.35–7.45
PCO_2	4.6–6kPa
PO_2	10–13.3kPa
HCO_3^-	22–26mmol/L
ABE	–2.4 to +2.2
Arterial O_2 saturation	95–98%
Mixed venous oxygen saturation	70–75%

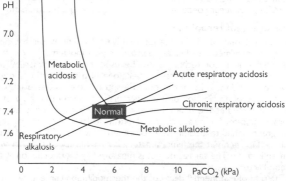

Fig. 8.4 Relationship between $PaCO_2$ and pH in various acid-base disturbances.

See also:

Oxygen therapy, p38; Ventilatory support—indications, p44; IPPV—adjusting the ventilator, p50; Pressure and stroke volume vatriation, p190; Respiratory failure, p350; General acid-base principles, p500; Metabolic acidosis, p502; Metabolic alkalosis, p504.

Extravascular lung water measurement

Standard methods of assessing pulmonary oedema are indirect. The chest X-ray allows only a qualitative assessment and is slow to change in response to clinical treatment. Assessment of cardiac filling pressures does not take into account the degree of capillary permeability or lymphatic adaptation. Consequently, a relatively low CVP or PAWP may be associated with pulmonary oedema formation. High filling pressures in chronic heart failure may be associated with no oedema and be entirely appropriate. Extravascular lung water (EVLW) measurement provides a technique for quantifying pulmonary oedema and monitoring the response to treatment.

Measurement technique

The normal value of 4–7mL/kg for extravascular lung water has been derived by gravimetric techniques performed post-mortem.

A double indicator technique can be used in patients whereby two indicators are injected via a central vein; one distributes within the vascular space and the other throughout the intra- and extra-vascular space. The volume of distribution of the indicators is derived from the dilution curves detected at the femoral artery. Cooled 5% glucose is used as a thermal indicator for intravascular and extravascular volume, and indocyanine green bound to albumin as a colorimetric indicator for intravascular volume. Detection at the femoral artery is by a fibreoptic catheter with a thermistor tip. The cardiac output is measured by thermodilution at the femoral artery.

The rate of exponential decay of the thermodilution curve allows derivation of the volume of distribution between the injection and detection sites (the heart and lungs).

> Pulmonary thermal volume = thermodilution cardiac output x rate of exponential decay of thermodilution curve (intravascular and extravascular volume)

Similar principles may be applied to the dye dilution curve produced on injection of indocyanine green which is assumed to distribute within the vascular space only.

> Pulmonary blood volume = dye dilution cardiac output x rate of exponential decay of dye dilution curve (intravascular volume)

EVLW may be calculated by subtracting pulmonary blood volume from pulmonary thermal volume.

Limitations of EVLW measurement

Since albumin can exchange across capillary membranes, pulmonary blood volume is over-estimated by this technique, and therefore, extravascular lung water is under-estimated. However, the corresponding error is small and not clinically significant. A more serious drawback is in the limitation of treatment options. Treatment of pulmonary oedema by diuresis and ultrafiltration have been shown to be less effective at reducing EVLW in capillary leak from inflammatory conditions compared to congestive heart failure. Similarly, the strategy of preventing oedema formation by diuresis while maintaining the circulation with catecholamine infusions appears to be futile; the vasoconstriction so produced increases EVLW.

See also:

Cardiac output—central thermodilution, p178; Cardiac output—peripheral thermodilution, p180;
Acute respiratory distress syndrome (1), p360; Acute respiratory distress syndrome (2), p362.

Respiratory imaging

Chest X-ray

The chest X-ray has the advantage that it can be performed at the bedside of a critically ill patient. It yields much useful information on pathologies within and outside the lung parenchyma (e.g. consolidation, pulmonary oedema, collapse, pleural effusion, pneumothorax); confirmation of suitable positioning of intra-tracheal, intravascular, and naso-gatric/oesophageal tubes and catheters; soft tissue and bony abnormalities; cardiac contour and size; vascular abnormalities (e.g. aortic diameter, oligaemic lung field suggestive of a pulmonary embolus); and free air under the diaphragm.

There are certain pitfalls that need to be appreciated:

- The position of the patient is usually supine (AP image) over-estimating ventricular dimensions and camouflaging the presence of a pneumothorax that sits in front of (or behind) normal lung tissue. Look for an 'inverted diaphragm' and increased lucency compared to the other lung.
- Underestimation of the size of pleural effusions or pneumothoraces.

Lateral chest X-rays may be useful in diagnosing a pneumothorax that is not obviously apparent on a supine film.

Ultrasound

Ultrasound can detect pleural or pericardial effusions, peripheral areas of consolidated lung, and peripheral pneumothorax. It can also assist with intravascular line placement to minimise risk of arterial or lung puncture and drainage of fluid collections.

CT scan

CT scan is the definitive imaging procedure for pathology within the thorax. Injection of contrast highlights vascular structures and the presence of pulmonary emboli in sub-segmental arteries (with high resolution scanning). It enables improved discrimination of pulmonary shadows, e.g. fluid, fibrosis, consolidation, atelectasis, abscess, empyema, and can be used to guide drainage procedures of air and fluid collections.

See also:
Airway obstruction, p348; Atelectasis and pulmonary collapse, p352; Acute chest infection (1),
p356; Acute respiratory distress syndrome (1), p360; Asthma—general management, p364;
Pneumothorax, p368; Haemothorax, p370; Pulmonary embolus, p376; Heart failure—assessment,
p392; Intrahospital transport, p644.

Cardiovascular monitoring

ECG monitoring

Continuous ECG monitoring is routinely used in every Critical Care Unit. The standard technique is to display a three-lead ECG (commonly lead II). Other limb leads may be used although the electrodes are placed at the shoulders and left side of the abdomen. Other lead configurations can be used for specific purposes:

- Chest–shoulder–V5: Early detection of left ventricular strain.
- Chest–manubrium–V5: Early detection of left ventricular strain.
- Chest–back–V5: p wave monitoring.

Modern monitors include alarm functions for bradycardia and tachycardia monitoring, and software routines for arrhythmia detection or ST segment analysis.

Causes of changes in heart rate or rhythm

Changes in heart rate or rhythm may be an indication of:
- Increased sympathetic/parasympathetic activity:
  - Circulatory insufficiency.
  - Pain.
  - Anxiety.
  - Hypoxaemia.
  - Hypercapnia.
  - Sepsis.
- Adverse drug effects:
  - Antiarrhythmics.
  - Sedatives.
- Electrolyte imbalance.
- Fever.

See also:
Tachyarrhythmias, p384; Bradyarrhythmias, p386; Acute coronary syndrome (1), p388;
Acute coronary syndrome (2), p390.

Blood pressure monitoring

Non-invasive techniques

Non-invasive techniques are intermittent but automated. They include oscillotonometry (detection of cuff pulsation as the systolic pressure), detection of arterial turbulence under the cuff, ultrasonic detection of arterial wall motion under the cuff, and detection of blood flow distal to the cuff. Any cuff system should use a cuff large enough to cover two thirds of the surface of the upper arm.

Invasive (direct) arterial monitoring

Blood pressure is most usefully monitored from larger limb arteries, e.g. femoral or brachial. However, because of the potential risk of damage to these arteries compromising the distal limb, it is generally safer to use radial, ulnar, or dorsalis pedis arteries. Pressure measured in a distal artery is higher than from a central vessel. The arterial cannula is connected to an appropriate transducer system via a short length of non-compliant manometer tubing. The transducer should be matched to the monitor, i.e. as recommended by the manufacturer of the monitor. The transducer must be zeroed to atmospheric pressure and be positioned at the level of the 4th intercostal space in the mid-axillary line. The transducer, manometer tubing, and cannula should be continuously flushed with 3mL/h saline or heparinised saline (1000IU/L).

Damping errors

A correctly damped system will return immediately to the pressure waveform after flushing. Return is slow in an over-damped system, and there is often resonance around the baseline before return to the pressure waveform in an under-damped system. An under-damped system will over-estimate systolic and under-estimate diastolic blood pressure. The converse is true for an over-damped system. Waveform shape cannot be correctly interpreted unless damping is correct.

Interpretation of waveform

The shape of the arterial pressure waveform gives useful qualitative information about the state of the heart and circulation (see figure 9.1):

Short systolic time	Hypovolaemia
	High peripheral resistance
Marked respiratory swing	Hypovolaemia
	Pericardial effusion
	Airways obstruction
	High intrathoracic pressure
Slow systolic upstroke	Poor myocardial contractility
	High peripheral resistance

Limitations of blood pressure monitoring

It is important not to rely on arterial blood pressure monitoring alone in the critically ill. A normal blood pressure does not guarantee adequate organ blood flow. Conversely, a low blood pressure may be acceptable if perfusion pressure is adequate for all organs and blood flow is high. Measurement of cardiac output and markers of organ perfusion, in addition to blood pressure, is necessary where there is doubt about the adequacy of the circulation.

Normal arterial waveform

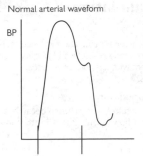

BP

Systolic time

Short systolic time

BP

Systolic time

Slow systolic upstroke

BP

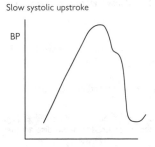

Fig. 9.1 Examples of arterial waveform shape.

See also:

Arterial cannulation, p166; Hypotension, p380; Hypertension, p382.

Arterial cannulation

Indications

Performed correctly, arterial cannulation is a safe technique allowing continuous monitoring of blood pressure and frequent sampling of blood. It is indicated in any patient with unstable or potentially unstable haemodynamic or respiratory status.

Radial artery cannulation

The radial artery is most frequently chosen because it is accessible and has good collateral blood flow. Allen's test, used to confirm the ulnar blood supply, is not reliable.

Technique of cannulation

Use aseptic technique. Hyperextend the wrist and abduct the thumb. After skin cleansing, local anaesthetic (1% plain lidocaine) is injected into the skin and subcutaneous tissue over the most prominent pulsation. The course of the artery is noted and a 20G Teflon cannula inserted along the line of the vessel. The vessel is usually entered in similar fashion to an intravenous cannula. There is usually some resistance to skin puncture. To avoid accidentally puncturing the posterior wall of the artery, the skin and artery should be punctured as two distinct manoeuvres. Alternatively, a small skin nick may be made to facilitate skin entry.

In the case of elderly patients with mobile, atheromatous vessels, a technique involving deliberate transfixation of the artery may be used. The cannula is passed through the anterior and posterior walls of the vessel, thus immobilising it. The needle is removed and the cannula withdrawn slowly into the vessel lumen before being advanced.

Seldinger-type kits are available for arterial cannulation. A guidewire is first inserted through a rigid steel needle. The indwelling plastic cannula is then placed over the guidewire.

The cannula should be connected to a continuous flushing device after successful puncture. Flushing with a syringe should be avoided since the high pressures generated may lead to a retrograde cerebral embolus.

Alternative sites for cannulation

Brachial artery

End artery supplying a large volume of tissue. Thus thrombosis has potentially severe consequences.

Ulnar artery

Should be avoided if the radial artery is occluded.

Femoral artery

May be difficult to keep clean. Also supplies a large volume of tissue. A longer catheter should be used to avoid displacement.

Dorsalis pedis artery

Blood pressure will be at ≥10–20mmHg higher than in central vessels.

Complications

- Digital ischaemia due to arterial spasm, thrombosis, or embolus.
- Bleeding (particularly in cases with altered coagulation status).
- Infection (with prolonged cannulation).
- False aneurysm.

See also:
Blood gas analysis, p154; Blood pressure monitoring, p164; Routine changes of disposables, p550.

Central venous catheter—insertion

Ultrasound-guided placement should be considered, especially for difficult placements. The technique with ultrasound guidance is different to the landmark technique; operators should be able to identify a patent vein and manipulate both probe and cannula simultaneously (see figure 9.2). There will be situations where an ultrasound device may be unavailable, so placement using anatomical landmarks alone should still be learnt.

Landmarks

Various landmarks have been described. For example:

- Internal jugular: Halfway between mastoid process and sternal notch, lateral to carotid pulsation, and inside medial border of sternocleidomastoid. Aim toward ipsilateral nipple, advancing under body of sternocleidomastoid until vein entered.
- Subclavian: 3cm below junction of lateral third and medial two thirds of clavicle. Turn head to contralateral side. Aim for point between jaw and contralateral shoulder tip. Advance needle to hit clavicle. Scrape needle around clavicle and advance further until vein entered.
- Femoral: Locate femoral artery in groin. Insert needle 3cm medially and angled rostrally. Advance until vein entered.

Insertion technique

The Seldinger technique (described below) is safer than the 'catheter-over-needle' technique and should generally be used in ICU patients.

1. Use aseptic technique throughout. Clean area with antiseptic (2% chlorhexidine) and surround with sterile drapes. Anaesthetise locally with 1% lidocaine. Flush lumen(s) of catheter with saline.
2. If available, use ultrasound to distinguish the vein from an adjacent artery by its compressibility, thinner wall and ovoid shape. The internal jugular and femoral veins are the easiest to locate by ultrasound.
3. Use needle to locate central vein. Confirm by aspiration of non-pulsatile blood into attached syringe or direct ultrasound visualisation of the needle entering the vein (with longitudinal probe position).
4. Pass wire (with 'J' or floppy end leading) through needle into vein. Only minimal resistance should be felt. If not, remove wire and confirm needle tip is still within vein lumen. If arrhythmias occur, the wire may be at the tricuspid valve and should be withdrawn a few cm.
5. Remove needle leaving wire extruding from skin puncture site.
6. Depending on size/type of catheter, a rigid dilator (± a prior scalpel nick to enlarge puncture site) may be passed over the wire to form a track through the subcutaneous tissues to the vein. Remove dilator.
7. Thread catheter over wire. Ensure end of wire extrudes from catheter to prevent accidental loss of wire in vein. Insert catheter into vein to depth of 15–20cm. Remove wire.
8. Aspirate and check respiratory swing, then flush with saline.
9. Attach catheter to skin using appropriate fixation device. Suturing is not generally recommended in view of increased risk of infection. Clean and dry area. A chlorhexidine-impregnated cuff may help avoid contamination. Use a sterile transparent semi-permeable dressing.
10. A chest X-ray verifies correct tip position (junction of superior vena cava and right atrium) and excludes pneumothorax. A satisfactory position should generally be confirmed before use of the catheter.

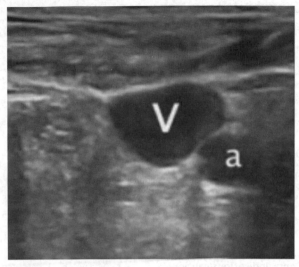

Fig. 9.2 Identification of internal jugular vein (v) and carotid artery (a) on transverse placement of probe.

See also:
Central venous catheter—use, p168; Central venous catheter—complications, p172.

Central venous catheter—use

Types of catheter

- Single, double, triple, or quadruple lumen.
- Sheaths for insertion of pulmonary artery catheter or pacing wire.
- Tunnelled catheter for long-term use.
- Multi-lumen catheters allow multiple infusions to be given separately ± continuous pressure monitoring. Minimises accidental bolus risk.
- Large-bore, double-lumen catheters for veno-venous dialysis/filtration.
- Common routes are internal jugular, subclavian, and femoral.
- 'Long' catheters can be inserted via brachial or axillary veins. Can be used for giving TPN and administering drugs that can cause phlebitis.

Uses

- Invasive haemodynamic monitoring.
- Infusion of drugs that can cause peripheral phlebitis or tissue necrosis if tissue extravasation occurs (e.g. TPN, epinephrine, amiodarone).
- Rapid volume infusion (NB. Rate of flow is inversely proportional to the length of the cannula).
- Access, e.g. for pacing wire insertion.
- Emergency access when peripheral circulation is 'shut down'.
- Renal replacement therapy, plasmapheresis, exchange transfusion.

Contraindications/cautions

- Coagulopathy.
- Undrained pneumothorax on contralateral side.
- Agitated, restless patient.

Central venous pressure measurement

An electronic pressure transducer is preferable to fluid manometry. The pressure transducer should be placed and 'zeroed' at the level of the left atrium (approximately mid-axillary line) rather than the sternum which is more affected by patient position (supine/semi-erect/prone). Venous pulsation and some respiratory swing should be seen in the trace but not a RV pressure waveform (i.e. catheter inserted too far).

See also:
Temporary pacing (1), p96; Parenteral nutrition, p130; Central venous catheter—insertion, p168;
Central venous catheter—complications, p172; Pulmonary artery catheter—insertion, p174; Routine
changes of disposables, p550.

Central venous catheter—complications

Infection

The incidence of local infection (usually coagulase negative *Staphylococcus* or *S. aureus*) rises after five days. The catheter site should be kept clean with an occlusive dressing which should be changed within seven days using 2% chlorhexidine in alcohol to clean the site. Strict asepsis should be used for dressing changes.

The need for maintaining the catheter *in situ* should be questioned daily. Unless the risk of new catheter insertion is very high (e.g. marked coagulopathy, anatomical issues), changing the catheter over a wire is not recommended.

Catheter-related sepsis should be considered if the patient develops an unexplained pyrexia or neutrophilia. Antibiotics may not be needed if mild, localised infection is present.

Removal of the catheter is necessary if the site is cellulitic or blood cultures taken through the catheter are positive. If the catheter is removed, the tip should be sent to the laboratory for culture.

Other complications

- Arterial puncture: Apply firm pressure directly over puncture site for 10–15mins (or longer). If continues, consider correcting any coagulopathy. Rarely, vascular surgical assistance may be needed.
- Haemorrhage: This may occur from around puncture site or from a previously failed attempt at insertion. Direct pressure for 5–10mins is usually successful though correction of coagulopathy may be needed if bleeding persists. If post-thrombolysis, consider tranexamic acid.
- Arrhythmias: Usually related to catheter tip 'tickling' tricuspid valve and normally resolves by withdrawing catheter by a few cm.
- Pneumothorax: If significant (e.g. >one third of hemithorax) or compromising cardiorespiratory status, drain air through catheter or chest drain. Otherwise, observe closely and drain subsequently, if necessary.
- Air embolism: Avoid by ensuring all Luer Lock connections are not loosely attached. If air embolism does occur, roll patient to left-hand side and place head down (Trendelenberg position) to prevent air entering pulmonary artery. Give FIO_2 1.0 to speed resorption of air. Try aspirating air through central line or consider angiography-guided aspiration if very large.
- Venous thrombosis: Suggested by unilateral swelling of distal limb; this can be confirmed by ultrasound. Remove catheter and anticoagulate (unless contraindicated).
- Haemothorax: Drain if necessary and monitor blood loss. Usually self-resolving. If bleeding persists, ensure coagulopathy is corrected. Seek a cardiothoracic surgical opinion if blood loss is substantial (>1L).
- Chylothorax (rare): Losses can exceed 1L/d. Often resolves spontaneously within 5–7d. If it persists, surgical ligation of the lymphatic duct may be necessary. The volume of loss may be reduced with TPN or a low-fat enteral diet.

See also:
Central venous catheter—insertion, p168; Central venous catheter—use, p170; Pneumothorax, p368; Haemothorax, p370; Routine changes of disposables, p550.

Pulmonary artery catheter—insertion

An 8Fr central venous introducer sheath must be inserted under strict aseptic technique. Pulmonary artery catheterisation is easier via internal jugular or subclavian veins.

1. Prepare catheter pre-insertion: 3-way taps on all lumens, flush lumens with crystalloid, inflate balloon with 1.6mL air and check for concentric inflation and leaks, place transparent sleeve over catheter to maintain future sterility, pressure transduce distal lumen and zero to reference point (usually mid-axillary line). Other pre-insertion calibration steps may be required, e.g. oxygen saturation.
2. Insert catheter beyond the length of the introducer sheath before inflating balloon. Advance catheter smoothly through the right heart chambers, pause to record pressures, and note waveform shape in RA, RV and PA (see figure 9.3). When a characteristic PAWP waveform is obtained, stop advancing catheter, deflate balloon, and ensure that PA waveform reappears. If not, withdraw catheter by a few cm.
3. Slowly re-inflate balloon, observing waveform trace. The wedge recording should not be obtained until at least 1.3mL of air has been injected into the balloon. If not, withdraw catheter 1–2cm and repeat. If 'overwedged' (pressure continues to climb on inflation), the catheter is inserted too far and the balloon has inflated forward over distal lumen. Immediately deflate, withdraw catheter 1–2cm and repeat.
4. After insertion, a chest X-ray is usually performed to verify catheter position and to exclude pneumothorax.

Contraindications/cautions
- Coagulopathy.
- Tricuspid valve prosthesis or disease.

Complications
- Problems of central venous catheterisation.
- Arrhythmias (especially when traversing tricuspid valve).
- Infection (including endocarditis).
- Pulmonary artery rupture.
- Pulmonary infarction.
- Knotting of catheter.
- Valve damage (do not withdraw catheter unless balloon deflated).

Troubleshooting
Excessive catheter length in a heart chamber causes coiling and a risk of knotting. No more than 15–20cm should be passed before the waveform changes. If not, deflate balloon, withdraw catheter, repeat. A knot can be managed by: (i) 'unknotting' with an intraluminal wire, (ii) pulling taut and removing catheter + introducer sheath together, or (iii) surgical or angiographic intervention.

If catheter fails to advance to next chamber, consider 'stiffening' catheter by injecting iced crystalloid through distal lumen, rolling patient to left lateral, or advancing catheter slowly with balloon deflated. The catheter should never be withdrawn with the balloon inflated.

Arrhythmias on insertion usually occur when the catheter tip is at the tricuspid valve. These usually resolve on withdrawing the catheter or, occasionally, after a slow bolus of 1.5mg/kg lidocaine.

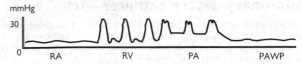

Fig. 9.3 Waveforms.

See also:
Pulmonary artery catheter—use, p176.

Pulmonary artery catheter—use

Several prospective multicentre studies in critically ill and decompensated heart failure patients found no impact on mortality with catheter use. As studies also reported an inadequate knowledge base regarding insertion and data interpretation, proper training in its use is mandated.

Uses

- Pressure monitoring—RA, RV, PA, PAWP.
- Flow monitoring—(right ventricular) cardiac output.
- Oxygen saturation—'mixed venous' (i.e. in RV outflow tract/PA), determination of left to right shunts (ASD, VSD).
- Derived variables—SVR, PVR, LVSW, RVSW, DO_2, VO_2, O_2ER.
- Temporary pacing.
- Right ventricular ejection fraction and end-diastolic volume.

Specialised catheters

- Continuous mixed venous oxygen saturation measurement.
- Continuous cardiac output measurement.
- RV end-diastolic volume, RV ejection fraction calculation.
- Ventricular (± atrial) pacing.

Management

Monitor PA pressure continuously to identify catheter migration and a wedged trace. If present, pull back catheter immediately to prevent pulmonary infarction due to arterial occlusion.

The risk of local infection rises after five days. Consider daily the need for the catheter. Removal ± change of site is needed if the site is cellulitic or positive cultures are grown from either line tip or blood.

Withdraw samples of pulmonary artery blood slowly from the distal lumen to prevent 'arterialisation', i.e. pulmonary venous sampling.

Wedge pressure measurements

- Inflate balloon slowly, monitoring the waveform to avoid potential vessel rupture, especially in elderly and/or pulmonary hypertension. The trace should only 'wedge' after ≥1.3mL air fills the balloon.
- Measure at end-expiration when intrathoracic pressure is closest to atmospheric pressure. For ventilated patients, end-expiration ≡ lowest wedge reading; during spontaneous breathing, end-expiration ≡ highest reading. Measurement is difficult in the dyspnoeic patient; a 'mean' wedge reading may be used in this instance.
- The PAWP cannot be higher than the PA diastolic pressure.
- CVP, PAWP, and cardiac output should not be measured during rapid volume infusion but after a period of equilibration (5–10min).
- The PAWP does not equal the LVEDP in mitral stenosis. In mitral regurgitation, measure PAWP at the end of the 'a' wave.

West's zones

The catheter tip should lie in a zone III region (where PA pressure > PV pressure > alveolar pressure) below left atrial level on a lateral CXR.

Suspect a non-zone III position if: (i) following a rise in PEEP, the PAWP rises by >50% of the increment, (ii) the wedge trace shows no detectable cardiac pulsation and/or excess respiratory variation.

A non-zone III position is more likely with PEEP and/or hypovolaemia.

Normal values

Stroke volume	70–100mL
Cardiac output	4–6L/min
Right atrial pressure	0–5mmHg
Right ventricular pressure	20–25/0–5mmHg
Pulmonary artery pressure	20–25/10–15mmHg
Pulmonary artery wedge pressure	6–12mmHg
Mixed venous oxygen saturation	70–75%

Derived variables

Variable	Calculation	Normal range
Cardiac index (CI)	$\dfrac{\text{Cardiac output}}{\text{Body surface area}}$	2.5–3.5L/min/m^2
Stroke index (SI)	$\dfrac{SV}{\text{Body surface area}}$	40–60mL/m^2
Systemic vascular resistance	$\dfrac{MAP - RAP}{\text{Cardiac output}} \times 79.9$	960–1400dyn.s/cm^5
Pulmonary vascular resistance	$\dfrac{PAP - PAWP}{\text{Cardiac output}} \times 79.9$	25–125dyn.s/cm^5
LV stroke work index	(MAP-PAWP) × SI × 0.0136	44–68g-m.m^2
RV stroke work index	(MPAP-RAP) × SI × 0.0136	4–8g-m.m^2
O$_2$ delivery	Cardiac output × 0.134 × Hb$_a$ × SaO$_2$	950–1300mL/min
O$_2$ consumption	Cardiac output × 0.134 × [(Hb$_a$ × SaO$_2$) − (Hb$_v$ × SvO$_2$)]	180–320mL/min
O$_2$ extraction ratio	$1 - \dfrac{SaO_2 - SvO_2}{SaO_2}$	0.25–0.30

Key papers

Richard C, Warszawski J, Anguel N, *et al.* for the French Pulmonary Artery Catheter Study Group. (2003) Early use of the pulmonary artery catheter and outcomes in patients with shock and acute respiratory distress syndrome: a randomised controlled trial. *JAMA* **290**: 2713–20.

Harvey S, Harrison DA, Singer M, *et al.* for the PAC-Man study collaboration. (2005) Assessment of the clinical effectiveness of pulmonary artery catheters in management of patients in intensive care (PAC-Man): a randomised controlled trial. *Lancet* **366**: 472–7.

Binanay C, Califf RM, Hasselblad V, *et al.* for the ESCAPE Investigators. (2005) Evaluation study of congestive heart failure and pulmonary artery catheterisation effectiveness: the ESCAPE trial. *JAMA* **294**: 1625–33.

See also:

Pulmonary artery catheter—insertion, p172; Cardiac output—central thermodilution, p178.

Cardiac output—central thermodilution

Thermodilution is utilised by the pulmonary artery catheter to measure right ventricular cardiac output. The principle is a modification of the Fick indicator dilution principle whereby a bolus of cooled 5% glucose is injected through the proximal lumen into the central circulation (right atrium), and the temperature change is detected by a thermistor at the catheter tip, some 30cm distal. A modification of the Hamilton–Stewart equation, utilising the volume, temperature, and specific heat of the injectate, enables cardiac output to be calculated by an online computer from a curve measuring temperature change in the pulmonary artery.

Continuous thermodilution measurement uses a modified catheter emitting heat pulses from a thermal filament lying 14–25cm from the tip. 7.5W of heat are added to the blood intermittently every 30–60s and these temperature changes are measured by a thermistor 4cm from the tip. Though updated frequently, the cardiac output displayed is usually an average of the previous 3–6min.

Thermodilution is also used by the PiCCO device, injecting cooled 5% glucose through a central vein, and measuring temperature change in the femoral artery.

Thermodilution injection technique

The computer constant must be set for the volume and temperature of the 5% glucose used. Ice-cold glucose (10mL) provides the most accurate measure. Room temperature injectate (5mL) is sufficiently precise for normal and high output states. However, its accuracy does worsen at low output values.
1. Press 'Start' button on computer.
2. Inject fluid smoothly over 2–3s.
3. Repeat at least twice more at random points in the respiratory cycle.
4. Average three measurements falling within 10% of each other. Reject outputs gained from curves that are irregular/non-smooth.

Erroneous readings

- Valve lesions: Tricuspid regurgitation will allow some of the injectate to reflux back into the right atrium. Aortic incompetence produces a higher left ventricular output; a proportion will regurgitate back into the left ventricle, thus the thermodilution-obtained value overestimates the effective forward flow from the left ventricle.
- Septal defects.
- Loss of injectate: Check that connections are tight and do not leak.

Disadvantages

- Non-continuous (by injection technique).
- 5–10% inter- and intra-observer variability.
- Erroneous readings with tricuspid regurgitation, intracardiac shunts.
- Frequently repeated measurements may result in considerable volumes of 5% glucose being injected.

See also:
Pulmonary artery catheter—insertion, p174; Pulmonary artery catheter—use, p176; Basic resuscitation, p338; Fluid challenge, p342; Hypotension, p380; Heart failure—assessment, p392.

Cardiac output—peripheral thermodilution

The PiCCO device utilises thermodilution measured peripherally. The most frequent artery used is the femoral into which a catheter (usually 5Fr in adults) is inserted. Specialised catheters are also available for axillary and radial artery insertion. A bolus of cold saline injected into a central vein is detected by a thermistor in the arterial catheter.

Advantages
- Reasonably accurate and less invasive than pulmonary artery placement.
- Other information derived.

Disadvantages
- Can underestimate low output values.
- Inaccurate with moderate/severe valvular regurgitation, intracardiac shunts, aortic aneurysm, aortic stenosis, pneumonectomy, pulmonary embolism, rapidly changing temperature, extracorporeal circulations.
- Large size of cannula can compromise distal leg perfusion.

Derived indices

As the injectate is administered centrally and the temperature difference is measured in a proximal artery, most of the temperature change occurs in the intrathoracic compartment. Hence, other volumetric variables such as intrathoracic blood volume and extravascular lung water can be estimated.

- Global end-diastolic volume (GEDV) = volume of blood within the four heart chambers.
- Intrathoracic blood volume (ITBV) = GEDV + blood volume within the pulmonary vessels.

ITBV and GEDV are measures of cardiac preload that studies suggest are comparable, if not superior, to standard cardiac filling pressures (CVP, PAWP), particularly as they are less influenced by mechanical ventilation.

- Extravascular lung water (EVLW) = water content in the lungs.
EVLW provides a bedside measure of the degree of pulmonary oedema. It correlates with the severity of ARDS and outcomes. There are little data at present showing its utility in guiding treatment and improving outcomes.

See also:
Extravascular lung water measurement, p156; Cardiac output - central thermodilution, p178; Basic resuscitation, p338; Fluid challenge, p342; Hypotension, p380; Heart failure - assessment, p392.

Cardiac output—indicator dilution

Dye dilution

Mixing of a given volume of indicator to an unknown volume of fluid allows calculation of this volume from the degree of indicator dilution. The time elapsed for the indicator to pass some distance in the cardiovascular system yields a cardiac output value, calculated as:

$$\frac{60 \times l}{C_m \times t}$$

... where l = amount of indicator injected, C_m = mean concentration of the indicator, and t = curve duration. Traditionally, indocyanine green was injected into a central vein with arterial blood repeatedly sampled to construct a time-concentration curve with a rapid upstroke and an exponential decay. Plotting the dye decay curve semi-logarithmically and extrapolating values to the origin produces cardiac output.

The LiDCO device is based on a similar principle, though using lithium as the 'dye'. This can be injected into a peripheral vein and sampled from the radial artery.

Advantages

- Reasonably accurate and less invasive than pulmonary artery placement.
- Other information derived.

Disadvantages

- Accumulation of lithium with multiple repeated measurements.
- Measurement/calibration takes >10min. Ideally, 2–3 lithium time-concentration curves should be performed per calibration to improve the coefficient of variation.
- Can underestimate low output values.
- Inaccurate with moderate/severe valvular regurgitation, major pulmonary embolism, intracardiac shunt.
- Paralysing agents and severe hyponatraemia interfere with lithium measurement.
- Lithium should not be used in pregnant patients.

See also:
Basic resuscitation, p338; Fluid challenge, p342; Hypotension, p380; Heart failure—
assessment, p398.

Cardiac output—Doppler ultrasound

Doppler ultrasound

An ultrasound beam of known frequency is reflected by moving blood corpuscles with a shift in frequency proportional to blood flow velocity. The actual velocity is calculated from the Doppler equation; this requires the cosine of the vector between the direction of the ultrasound beam and that of blood flow. This has been applied to blood flow in the ascending aorta and aortic arch (via a suprasternal approach), descending thoracic aorta (oesophageal approach), and intracardiac flow (e.g. transmitral from an apical approach). Spectral analysis of the Doppler frequency shifts produces velocity-time waveforms, the area of which represents 'stroke distance', i.e. the distance travelled by a column of blood with each left ventricular systole. (See figure 9.4). The product of stroke distance and aortic (or mitral valve) cross-sectional area is stroke volume. Cross-sectional area can be measured echocardiographically. However, as both operator expertise and equipment is required, this additional measurement can be either ignored or assumed from nomograms to provide a reasonable *estimate* of stroke volume.

Advantages
- Quick and minimally invasive.
- Reasonably accurate if performed properly.
- Measures left heart output, unaffected by mitral (unless measured transmitrally) or tricuspid regurgitation, or by intracardiac shunts.
- Continuous (via oesophageal approach)—but may need repositioning.
- Other information on contractility, preload, and afterload from waveform shape (see figure 9.5).
- Multiple studies showing outcome benefit in high-risk surgical patients from guided fluid optimisation intra-operatively or post-operatively.

Disadvantages
- Non-continuous (unless via oesophagus).
- Learning curve to ensure correct signal is insonated (≈5–10 oesophageal, ≈15–20 with suprasternal and 30+ with intracardiac).
- Not reliable with turbulent flow conditions, e.g. intra-aortic balloon counterpulsation (oesophageal), aortic stenosis or regurgitation (suprasternal or intracardiac from aortic outflow tract), mitral regurgitation (transmitral).
- Oesophageal approach assumes proportionality of flow going to upper and lower body is maintained (approximately 30:70)—this will change during aortic cross-clamping (vascular surgery) or use of epidural.
- Suprasternal measurements can be hampered by short neck or obesity (probe has to get behind sternum to insonate ascending aorta or arch correctly), mediastinal air (e.g. post-cardiac surgery), and co-located vessels, e.g. innominate artery.

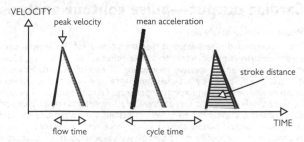

Fig. 9.4 Doppler velocity-time waveform.

- Corrected flow time (FTc) = flow time corrected to heart rate of 60bpm. Normal range is 330–360ms. The FTc is inversely related to systemic vascular resistance. Thus, FTc falls with decreased preload or increased afterload (e.g. hypovolaemia, vasoconstriction, obstruction such as PE or tamponade) while FTc increases with vasodilatation.
- Peak velocity (and acceleration) are markers of left ventricular contractility and are age-dependent (see table below). Values increase with positive inotropy and fall with negative inotropic states (e.g. heart failure, beta-blockade).

Age	Normal range of peak velocity (cm/s)
20	90–120
50	60–80
70	50–70

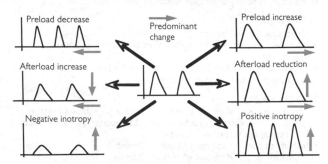

Fig. 9.5 Effect of haemodynamic changes on Doppler velocity-time waveform shape.

See also:
Basic resuscitation, p338; Fluid challenge, p342; Hypotension, p380; Heart failure—assessment, p398.

Cardiac output—pulse contour analysis

Pulse contour analysis

The concept of this technique is that the contour of the arterial pressure waveform is proportional to stroke volume. This, in theory, allows continuous, minimally invasive monitoring of cardiac output. However, it is greatly influenced by arterial compliance (the relationship between pressure and volume) and aortic impedance. Thus, the major challenges for technologies using this approach are to assess arterial compliance consistently and accurately in an individual patient and to be able to track changes in cardiac output closely when there are concurrent changes in compliance, e.g. during rapid blood loss, vasodilatation, or changes in temperature.

This is complicated further by the changing morphology of the blood pressure waveform as it travels down peripheral arteries, especially during alterations in blood flow redistribution, e.g. with severe vasoconstriction. It is also essential to ensure a correctly damped pressure waveform and non-kinking of the arm (radial) or groin (femoral).

There are several commercial devices which use their own proprietary algorithms to estimate stroke volume. The LiDCOplus and PiCCO systems use an alternative cardiac output measuring technique (lithium dye dilution and peripheral thermodilution, respectively) in tandem for initial calibration and subsequent re-calibration. The Flotrac and LiDCOrapid systems derive an estimate of cardiac output without a calibrating device using the patient's blood pressure, gender, age, and body surface area. There are significant concerns regarding the overall accuracy of these systems and their ability to follow trends, especially those devices not calibrated against a reference technique. Even in calibrated systems, the literature suggest the need for frequent routine recalibration (1–4 hourly) or earlier if circulatory status changes to any significant extent.

Advantages

- Continuous flow monitoring.
- Uses data from an arterial cannula already *in situ* for pressure monitoring.
- Assessment of fluid responsiveness using pulse pressure, systolic pressure, or stroke volume variation.

Disadvantages

- Changes in vascular compliance (e.g. with changes in blood pressure, cardiac output, vascular resistance, body temperature) affect accuracy, thus regular recalibration is needed.
- Inability to confirm accuracy of non-calibrated devices (stroke volume estimation or trend following) unless a reference technique is used.
- Requires a good quality, non-obstructed, non-damped waveform.
- Ongoing debate about relative signal quality from radial vs femoral.
- Unreliable with arrhythmias.
- Unreliable with aortic stenosis and severe peripheral vascular disease.
- Cannot be used with intra-aortic balloon counterpulsation.

See also:

Basic resuscitation, p338; Fluid challenge, p342; Hypotension, p380; Heart failure—assessment, p392.

Cardiac output—other techniques

Thoracic bio-impedance

Impedance changes originate in the thoracic aorta when blood is ejected from the left ventricle. This effect is used to determine stroke volume from formulae utilising the electrical field size of the thorax, baseline thoracic impedance, and fluctuation related to systole and ventricular ejection time. A correction factor for sex, height, and weight is also used. The technique simply utilises four pairs of electrodes placed in proscribed positions on the neck and thorax; these are connected to a dedicated monitor which measures thoracic impedance to a low amplitude, high (70kHz) frequency 2.5mA current applied across the electrodes.

Advantages

Quick, safe, totally non-invasive, reasonably accurate in normal, spontaneously breathing subjects.

Disadvantages

Discrepancies in critically ill patients, (especially those with arrhythmias, tachycardias, intrathoracic fluid shifts, anatomical deformities, aortic regurgitation, metal within the thorax, inability to verify signal).

Thoracic bioreactance

This novel technology increases the signal-to-noise ratio by ~100-fold over bio-impedance. Four pairs of double electrodes are sited on the thorax (just below the sternum) and the mid-axial line just below the shoulders. The upper electrodes emit a low-level electrical current that is sensed by their lower pairs. The signal utilises both bioimpedance and the relationship between the amount of thoracic fluid at any given time-point, and frequency shifts occurring as the electric current crosses the thorax. This produces the haemodynamic reactance waveform. Clinical experience of its accuracy and reliability, particularly in critically ill patients, is limited at present.

Direct Fick

The amount of substance passing into a flowing system equals the difference in concentration of the substance on each side of the system multiplied by flow within the system. Cardiac output is usually calculated by dividing total body O_2 consumption by the difference in O_2 content between arterial and mixed venous blood. Alternatively, CO_2 production can be used as the indicator. Arterial CO_2 can be derived non-invasively from end-tidal CO_2 while mixed venous CO_2 can be determined by rapid rebreathing into a bag until CO_2 levels have equilibrated.

Advantages

'Gold standard' for cardiac output estimation.

Disadvantages

For VO_2: Invasive (requires measurement of mixed venous blood), requires leak-free, open circuit or an unwieldy, closed circuit technique, oxygen consumption measurements via metabolic cart unreliable if FIO_2 is high, lung oxygen consumption not measured by pulmonary artery catheter technique (may be high in ARDS, pneumonia ...).

For CO_2: Non-invasive but requires normal lung function, and is thus not generally applicable in ICU patients.

See also:
Basic resuscitation, p338; Fluid challenge, p342; Hypotension, p380; Heart failure—
assessment, p392.

Pressure and stroke volume variation

These can be used, within strict limitations (see below), to assess the likelihood of responsiveness of the circulation to a fluid challenge. It is based on the variation in size and height of the arterial pressure waveform during the respiratory cycle (see figure 9.6). In spontaneously breathing subjects, BP decreases on inspiration due to decreased left heart output. The range in normal subjects is 5–10mmHg. The reverse is seen during positive pressure ventilation where BP decreases on expiration. Pulsus paradoxus is an exaggeration of this phenomenon seen with marked changes in intrathoracic pressure (e.g. severe asthma) or impaired left heart filling (e.g. pericardial tamponade).

Stroke volume variation (SVV)

$$\frac{SVmax - SVmin}{0.5\,(SVmax + SVmin)}$$

Pulse pressure variation (PPV)

$$\frac{PPmax - PPmin}{0.5\,(PPmax + PPmin)}$$

Variation >10–15% (the optimal positive and negative predictive values vary between studies) suggests a high likelihood of preload responsiveness. It can also indicate deleterious effects of PEEP on the circulation.

Systolic pressure variation (SPV)

The difference between maximal and minimal values of systolic pressure during one breath. As well as SPV, the delta down (Δdown) component (difference between systolic pressure during a short period of apnoea and the lowest value during a breath) >5mmHg also predicts volume responsiveness.

Advocates for the different measurements all claim superiority of their favoured techinque over the others. Pulse pressure depends on stroke volume and arterial compliance while systolic pressure depends on stroke volume, arterial compliance, and diastolic pressure.

Limitations of PPV, SPV, and SVV
- Use only in mechanically ventilated, deeply sedated ± paralysed patients in full control mode ventilation (i.e. no spontaneous triggered breaths) receiving fixed rate tidal volumes (generally ≥10mL/kg).
- Not reliable with arrhythmias.
- Unreliable in spontaneously breathing, non-intubated patients where tidal volumes are smaller and variable.
- Major risk of volume overload in conditions which also result in LV underfilling, e.g. obstruction (e.g. pulmonary embolus, tamponade, atrial myxoma) or right heart failure (e.g. right ventricular infarction).
- Vasodilatation may increase SVV.
- Recruitment of abdominal muscles and forced expiration is a common finding in ICU patients, resulting in a large rise in BP during expiration ± changes in SV, thus rendering unreliable results.

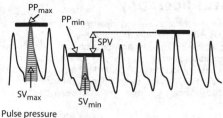

PP Pulse pressure
SV Stroke volume
SPV Systolic pressure variation

Fig. 9.6 Pulse pressure, systolic pressure, and stroke volume variation.

See also:
Fluid challenge, p342.

Echocardiography

Combines structural as well as dynamic assessment of the heart using ultrasound reflected off various interfaces.

Transthoracic or transoesophageal probes provide information on valve integrity, global (diastolic and systolic) and regional ventricular function, wall thickness, pericardial fluid or thickening, aortic dissection, ventricular volumes, ejection fraction, and pulmonary pressures. It can also diagnose intracardiac masses (e.g. myxoma, clot), endocarditis, and pulmonary embolism.

Different parts of the heart can be best imaged from different approaches, e.g. apical four-chamber (see figure 9.7), left parasternal long axis (see figure 9.8), subcostal. Echocardiography can be used in single (M-mode) or 2-dimensional modes.

Echocardiography is often combined with integral Doppler ultrasound for cardiac output estimation derived from combined measurement of aortic diameter plus flow at various sites, e.g left ventricular outflow tract, aorta, transmitral. Analytical software or formulae can also enable computation of cardiac output from estimations of ventricular volumes.

Advantages
- Non-invasive, safe.
- Relatively quick.
- Provides other useful information on cardiac structure and function.

Disadvantages
- Expensive equipment.
- Lengthy learning curve and inter-observer variability.
- Body habitus or pathology (e.g. emphysema) may impair image quality.

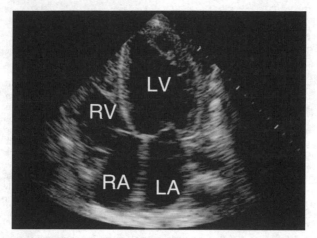

Fig. 9.7 Apical four-chamber view.

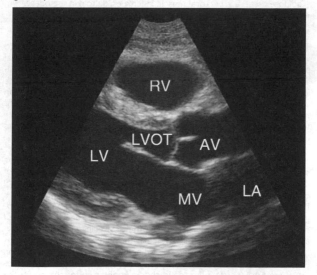

Fig. 9.8 Parasternal long axis view. RV right ventricle; LVOT left ventricular outflow tract; AV aortic valve; MV mitral valve; LA left atrium; RA right atrium.

See also:
Cardiac output—Doppler ultrasound, p184.

Tissue perfusion monitoring

Near-infrared spectroscopy (NIRS)

This non-invasive technique utilises near-infrared light to quantitate tissue oxyhaemoglobin concentration (StO_2) or, more accurately, microvascular oxygenation in arterioles, capillaries, and venules. It may measure oxymyoglobin, though to what extent this influences the measurement is uncertain. It is usually measured in a peripheral muscle, such as the thenar eminence or deltoid. As resting values vary widely in normal subjects (70–95%), it is a poor indicator of mild to moderate shock states. It can be useful in detecting peripheral compartment syndrome. More utility can be gained from the rate of fall in StO_2 during proximal arterial occlusion (and/or rise in StO_2 on release of occlusion). A reduced rate of fall on occlusion suggests decreased tissue O_2 utilisation ± microvascular perfusion.

Specialised spectrophotometers have the ability to detect mitochondrial cytochrome oxidase redox states—this has been studied predominantly in neonatal brains, though there is potential for extrapolation to other organs. StO_2 has been shown to relate to interstitial tissue PO_2.

Cautions
- Reliability poor if used in muscle groups with significant overlying adipose tissue, e.g. pectoral muscle in females, deltoid in the obese.
- Dark skin pigmentation may affect the readings.

Microvascular circulation visualisation

This non-invasive technique uses sidestream darkfield imaging (SDF) to visualise the microcirculation. An earlier technique used orthogonal polarisation spectroscopy (OPS), but this is no longer commercially available. Briefly, OPS utilised polarised light scattered by the tissue and collected by the objective lens. High quality images of the microcirculation were obtained by absorbing surface structures lit up by depolarised light returning from deeper structures. SDF uses the same principle but, rather than polarised light, uses light-emitting diodes that are isolated from its inner image-conducting core.

The technique is mainly used sublingually, but can be applied to other areas, e.g. rectum, bowel stoma, or directly to internal organs during surgery. The device software enables offline semi-quantitative analysis of microcirculatory alterations affecting capillary density and heterogeneity of blood flow. The proportion of perfused capillaries may vary as may flow characteristics within separate capillaries, e.g. continuous or stop-go. Plasma and cellular factors, e.g. viscosity, red cell rheology, degree of platelet and neutrophil rolling, and endothelial swelling—all affect microvascular flow characteristics. Microvascular thrombosis is rare.

It is a research tool at present providing images of the microcirculation in different organ beds in a variety of conditions. Persisting abnormalities are a good prognostic indicator in shock. Applicability of changes in the sublingual circulation to other beds is uncertain at present; discrepancy was shown with the intestinal microcirculation in sepsis.

Cautions
- Excess probe pressure will affect the microcirculation.

See also:
Other neurological monitoring, p206.

Gut tonometry

A gas permeable silicone balloon attached to a sampling tube is passed into the lumen of the gut nasogastrically. Devices exist for tonometry in the stomach or sigmoid colon although they are now rarely used. The tonometer allows indirect measurement of the PCO_2 of the gut mucosa and calculation of the pH of the mucosa.

Indications

Gut mucosal hypoperfusion is an early consequence of hypovolaemia. Covert circulatory inadequacy due to hypovolaemia may be detected as gut mucosal acidosis and has been related to post-operative complications after major surgery. In critically ill patients, there is some evidence that prevention of gut mucosal acidosis improves outcome. The sigmoid colon tonometer is useful to detect ischaemic colitis early (e.g. after abdominal vascular surgery).

Technique

Saline tonometry

In the original technique, the tonometer balloon was prepared by degassing and filling with 2.5mL 0.9% saline. The saline was withdrawn into a syringe connected to the sampling tube prior to insertion. After insertion, the saline was passed back into the balloon. The PCO_2 of the saline in the balloon equilibrated with the PCO_2 of the gut lumen over a period of 30–90min. At steady state, it was assumed that the PCO_2 of the gut lumen and gut mucosa were in equilibrium. Time correction factors were derived for partial equilibration between the balloon saline and the gut lumen. The measurement was completed by sampling the saline from the balloon and an arterial blood sample for measurement of $[HCO_3^-]$.

Gas tonometry

Using air in the tonometry balloon allows more rapid equilibration between the tonometer and the luminal PCO_2. A modified capnometer automatically fills the balloon with air and samples the PCO_2 after 5–10min equilibration. Subsequent cycles of balloon filling do not use fresh air so CO_2 equilibration is quicker. Tonometric PCO_2 may be compared with end-tidal PCO_2 (measured with the same capnometer)

$$pHi - 6.1 + \log_{10} \frac{arterial\left[HCO_3\right]}{tonometer\ PCO_2 \times K}$$

as an estimate of arterial PCO_2. With a normal capnogram, a balloon PCO_2 significantly higher than end-tidal PCO_2 implies gut mucosal hypoperfusion.

pH vs regional PCO_2

The pH of the gut mucosa (pHi) may be calculated using a modified Henderson–Hasselbach equation, where K is the time-dependent equilibration constant. However, most of the variation in the measurement is due to variation in regional PCO_2.

Comparing regional PCO_2 with $PaCO_2$ gives as much information as making the calculation of pHi, and overcomes the problematic assumption that arterial $[HCO_3^-]$ is equivalent to mucosal capillary $[HCO_3^-]$.

See also:
Blood gas machine, p152; Blood gas analysis, p154; Tissue perfusion monitoring, p198.

Neurological monitoring

Intracranial pressure monitoring

Indications
To confirm the diagnosis of raised intracranial pressure (ICP) and monitor treatment. May be used in cases of head injury, particularly if ventilated, Glasgow coma score ≤8, or with an abnormal CT scan. Also used in encephalopathy, post-neurosurgery, and in selected cases of intracranial haemorrhage. Although a raised ICP can be related to poor prognosis after head injury, the converse is not true. Sustained reduction of raised ICP (or maintenance of cerebral perfusion pressure) in head injury may improve outcome although large controlled trials are lacking.

Methods of monitoring intracranial pressure

Ventricular monitoring
A catheter is inserted into the lateral ventricle via a burr hole. The catheter may be connected to a pressure transducer or may contain a fibreoptic pressure monitoring device. Both catheters require regular calibration according to the manufacturers' instructions. Both systems should be tested for patency and damping by temporarily raising intracranial pressure (e.g. with a cough or by occluding a jugular vein). CSF may be drained through the ventricular catheter to reduce intracranial pressure.

Subdural monitoring
The dura is opened via a burr hole and a hollow bolt inserted into the skull. The bolt may be connected to a pressure transducer or admit a fibreoptic or high-fidelity pressure monitoring device. A subdural bolt is easier to insert than ventricular monitors. The main disadvantages of subdural monitoring are a tendency to underestimate ICP and damping effects. Again calibration and patency testing should be done regularly.

Complications
• Infection, particularly after five days.
• Haemorrhage, particularly with coagulopathy or difficult insertion.

Using ICP monitoring
Normal ICP is <10mmHg. A raised ICP is usually treated when >25mmHg in head injury. As ICP increases, there are often sustained rises in ICP to 50–100mmHg lasting for 5–20min, increasing with frequency as the baseline ICP rises. This is associated with 60% mortality. Cerebral perfusion pressure (CPP) is the difference between mean BP and mean ICP. Treatment aimed at reducing ICP may also reduce mean BP. It is important to maintain CPP at >50–60mmHg.

See also:
Intracranial haemorrhage, p448; Subarachnoid haemorrhage, p450; Raised intracranial pressure, p454; Head injury (1), p586.

Jugular venous bulb saturation

Retrograde passage of a fibreoptic catheter from the internal jugular vein into the jugular bulb enables continuous monitoring of jugular venous bulb saturation (SjO_2). This can be used in conjunction with other monitors of cerebral haemodynamics such as middle cerebral blood flow, cerebral arterio-venous lactate difference, and intracranial pressure to direct management.

Principles of SjO_2 management

- Normal values are approximately 65–70%.
- In absence of anaemia and with normal SaO_2, SjO_2 >75% suggests luxury perfusion or global infarction.
- SjO_2 <54% corresponds to cerebral hypoperfusion while values <40% suggest global ischaemia, and are usually associated with increased cerebral lactate production.
- Knowledge of SjO_2 allows optimisation of brain blood flow to avoid: (i) excessive or inadequate perfusion, and (ii) iatrogenically-induced hypoperfusion through treating raised intracranial pressure aggressively with diuretics and hyperventilation.
- Studies in trauma patients have found higher mortality with episodes of jugular venous desaturation and a significant relationship between CPP and SjO_2 when CPP is <70mmHg. A falling SjO_2 may be an indication to increase CPP, though no prospective randomised trial has yet been performed to study the effect on outcome.
- Approximately 85% of cerebral venous drainage passes down one of the internal jugular veins (usually right). SjO_2 usually represents drainage from both hemispheres and is equal on both sides. However, after focal injury, this pattern of drainage may alter.

Insertion technique

1. Insert introducer sheath rostrally in internal jugular vein.
2. Calibrate fibreoptic catheter pre-insertion.
3. Insert catheter via introducer sheath; advance to jugular bulb.
4. Withdraw introducer sheath.
5. Confirm: (i) free aspiration of blood via catheter, (ii) satisfactory light intensity reading, (iii) satisfactory positioning of catheter tip by lateral cervical X-ray (high in jugular bulb, above level of 2nd cervical vertebra).
6. Perform *in vivo* calibration, repeat calibration 12-hourly.

Troubleshooting

If the catheter is sited too low in the jugular bulb, erroneous SjO_2 values may result from mixing of intracerebral and extracerebral venous blood. This could be particularly pertinent when cerebral blood flow is low.

- Ensure light intensity reading is satisfactory; if too high, the catheter may be abutting against a wall, and if low, the catheter may not be patent or have a small clot over the tip. Before treating the patient, always confirm the veracity of low readings against a blood sample drawn from the catheter and measured in a co-oximeter.

Formulae

$$CMRO_2 = CBF \times 1.34 \times \left[Hb\right] \times \left(SaO_2 - SjO_2\right)$$

… where $CMRO_2$ = cerebral metabolism of oxygen
CBF = cerebral blood flow
SjO_2 = jugular bulb oxygen saturation
$SaO_2(\%)$ = arterial oxygen saturation

$$\text{Cerebral oxygen extraction ratio} = \left(\frac{SaO_2 - SjO_2}{SjO_2}\right)$$

Cerebral perfusion pressure = systemic BP − intracranial pressure

See also:

Intracranial pressure monitoring, p200; Other neurological monitoring, p206; Intracranial haemorrhage, p448; Subarachnoid haemorrhage, p450; Raised intracranial pressure, p454; Head injury (1), p586.

EEG/CFM monitoring

EEG monitoring

The EEG reflects changes in cortical electrical function. This, in turn, is dependent on cerebral perfusion and oxygenation. EEG monitoring can be useful to assess epileptiform activity as well as cerebral well-being in patients who are sedated and paralysed. The conventional EEG can be used intermittently, but data reduction and artefact suppression are necessary to allow successful use of EEG recordings in the ICU.

Bispectral index (BIS) monitor

BIS is a statistical index derived from the EEG and expressed as a score between 0–100. Scores below 50 have been reliably associated with anaesthesia-induced unconsciousness. Assessment in the critically ill patient may be complicated by various confounding factors such as septic encephalopathy, head trauma, and hypoperfusion. A low score is related to deep or excessive sedation, and may allow dose reduction (or cessation) of sedative agents, especially in paralysed patients.

Cerebral function monitor (CFM)

The CFM is a single channel, filtered trace from two recording electrodes placed over the parietal regions of the scalp. A third electrode may be used in the midline to help with interference detection. The parietal recording electrodes are usually placed close to watershed areas of the brain in order to allow maximum sensitivity for ischaemia detection. Voltage is displayed against time on a chart running at 6–30cm/h.

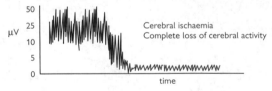

Fig. 10.1a Typical CFM recording in cerebral ischaemia.

Use of CFM

The CFM may detect cerebral ischaemia; burst suppression (periods of increasingly prolonged electrical silence) provides an early warning (see figure 10.1a).

Sedation produces a fall in baseline to <5μV, equivalent to burst suppression. This is equivalent to maximum reduction in cerebral VO$_2$ and no further benefit would be gained from additional sedation (see figure 10.1b).

Seizure activity may be detected in patients despite apparently adequate clinical control or where muscle relaxants have been used (see figure 10.1c).

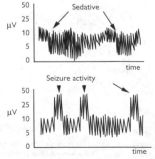

Fig. 10.1b-c Typical CFM recordings in sedation (b) or during seizure activity (c).

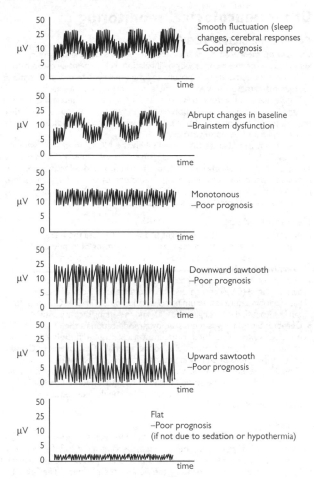

Fig. 10.2 Typical CFM patterns.

See also:
Sedatives and tranquilisers, p308; Coma, p438; Generalised seizures, p444; Head injury (1), p586;
Head injury (2), p588; Hypothermia, p606; Brain stem death, p652.

Other neurological monitoring

Cerebral blood flow (CBF)

CBF can be measured by radioisotope techniques utilising tracers such as xenon-133 given intravenously or by inhalation. This remains a research tool in view of the radioactivity exposure and the usual need to move the patient to a gamma-camera. However, portable monitors are now available.

Middle cerebral artery (MCA) blood flow can be determined non-invasively by transcranial Doppler ultrasonography. The pulsatility index (PI) relates to cerebrovascular resistance, with a rise in PI indicating a rise in resistance and cerebral vasospasm.

Vasospasm can also be diagnosed when the MCA blood flow velocity exceeds 120cm/s and severe vasospasm when velocities >200cm/s. Low values of common carotid end-diastolic blood flow and velocity have been shown to be highly discriminating predictors of brain death. Impaired reactivity of CBF to changes in PCO_2 (in normals 3–5% per mmHg PCO_2 change) is another marker of poor outcome.

Near-infrared spectroscopy (NIRS)

- Near-infrared (700–1000nm) light propagated across the head is absorbed by haemoglobin (oxy- and deoxy-), myoglobin, and oxidised cytochrome aa_3 (the terminal part of the respiratory chain involved in oxidative phosphorylation).
- The sum of (oxy- + deoxy-) haemoglobin is considered an index of cerebral blood volume (CBV) change, and the difference as an index of change in haemoglobin saturation assuming no variation occurs in CBV. CBV and flow can be quantified by changing the FIO_2 and measuring the response.
- Cerebral blood flow is measured by a modification of the Fick principle. Oxyhaemoglobin is the intravascular non-diffusible tracer, its accumulation being proportional to the arterial inflow of tracer. Good correlations have been found with the xenon-133 technique.
- Cytochrome aa_3 cannot be quantified by NIRS, but its redox status may be followed to provide some indication of mitochondrial function.
- Movement artefact must be avoided and some devices require shielding from ambient lighting.

Lactate

The brain normally utilises lactate as a fuel. However, in states of severely impaired cerebral perfusion, the brain may become a net lactate producer with the venous lactate rising above the arterial value. A lactate oxygen index can be derived by dividing the veno-arterial lactate difference by the arterio-jugular venous oxygen difference. Values >0.08 are consistently seen with cerebral ischaemia.

Cerebral microdialysis

Microdialysis catheters may be placed in the brain during surgery to assess brain metabolism. Extracellular fluid chemicals diffuse into the catheter and are sampled for bedside analysis of, e.g. glucose, lactate, and pyruvate. An elevated extracellular fluid lactate:pyruvate ratio is a sensitive marker of ischemia following acute brain injury. The technique can monitor tissue at risk of ischaemia, e.g. due to vasospasm, or to determine the safe lower limit of cerebral perfusion pressure.

See also:
Tissue perfusion monitoring, p194; Lactate, p236.

Laboratory monitoring

Urea and creatinine

Measured in blood, urine and, occasionally, in other fluids such as abdominal drain fluid (e.g. ureteric disruption, fistulae).

Urea

A product of the urea cycle resulting from ammonia breakdown, it depends upon adequate liver function for synthesis and adequate renal function for excretion. Low levels are seen in cirrhosis and high levels in renal failure.

Uraemia is a clinical syndrome, including lethargy, drowsiness, confusion, pruritus, and pericarditis resulting from high plasma levels of urea (or, more correctly, nitrogenous waste products—azotaemia).

The ratio of urine:plasma urea may help to distinguish oliguria of renal or pre-renal origins. Higher ratios (>10:1) occur in pre-renal conditions e.g. hypovolaemia, while low levels (<4:1) occur with direct renal causes.

24h measurement of urinary urea (or nitrogen) excretion has been previously used as a guide to nutritional protein replacement, but is currently not considered a useful routine tool.

Creatinine

A product of creatine breakdown, it is predominantly derived from skeletal muscle and is also renally excreted. Low levels are found with malnutrition and high levels with muscle breakdown (rhabdomyolysis) and impaired excretion (renal failure). In the latter case, a creatinine value >120µmol/L suggests a creatinine clearance <25mL/min.

The usual ratio for plasma urea (mmol/L) to creatinine (µmol/L) is approximately 1:10. A much lower ratio in a critically ill patient is suggestive of rhabdomyolysis whereas higher ratios are seen in cirrhosis, malnutrition, hypovolaemia, and hepatic failure.

The ratio of urine:plasma creatinine may help distinguish between oliguria of renal or pre-renal origins. Higher ratios (>40) are seen in pre-renal conditions and low levels (<20) with direct renal causes.

Creatinine clearance

Creatinine clearance is a measure of glomerular filtration. Once filtered, only small amounts of creatinine are re-absorbed.

$$\text{Creatinine clearance} = \frac{U \times V \times 1000}{P \times T}$$

... where   U is urine creatinine (mmol/L)
                        V is urine volume (mL)
                        P is plasma creatinine (µmol/L)
                        T is time of urine collection (min)

Normal plasma ranges

Urea	2.5–6.5mmol/L
Creatinine	70–120µmol/L (depends on lean body mass)
Creatinine clearance male	85–125mL/min
Creatinine clearance female	75–115mL/min

See also:

Oliguria, p398; Acute renal failure—diagnosis, p400.

Electrolytes (Na^+, K^+, Cl^-, HCO_3^-)

Measured accurately by direct-reading, ion-specific electrodes from plasma or urine, though they are sensitive to interference by excess liquid heparin.

Sodium, potassium

Plasma levels may be elevated, but poorly reflect intracellular (approximately 3–5mmol/L for Na^+, 140–150mmol/L for K^+) or total body levels. Plasma potassium levels are affected by plasma H^+ levels; a metabolic acidosis reduces urinary potassium excretion while an alkalosis will increase excretion.

Older measuring devices such as flame photometry or indirect-reading, ion-specific electrodes gave spuriously low plasma Na^+ levels with concurrent hyperproteinaemia or hypertriglyceridaemia.

Urinary excretion depends on intake, total body balance, acid-base balance, hormones (including antidiuretic hormone, aldosterone, corticosteroids, atrial natriuretic peptide), drugs (particularly diuretics, non-steroidal anti-inflammatories, and ACE inhibitors), and renal function.

In oliguria, a urinary Na^+ level <10mmol/L suggests a pre-renal cause whereas >20mmol/L is seen with direct renal damage. This does not apply if diuretics have been given previously.

Chloride, bicarbonate

Bicarbonate levels vary with acid-base balance.

In the kidney, Cl^- reabsorption is increased when HCO_3^- reabsorption is decreased, and vice versa. Plasma $[Cl^-]$ thus tends to vary inversely with plasma $[HCO_3^-]$, keeping the total anion concentration normal. A raised $[Cl^-]$ (producing a hyperchloraemic metabolic acidosis) may be seen with administration of large volumes of isotonic saline or isotonic, saline-containing colloid solutions. Hyperchloraemia is also found with experimental salt water drowning but rarely seen in actual cases.

Anion gap

The anion gap is the difference between unestimated anions (e.g. phosphate, ketones, lactate) and cations.

In metabolic acidosis, an increased anion gap occurs with renal failure, ingestion of acid, ketoacidosis, and hyperlactataemia whereas a normal anion gap (usually associated with hyperchloraemia) is found with decreased acid excretion (e.g. Addison's disease, renal tubular acidosis) and loss of base (e.g. diarrhoea, pancreatic/biliary fistula, acetazolamide, ureterosigmoidostomy).

Normal plasma ranges

Sodium	135–145mmol/L
Potassium	3.5–5.3mmol/L
Chloride	95–105mmol/L
Bicarbonate	23–28mmol/L

Anion gap = plasma [Na$^+$] + [K$^+$] – [HCO$_3$$^-$] – [Cl$^-$].
Normal range 8–16mmol/L

See also:

Blood gas analysis, p154; Electrolyte management, p482; Hypernatraemia, p484;
Hyponatraemia, p486; Hyperkalaemia, p488; Hypokalaemia, p490; General acid-base principles,
p500; Metabolic acidosis, p502.

Calcium, magnesium, and phosphate

Calcium

Plasma calcium levels have been traditionally corrected to plasma albumin levels; this is now considered irrelevant, particularly at the low albumin levels seen in critically ill patients. Measurement of the ionised fraction is now considered more pertinent since it is the ionised fraction that is responsible for the extracellular actions of calcium, with changes in the ionised fraction being responsible for the symptomatology.

High calcium levels occur with hyperparathyroidism, certain malignancies, and sarcoidosis, while low levels are seen in renal failure, severe pancreatitis, and hypoparathyroidism.

Magnesium

Plasma levels poorly reflect intracellular or whole body stores, 65% of which is in bone and 35% in cells. The ionised fraction is approximately 50% of the total level.

High magnesium levels are seen with renal failure and excessive administration; this rarely requires treatment unless serious cardiac conduction problems or neurological complications (respiratory paralysis, coma) intervene.

Low levels occur following severe diarrhoea, diuretic therapy, alcohol abuse, and accompany hypocalcaemia.

Magnesium is used therapeutically for a number of conditions, including ventricular and supraventricular arrhythmias, eclampsia, seizures, asthma, and after myocardial infarction. Supranormal plasma levels of 1.5–2.0mmol/L are often sought.

Magnesium levels tend to follow potassium levels. Hypokalaemia is resistant to treatment unless magnesium is corrected first.

Phosphate

High levels are seen with renal failure and in the presence of an ischaemic bowel. Low levels (sometimes <0.1mmol/L) occur with critical illness, chronic alcoholism, and diuretic usage, and may possibly result in muscle weakness, failure to wean, and myocardial dysfunction.

Normal plasma ranges

Calcium	2.2–2.6mmol/L
Ionised calcium	1.05–1.2mmol/L
Magnesium	0.7–1.0mmol/L
Phosphate	0.7–1.4mmol/L

See also:

Hypomagnesaemia, p492; Hypercalcaemia, p494; Hypocalcaemia, p496; Hypophosphataemia, p498; Pre-eclampsia and eclampsia, p634.

Cardiac function tests

The diagnosis of myocardial infarction has been redefined as a typical rise, then fall in troponin, or a more rapid rise and fall in CK–MB, with at least one of the following:

- Ischaemic symptoms.
- Development of pathological Q waves on ECG.
- ECG ST elevation or depression.
- Coronary intervention.

Troponins

Troponins are bound to the actin filament within muscles and are involved in excitation-contraction coupling. Both cardiac troponin T and troponin I are coded by specific genes and are immunologically distinct from those in skeletal muscle. Neither is detectable in normal healthy individuals, but both are released into the bloodstream from cardiomyocytes damaged by necrosis, toxins, and inflammation. They become detectable by 4–6h after myocardial injury, peak at 14–18h, and persist for up to 12 days. Current assays are highly specific as they use recombinant human cardiac tropinin T as a standard.

Due to their high sensitivity, plasma levels rise with other cardiac insults, e.g. tachycardia (SVT/VT), pericarditis, myocarditis, sepsis, heart failure, severe exertion, and pulmonary embolism. The degree of rise post-MI or during critical illness correlates with a worse outcome.

A positive test is when the cardiac troponin T or I exceeds the 99th percentile of values for a control group on ≥1 occasion during the first 24h after the index clinical event. For cardiac troponin T, this is quoted as 0.05–0.1ng/mL though many labs now consider values >0.03ng/mL as positive. Values for cardiac troponin I depend on the particular assay used (usually >0.5–1.5ng/mL). The negative predictive value after an acute MI is probably strongest after 6h. Sensitivity peaks at 12h but at the expense of a lower specificity. With renal dysfunction, higher levels are needed to diagnose myocardial damage due to impaired excretion.

Cardiac enzymes

Creatine kinase (CK) is detectable in plasma within a few hours of myocardial injury. The cardiac-specific isoform (CK-MB) can be measured if there is concurrent skeletal muscle injury. CK and aspartate aminotransferase (AST) peak by 24h and fall over 2–3 days whereas the rise and subsequent fall in plasma lactate dehydrogenase takes 1–2 days longer (see figure 11.1).

Brain (or B-type) natriuretic peptide (BNP)

Cardiomyocytes produce and secrete cardiac natriuretic peptides. Plasma levels rise in a variety of conditions, but high levels are predominantly associated with heart failure and increase in relation to severity. A sensitivity of 90–100% is claimed, whereas specificity is approximately 70–80%. Numerous commercial assays for BNP or proBNP are now available, each with their own diagnostic range. They are useful as a screening tool for patients presenting with dyspnoea, for prognostication, and for titration of therapy. Levels rise in the elderly, in renal failure, and in pulmonary diseases causing right ventricular overload (e.g. pulmonary embolus).

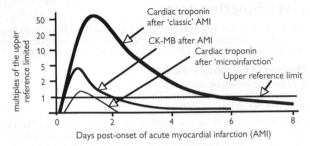

Fig. 11.1 Pattern of troponin and cardiac isoenzyme change after myocardial infarction.

Key papers

Alpert JS, Thygesen K, Antman E, et al. (2000) Myocardial infarction redefined—a consensus document of The Joint European Society of Cardiology/American College of Cardiology committee for the redefinition of myocardial infarction. *J Am Coll Cardiol* **36**: 959–69.

McCullough PA, Nowak RM, McCord J, et al. (2002) B-type natriuretic peptide and clinical judgment in emergency diagnosis of heart failure: analysis from Breathing Not Properly (BNP) Multinational Study. *Circulation* **106**: 416–22.

McLean AS, Huang SJ, Salter M. (2008) Bench-to-bedside review: The value of cardiac biomarkers in the intensive care patient. *Crit Care* **12**: 215.

See also:

Acute coronary syndrome (1), p388; Acute coronary syndrome (2), p390; Heart failure—assessment, p392.

Liver function tests

Hepatic metabolism proceeds via phase I enzymes (oxidation and phosphorylation), and subsequently, phase II enzymes (glucuronidation, sulphation, acetylation). Phase I enzyme reactions involve cytochrome P450.

Markers of hepatocyte damage
- Alanine aminotransferase (ALT).
- Aspartate aminotransferase (AST).
- Lactate dehydrogenase (LDH).

Patterns and ratios of various enzymes are variable and unreliable diagnostic indicators. Measurement of ALT alone is usually sufficient. It is more liver-specific, but less sensitive than AST and has a longer half-life.

AST is not liver-specific, but is a sensitive indicator of hepatic damage. The plasma level is proportional to the degree of hepatocellular damage. Low levels occur in extrahepatic obstruction and inactive cirrhosis.

LDH is insensitive and non-specific. Isoenzymes are needed to distinguish cardiac, erythrocyte, skeletal muscle, and liver injury.

Acute phase reactants such as C-reactive protein (CRP) produced by the liver increase during critical illness and following hepatocellular injury.

Markers of cholestasis
- Bilirubin.
- Alkaline phosphatase.
- Gamma-glutamyltransferase (γ-GT).

Bilirubin is conjugated with glucuronide by the hepatocytes. The conjugated fraction is water-soluble whereas the unconjugated fraction is lipid-soluble. Levels are increased with intra- and extra-hepatic biliary obstruction (predominantly conjugated), hepatocellular damage, and haemolysis (usually mixed picture). Jaundice is detected when levels >45μmol/L.

Alkaline phosphatase is released from bone, liver, intestine, and placenta. In the absence of bone disease (check Ca^{2+} and PO_4^{3-}) and pregnancy, raised levels usually indicate biliary tract dysfunction.

A raised γ-GT is a highly sensitive marker of hepatobiliary disease. Increased synthesis is induced by obstructive cholestasis, alcohol, various drugs and toxins, acute and chronic hepatic inflammation.

Markers of reduced synthetic function
- Albumin.
- Clotting factors.
- Cholinesterase.

Albumin levels fall during critical illness due to protein catabolism, capillary leak, decreased synthesis, dilution with artificial colloids.

Coagulation factors II, VII, IX, and X are liver-synthesised. Over 33% of functional hepatic mass must be lost before any abnormality is seen.

Indicators of function
- Lidocaine metabolites (MegX).

Indicators of hepatic blood flow
- Indocyanine green clearance.
- Bromosulphthalein clearance.

Normal plasma ranges

Albumin	35–53g/L
Bilirubin	3–17µmol/L
Conjugated bilirubin	0–6µmol/L
Alanine aminotransferase	5–50U/L
Alkaline phosphatase	100–280U/L
Aspartate aminotransferase	11–55U/L
Cholinesterase	2.3–9.0kU/L
γ-glutamyltransferase	5–37U/L
Lactate dehydrogenase	230–460U/L

See also:

Jaundice, p428; Acute liver failure, p430; Hepatic encephalopathy, p432; Chronic liver failure, p434; Paracetamol poisoning, p524; HELP syndrome, p636.

Full blood count

Haemoglobin

A raised haemoglobin occurs in polycythaemia (primary and secondary to chronic hypoxaemia) and in haemoconcentration. Anaemia may be due to reduced red cell mass (decreased red cell production or survival) or haemodilution. The latter is common in critically ill patients. In severe anaemia, there may be a hyperdynamic circulation which, if severe, may decompensate to cardiac failure. In this case, blood transfusion must be performed with extreme care to avoid fluid overload or in association with plasmapheresis. Differential diagnosis of anaemia includes:

Reduced MCV	Iron deficiency (anisocytosis and poikilocytosis)
Raised MCV	Vitamin B12 or folate deficiency
	Alcohol excess or liver disease
	Hypothyroidism
Normal MCV	Anaemia of chronic disease
	Bone marrow failure (e.g. acute folate deficiency)
	Hypothyroidism
	Haemolysis (increased reticulocytes and bilirubin)

White blood cells

A raised white cell count is extremely common in critical illness. Causes of changes in the differential count include:

Neutrophilia	Lymphocytosis	Eosinophilia
Bacterial infection	Brucellosis	Asthma
Trauma, surgery and burns	Typhoid	Allergic conditions
Haemorrhage	Myasthenia gravis	Parasitaemia
Inflammation	Hyperthyroidism	
Corticosteroid therapy	Leukaemia	
Leukaemia		
Neutropaenia	**Lymphopaenia**	
Viral infections	Corticosteroid therapy	
Tuberculosis	SLE	
Sulphonamide treatment	Legionnaire's disease	
Severe sepsis	AIDS	
Hypersplenism		
Bone marrow failure		

Platelets

Correct interpretation of platelet counts requires venous (not capillary) blood. Arterial blood from an indwelling cannula is not ideal. Thrombocytopaenia is due to decreased platelet production (bone marrow failure, vitamin B12, or folate deficiency), decreased platelet survival (ITP, TTP, infection, hypersplenism, heparin therapy), increased platelet consumption (haemorrhage, DIC), or *in vivo* aggregation giving an apparent thrombocytopaenia; this should be checked on a blood film. Spontaneous bleeding is associated with platelet counts <10x10^9/L and platelet cover is required for procedures or traumatic bleeds at counts <50x10^9/L.

Normal ranges

Haemoglobin	13–17g/dL (men), 12–16g/dL (women)
MCV	76–96fL
White cell count	4–11x10^9/L
Neutrophils	2–7.5x10^9/L
Lymphocytes	1.3–3.5x10^9/L
Eosinophils	0.04–0.44x10^9/L
Basophils	0–0.1x10^9/L
Monocytes	0.2–0.8x10^9/L
Platelets	150–400x10^9/L

See also:
Anaemia, p472; Sickle cell disease, p474; Haemolysis, p476; Platelet disorders, p478.

Coagulation monitoring

Basic coagulation screen

The basic screen consists of a platelet count, prothrombin time, activated partial thromboplastin time, and thrombin time. Close attention to blood sampling technique is very important for correct interpretation of coagulation tests. Drawing blood from indwelling catheters should ideally be avoided since samples may be diluted or contaminated with heparin. The correct volume of blood must be placed in the sample tube to avoid dilution errors. Laboratory coagulation tests are usually performed on citrated plasma samples taken into glass tubes.

Specific coagulation tests

Activated clotting time (ACT)

Sample tube contains celite which activates the contact system; thus, the ACT predominantly tests the intrinsic pathway. The ACT is prolonged by heparin therapy, thrombocytopaenia, hypothermia, haemodilution, fibrinolysis, and high-dose aprotinin. Normal is 100–140s.

Thrombin time (TT)

Sample tube contains lyophilised thrombin and calcium. Thrombin bypasses the intrinsic and extrinsic pathways such that the coagulation time tests the common pathway with conversion of fibrinogen to fibrin. The TT is prolonged by fibrinogen depletion, e.g. fibrinolysis or thrombolysis and heparin via antithrombin III-dependent interaction with thrombin. A high-dose TT is more sensitive to heparin anticoagulation than fibrinogen levels. Normal is 12–16s.

Prothrombin time (PT)

Sample tube contains tissue factor and calcium. Tissue factor activates the extrinsic pathway. The PT is prolonged with coumarin anticoagulants, liver disease, and vitamin K deficiency. Normal is 12–16s. The international normalised ratio (INR) relates PT to control and is normally 1.

Activated partial thromboplastin time (APTT)

Sample tube contains kaolin and cephalin as a platelet substitute to activate the intrinsic pathway. The APTT is prolonged by heparin therapy, DIC, severe fibrinolysis, von Willebrand factor, factor VIII, factor XI, or factor XIII deficiencies. Normal is 30–40s.

D-dimers and fibrin degradation products (FDPs)

Fibrin fragments are released by plasmin lysis. FDPs can be assayed by an immunological method; they are often measured in the critically ill to confirm disseminated intravascular coagulation. A level of 20–40mcg/mL is common post-operatively, in sepsis, trauma, renal failure, pulmonary embolus, and DVT. Raised levels do not distinguish fibrinogenolysis and fibrinolysis. Assay of the D-dimer fragment is more specific for fibrinolysis, e.g. in DIC, since it is only released after fibrin is formed.

Coagulation factor assays

Assays are available for all coagulation factors and may be used for diagnosis of specific defects. As heparins inhibit factor Xa activity, the factor Xa assay is the most specific method of controlling low molecular weight heparin therapy.

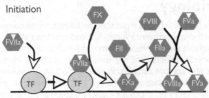

Initiation

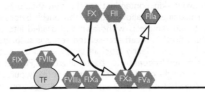

Amplification/thrombin (FIIa) formation

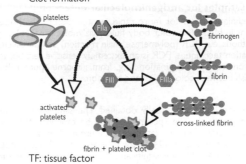

Clot formation

TF: tissue factor

Fig. 11.2 The coagulation cascade.

The traditional coagulation cascade consisting of extrinsic, intrinsic, and common pathways is now considered outmoded, inconsistent with clinical observations, and inadequate to explain the pathways leading to haemostasis *in vivo*. This schema has been replaced recently by a cell-based model with the major initiating haemostasis event *in vivo* being the action of factor VIIa and tissue factor at the site of injury.

See also:

Intra-aortic balloon counterpulsation, p102; Haemo(dia)filtration (1), p108; Haemo(dia)filtration (2), p110; Plasma exchange, p114; Anticoagulants, p318; Thrombolytics, p320; Coagulants and antifibrinolytics, p322; Pulmonary embolus, p376; Acute liver failure, p430; Bleeding disorders, p468; Clotting disorders, p470.

Bacteriology

Microbiology samples should, if possible, be taken prior to commencement of antimicrobial therapy. In severe infections, broad-spectrum antimicrobials should be started without awaiting results. Sampling sites include those suspected clinically of harbouring infection or, if a specific site cannot be identified clinically, blood, urine, and sputum samples. In severe infection, indwelling intravascular catheters should be replaced and the tips sent for culture. Samples should be sent to the laboratory promptly for early incubation and to prevent potentially misleading growth. Swabs must be sent in appropriate transport media.

Blood cultures

In order to avoid skin contamination, the skin should be cleaned with alcohol/chlorhexidine and allowed to dry thoroughly before venepuncture. A 10–20mL blood sample is withdrawn and divided into anaerobic and aerobic culture bottles. If catheter-related sepsis is suspected, a catheter sample may be taken. Clearly label all samples. Culture bottles are incubated and examined frequently for bacterial growth. Positive cultures must be interpreted in light of the clinical picture; an early, pure, heavy growth from multiple bottles is probably significant. Cultures from the critically ill may grow later or not at all due to antibiotic therapy. Any Gram-negative isolates or *Staphylococcus aureus* are taken as significant.

Blood samples for antigen/molecular detection

New techniques allow for more rapid identification of the presence of organisms in blood (or other body fluids) via molecular DNA amplification methods, e.g. PCR (polymerase chain reaction) or fluorescent *in situ* hybridisation techniques. PCR is an extremely sensitive test but is prone to environmental contamination (e.g. from airborne spores). It cannot distinguish between colonisation and infection.

Urine

Catheter specimens are usually obtained. The sampling site should be prepared aseptically. The specimen should be examined for organisms, casts, and crystals. Urine is plated onto culture medium with a calibrated loop and incubated for 18–24h prior to examination. Bacteria $>10^8$/L (or a pure growth $\geq10^5$/L) are significant. If the catheter has been in place for >2d, all urine specimens show bacterial growth. Isolation of the same organism from blood confirms a significant culture. Urine can also be used for antigen testing (e.g. Pneumococcus, *L. pneumophilia*).

Sputum/bronchial samples

Sputum samples are easily contaminated during collection, particularly from non-intubated patients. Suction specimens from intubated patients can be taken via a sterile suction catheter, protected catheter brush, or from specific lung segments via a bronchoscope. Gram-negative bacteria are frequently isolated from tracheal aspirates of intubated patients; only deep suction specimens are significant. Blood cultures should accompany sputum specimens if pneumonia is suspected.

Pus samples and wound swabs

Aspirated pus must be sent to the lab immediately, or a swab taken and sent in transport medium. Pus is preferable for bacterial isolation.

Typical ICU-acquired infections

Pneumonia	*Ps. aeruginosa, S. aureus, Klebsiella* spp., *Enterobacter* spp.
Urinary infection	*E. coli, Ps. aeruginosa, Klebsiella* spp., *Proteus* spp.
Catheter-related sepsis	*S. aureus*, coagulase-negative *Staphylococci*

See also:
Pleural aspiration, p86; Fibreoptic bronchoscopy, p88; Chest physiotherapy, p90; Virology, serology and assays, p226; Urinalysis, p232; Acute chest infection (1), p356; Acute chest infection (2), p358; Infection—diagnosis, p552.

Virology, serology, and assays

Antibiotic assays

Antibiotic assays are usually performed for drugs with a narrow therapeutic range such as aminoglycosides and vancomycin. It is not usual to request an assay on day 1 of treatment. Thereafter, samples are taken daily prior to giving a dose and at 1h after an IV injection or infusion.

Serology

A clotted blood specimen allows antibodies to viral and atypical antigens to be assayed. It is usual to send acute and convalescent (14 days) serum to determine rising antibody titres. Single sample titres may be used to determine previous exposure and carrier status.

Hepatitis B

Serology includes hepatitis B surface antigen as a screening test and hepatitis B core antigen to determine infectivity. There is a 10% carrier rate in South East Asians. Serology should be sent in all high-risk patients, e.g. jaundice, IV drug abuse, homosexuals, prostitutes, those with tattoos or unexplained hepatic enzyme abnormalities. Serology should be sent in staff who suffer accidental exposure to body fluids, e.g. needlestick injury. Those who are not immune may be treated with immunoglobulin.

HIV

Since HIV positive status carries consequences for lifestyle and insurance, it should rarely be assessed without prior counselling and consent. The viral load (measure of activity) and CD4 count may be used to assess the likelihood of symtomatology being AIDS-related, although the CD4 will fall with acute critical illness; again, consent should usually be sought pre-testing. High-risk patients should be considered for testing, e.g. homosexual males, intravenous drug abusers, haemophiliacs, those of Central African origin. In critically ill patients, such consent can rarely be obtained and unconsented testing may be used where management may change significantly with knowledge of the HIV status or where organ donation is being considered. Most AIDS-related infections can be adequately treated without knowledge of HIV status. However, patients or staff who are recipients of a needlestick injury can be treated with anti-retroviral therapies if the donor is known to be HIV-positive; unconsented testing may be reasonable in this situation.

Viral culture

Most commonly used for CMV. Samples of blood, urine, or bronchial aspirate may be sent for DEAFF (detection of early antigen fluorescent foci). Herpes virus infections may be detected by electron microscopy of samples (including pustule fluid) and adenovirus in immunosuppressed patients with a chest infection.

Fungi

Candida and *Aspergillus spp.* can be assessed by culture, PCR, or antigen tests. Cryptococcus can be detected by Indian ink stain in biopsy samples. Detection in blood of galactomannan, a component of the Aspergillus cell wall is an alternative means of diagnosis.

Common serology for critically ill patients

- Hepatitis A.
- Hepatitis B.
- Hepatitis C.
- HIV.
- CMV.
- *Mycoplasma pneumoniae.*
- *Legionella pneumophilia.*

Antibiotic therapeutic levels

	Trough (mg/L)	Peak (mg/L)
Amikacin	<8	30
Gentamicin	<2	4–10*
Tobramycin	<2	4–10
Vancomycin	<8	20–30

* Seek microbiological advice if once-daily gentamicin is used

See also:
Bacteriology, p224; Urinalysis, p232; Acute chest infection (1), p356; Acute chest infection (2), p358;
Infection—diagnosis, p552; HIV related disease, p566; SARS, VHF and H5N1, p570.

Toxicology

Purpose

Samples taken from blood, urine, vomitus, or gastric lavage (depending on drug or poison ingested) for:

- Monitoring of therapeutic drug levels (usually plasma) and avoidance of toxicity, e.g. digoxin, aminoglycosides, lithium, phenytoin, theophylline.
- Identification of unknown toxic substances (e.g. cyanide, amphetamines, opiates) causing symptomatology and/or pathology. Always take a urine sample for analysis.
- Confirmation of toxic plasma levels and monitoring of treatment effect, e.g. paracetamol, aspirin.
- Medicolegal, e.g. alcohol, recreational drugs following road trauma.

Samples

Confirm with chemistry laboratory ± local Poisons Unit as to which, how, and when body fluid samples should be taken for analysis, e.g. peak/trough levels for aminoglycosides, urine samples for out-of-hospital poisoning, repeat paracetamol levels to monitor efficacy of treatment.

See also:
Virology, serology, and assays, p226; Poisoning—general principles, p520.

Miscellaneous monitoring

Urinalysis

Techniques

- Biochemical/metabolic:
  - Colorimetric 'dipsticks' read manually from reference chart or by automated machine within 15s–2min of dipping in urine (see manufacturers' instructions). Usually performed at the bedside.
  - Sodium and potassium levels can be measured in many analysers used for plasma electrolyte measurement. Re-calibration of the machine or special dilution techniques may be required.
  - Laboratory analysis, e.g. for urea, osmolality, electrolytes, creatinine, myoglobin, urate.
- Haematological—either by dipstick or laboratory testing.
- Microbiological—microscopy, culture, sensitivity; antigen tests.
- Renal disease—usually by microscopy + laboratory testing.

Associated tests

Some of the above investigations are performed in conjunction with a blood test, e.g. urine:plasma ratios of urea, creatinine, and osmolality to distinguish renal from pre-renal causes of oliguria, 24h urine collection plus plasma creatinine for creatinine clearance estimation.

Cautions

- White blood cells, proteinuria, and mixed bacterial growths are routine findings in catheterised patients and do not necessarily indicate infection.
- Urinary nitrite is a useful indicator of infection.
- A 'positive' dipstick test for blood does not differentiate between haematuria, haemoglobinuria, or myoglobinuria.
- Only conjugated bilirubin is excreted into the urine.
- Urinary sodium and potassium levels are increased by diuretic usage.

Urinalysis tests
Biochemical/metabolic:

pH	Dipstick
Glucose	Dipstick
Ketones	Dipstick
Protein	Dipstick, laboratory
Bilirubin	Dipstick
Nitrite	Dipstick
Sodium, potassium	Electrolyte analyser, laboratory
Urea, creatinine, nitrogen	Laboratory
Osmolality	Laboratory
Specific gravity	Bedside gravimeter, laboratory
Myoglobin	Laboratory, positive dipstick to blood
Drugs, poisons	Send to Poisons Reference Laboratory

Haematological:

Red blood cells	Microscopy, positive dipstick to blood
Haemoglobin	Laboratory, positive dipstick to blood
Neutrophils	Dipstick, laboratory

Microbiological:

Bacteriuria	Microscopy, culture
TB	Microscopy, culture (early morning specimens)
Legionnaire's disease	Laboratory

Nephro-urological:

Haematuria	Microscopy
Granular casts	Microscopy
Protein	Laboratory
Sodium, potassium	Electrolyte analyser, laboratory
Malignant cells	Cytology

See also:
Virology, serology, and assays, p226; Diabetic ketoacidosis, p510; Hyperosmolar diabetic emergencies, p512.

Indirect calorimetry

Calorimetry refers to the measurement of energy production. Direct calorimetry is the measurement of heat production in a sealed chamber but is impractical for critically ill patients. Indirect calorimetry measures the rate of oxidation of metabolic fuels by detecting the volume of O_2 consumed and CO_2 produced. The ratio of CO_2 production to O_2 utilisation (respiratory quotient or RQ) defines which fuels are being utilised (see table 10.1). Knowledge of the oxygen utilisation by the various fuels allows calculation of energy production. Carbohydrate and fat are oxidised to CO_2 and water producing 15–17 and 38–39kJ/g, respectively. Protein is oxidised to CO_2, water, and nitrogen (subsequently excreted as urea), producing 15–17kJ/g.

Technique of indirect calorimetry

Inspiratory and mixed expiratory gases must be sampled. O_2 concentration may be measured by a fuel cell sensor or a fast response, paramagnetic sensor. CO_2 is usually measured by infrared absorption. Sensors may be calibrated with reference to known concentrations of standard gas or by burning a pure fuel with a predictable O_2 consumption. Measurements are usually made at ambient temperature, pressure, and humidity prior to conversion to standard temperature, pressure, and humidity. To calculate metabolic rate (energy expenditure), inspired and expired minute volumes are required. It is common for one minute volume to be measured and the other derived from a Haldane transformation:

$$V_I = V_E \times \frac{N_E}{N_I}$$

The nitrogen concentrations are assumed to be the concentration of gas which is not O_2 or CO_2. Calculation of energy expenditure utilises a modification of the de Weir formula:

$$\text{Energy expenditure} = (3.94VO_2 + 1.11VCO_2) \times 1.44$$

Although it is possible to calculate the rate of protein metabolism by reference to the urinary urea concentration, and therefore, to separate non-protein from protein energy expenditure, the resulting modification of the above formula is not usually clinically significant.

Errors associated with indirect calorimetry

Underestimate VCO_2 H^+ ion loss, haemodialysis, haemofiltration.
Overestimate VCO_2 Hyperventilation, HCO_3^- infusion.
Underestimate VO_2 Free radical production, unmeasured O_2 supply.
FIO_2 >0.6   Small difference between inspired and expired O_2.
Loss of volume   Circuit leaks, bronchopleural fistula.

Use of indirect calorimetry

Helps to match nutritional intake to energy expenditure. It is important to feed critically ill patients appropriately, avoiding both underfeeding and overfeeding (see table opposite). Indirect calorimetry may also be used to assess work of breathing by assessing the change in VO_2 during weaning from mechanical ventilation. The VO_2 change may also be used to assess appropriate levels of sedation and analgesia.

Respiratory quotients for various metaboliic fuels

Ketones	0.63
Fat	0.71
Protein	0.80
Carbohydrate	1.00

The whole body RQ depends on the fuel or combination of fuels being utilised. Normally, a combination of fat and carbohydrate are utilised with an RQ of 0.8. Lipogenesis associated with both sepsis and overfeeding may give a RQ of 1.1–1.3.

See also:
Nutrition—use and indications, p126; Enteral nutrition, p128; Parenteral nutrition, p130.

Lactate

Pyruvate, the end-product of glycolysis, is taken up from the cytosol into the mitochondria by pyruvate dehydrogenase and metabolised to acetyl CoA, the entry point into the Krebs's cycle (see figure 12.1). Electrons are donated from the Krebs's cycle to the electron transport chain via NADH and $FADH_2$. Pyruvate not taken up by mitochondria goes into equilibrium with lactate. This reaction is catalysed in either direction by lactate dehydrogenase (see figure 12.2)

Causes of lactic acidosis

Increased lactate production is not due simply to tissue hypoxia. It can be generated either by excess glycolysis in relation to downstream requirements (e.g. excess stimulation by exogenous or endogenous epinephrine) or by a downstream block, e.g. of pyruvate dehydrogenase (sepsis), oxygen insufficiency (any cause of tissue hypoxia), or mitochondrial electron transport chain dysfunction (e.g. sepsis, CO poisioning). In sepsis, blood lactate levels rise in part due to increased activity of the skeletal muscle Na^+ pump driven by epinephrine-stimulated glycolysis.

A further cause of hyperlactataemia is decreased utilisation. This is particularly apparent with liver (± kidney) dysfunction, especially when exogenous lactate is being administered, e.g. lactate-buffered renal replacement fluid. Lactate is a buffer, not an acid, so a high blood lactate is not, therefore, synonymous with lactic acidosis; there needs to be a concurrent metabolic acidosis for diagnosis.

Lactic acidosis is traditionally classified as type A or type B. Type A refers to excess production when tissue oxygenation is inadequate. Type B occurs where there is no systemic tissue hypoxia. A severe and persistent type A lactic acidosis is associated with a poor outcome.

Measurement of blood lactate

Analysers are available to allow rapid measurement of blood or plasma lactate on small samples using enzyme-based methods. The enzymatic conversion of lactate to pyruvate is an oxygen-utilising reaction. The extraction of oxygen from the sample can be detected by a sensitive oxygen fuel cell sensor and is directly proportional to the sample lactate concentration. A whole blood sample (venous or arterial since there is no practical difference) is collected into a heparin fluoride tube to prevent coagulation and glycolysis (lactate-producing). Nitrite may be used in the sample tube to convert haemoglobin to the met-form, thus avoiding uptake of oxygen during the enzyme reaction.

The enzymatic method is specific for the L-isomer and will not detect D-lactate (seen, for example, in short bowel syndrome). Lactate may also be measured from regional sites to aid assessment of regional perfusion (e.g. arterial jugular venous bulb difference).

Normal blood lactate <1.8mmol/L.

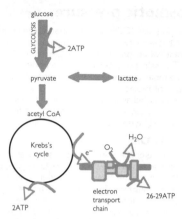

Fig. 12.1 Bioenergetic pathway from oxidation of glucose.

$$HOH - \overset{\displaystyle COO^-}{\underset{\displaystyle COO^-}{\overset{|}{\underset{|}{C}}}} - + NAD^+ \quad \underset{\overset{\displaystyle lactate}{\displaystyle dehydrogenase}}{\rightleftharpoons} \quad \overset{\displaystyle COO^-}{\underset{\displaystyle CH_3}{\overset{|}{\underset{|}{C=O}}}} + NADH + H^+$$

lactate   pyruvate

Fig. 12.2 Pyruvate–lactate equilibrium.

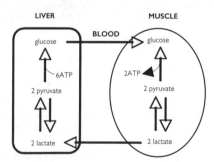

Fig. 12.3 Cori cycle (lactate–glucose between liver and muscle).

Key papers

Levy B, Gibot S, Franck P, et al. (2005) Relation between muscle Na^+K^+ ATPase activity and raised lactate concentrations in septic shock: a prospective study. *Lancet* **365**: 871–5.

Totaro RJ, Raper RF. (1997) Epinephrine-induced lactic acidosis following cardiopulmonary bypass. *Crit Care Med* **25**:1693–9.

See also:

Blood gas analysis, p154; Jugular venous bulb saturation, p202; Other neurological monitoring, p206; Metabolic acidosis, p502.

Colloid osmotic pressure

Colloid osmotic pressure (COP) is the pressure required to prevent net fluid movement between two solutions separated by a selectively permeable membrane when one contains a greater colloid concentration than the other. The selectively permeable membrane should impede the passage of colloid molecules, but not small ions and water. COP is determined by number of molecules rather than type. However, most solutions exhibit non-ideal behaviour due to intermolecular interactions and electrostatic effects. Hence, COP cannot be inferred from plasma protein concentrations; it must be measured.

Measurement of COP

In a membrane oncometer, the plasma sample is separated from a reference 0.9% saline solution by a membrane with a molecular weight exclusion between 10,000 and 30,000 dalton. The reference solution is in a closed chamber containing a pressure transducer. Saline will pass to the sample chamber by colloid osmosis, creating a negative pressure in the reference chamber. When the negative pressure prevents any further flow across the membrane, it is equal to the COP of the sample. Normal plasma COP is 25–30mmHg.

Clinical use of COP measurement

Assessing significance of reduced plasma proteins

Plasma albumin levels are almost invariably reduced in critically ill patients. Causes include interstitial leakage, failed synthesis, and increased metabolism. However, the same group of patients often has raised levels of acute phase proteins which contribute to COP. Since there is no evidence that correction of plasma albumin levels is beneficial, many clinicians correct plasma volume deficit with artificial colloid. These will contribute to COP while also reducing hepatic albumin synthesis. If COP is maintained >20mmHg, it is likely that reduced plasma albumin levels are of no significance.

Avoiding pulmonary oedema

It has been suggested that a difference between COP and pulmonary artery wedge pressure >6mmHg minimises the risk of pulmonary oedema. However, in the face of severe capillary leak, it is unlikely that pulmonary oedema can be avoided if plasma volumes are to be maintained compatible with circulatory adequacy. Conversely, a normal COP would not necessarily prevent pulmonary oedema in severe capillary leak; the contribution of COP to fluid dynamics in this situation is much reduced.

Selection of appropriate fluid therapy

It is difficult not to support the use of colloid fluids in hypo-oncotic patients. In patients with renal failure, the repeated use of colloid fluid may lead to a hyper-oncotic state. This is associated with tissue dehydration and failure of glomerular filtration (thus prolonging the renal failure). Measurement of a high COP in patients who have been treated with artificial colloids should direct the use of crystalloid fluids. It is important to note that excessive diuresis may also lead to a hyper-oncotic state for which crystalloid replacement may be necessary.

See also:
Colloids, p246.

Fluids

Crystalloids

Types
- Balanced electrolyte: e.g. Ringer's lactate, Hartmann's solution.
- Saline: e.g. 0.9% saline, 0.18% saline in 4% glucose.
- Glucose: e.g. 5%, 10%, 20%, 50%.
- Sodium bicarbonate: e.g. 1.26%, 8.4%.

Uses
- Crystalloid fluids to provide daily requirements of water and electrolytes. They should be given to critically ill patients as a continuous background infusion to supplement fluids given during feeding or to carry drugs.
- Higher concentration glucose infusions may be used to prevent hypoglycaemia.
- Crystalloid fluids may contain potassium chloride supplements.
- Sodium bicarbonate may be used to correct metabolic acidosis, for urinary alkalinisation, etc.

Routes
- IV.

Notes
- Significant plasma volume deficit should be replaced with colloid solutions since crystalloids are rapidly lost from the plasma, particularly during periods of increased capillary leak, e.g. sepsis.
- As most plasma substitutes are carried in saline solutions, any additional salt containing crystalloid infusion is only needed to replace excess sodium losses.
- The sodium content of 0.9% saline is equivalent to that of extracellular fluid. Therefore, salt-containing solutions distribute throughout the extracellular fluid space.
- Ringer's lactate or Hartmann's solution avoid hyperchloraemic acidosis caused by the relative excess chloride infused with 0.9% saline. Hyperchloraemic acidosis may adversely affect coagulation and renal function though human data are lacking.
- A daily requirement of 70–80mmol sodium is normal although there may be excess loss in sweat and from the gastrointestinal tract. This can be provided as saline or balanced electrolyte solution.
- 5% glucose is used to supply intravenous water requirements. Since there are no electrolytes to favour distribution to one space or another, water distributes uniformly throughout the extracellular and intracellular spaces. The 50g/L glucose content ensures an isotonic solution, but only provides 200Cal/L. Normal requirement is approximately 1.5–2L/d.
- Water loss in excess of electrolytes is uncommon but occurs in excess sweating, fever, hyperthyroidism, diabetes insipidus, and hypercalcaemia. 5% glucose is an appropriate replacement fluid for water loss.
- Potassium chloride must be given slowly since rapid injection may cause fatal arrhythmias. No more than 40mmol/h should be given and even this may be dangerous in some patients. Up to 20mmol/h is safer. The frequency of infusion is dictated by plasma potassium measurements.

Ion content of crystalloids (mmol/L)

	Na$^+$	K$^+$	HCO$_3^-$	Cl$^-$	Ca^{2+}
0.9% saline	150			150	
Hartmann's	131	5	29	111	2
0.18% saline in 4% glucose	30			30	

Ion content of gastrointestinal fluids (mmol/L)

	H$^+$	Na$^+$	K$^+$	HCO$_3^-$	Cl$^-$
Gastric	40–60	20–80	5–20	150	100–150
Biliary		120–140	5–15	30–50	80–120
Pancreatic		120–140	5–15	70–110	40–80
Small bowel		120–140	5–15	20–40	90–130
Large bowel		100–120	5–15	20–40	90–130

See also:

Nutrition—use and indications, p126; Electrolytes (Na$^+$, K$^+$, Cl, HCO$_3^-$), p212; Sodium bicarbonate, p244; Colloids, p246; Electrolyte management, p482; Hyponatraemia, p486; Hypokalaemia, p490; Metabolic acidosis, p504; Hypoglycaemia, p506.

Sodium bicarbonate

Types
- Isotonic sodium bicarbonate 1.26%.
- Hypertonic sodium bicarbonate 8.4%.

Uses
- Correction of metabolic acidosis.
- Alkalinisation of urine, e.g. for salicylate overdose, treatment of rhabdomyolysis.
- Alkalinisation of blood, e.g. for treatment of tricyclic antidepressant overdose.

Routes
- IV.

Notes
- Isotonic (1.26%) sodium bicarbonate may be used to correct acidosis associated with renal failure or to induce a forced alkaline diuresis.
- The hypertonic (8.4%) solution (1mEq HCO_3^-/mL) is rarely required in intensive care practice to raise blood pH in severe metabolic acidosis.
- Bicarbonate therapy is inappropriate when tissue hypoperfusion or necrosis is present.
- Administration may be indicated as either specific therapy (e.g. alkaline diuresis for salicylate overdose) or if the patient is dyspnoeic in the absence of tissue hypoperfusion (e.g. renal failure).
- The $PaCO_2$ may rise if minute volume is not increased.
- Bicarbonate cannot cross the cell membrane without dissociation so the increase in $PaCO_2$ may result in intracellular acidosis and depression of myocardial cell function.
- A decrease in plasma ionised calcium as a result of alkalinisation may also cause a decrease in myocardial contractility. Significantly worse haemodynamic effects have been reported with bicarbonate compared to equimolar saline in patients with severe heart failure.
- Convincing human data that bicarbonate improves myocardial contractility or increases responsiveness to circulating catecholamines in severe acidosis are lacking. Acidosis secondary to myocardial depression is related to intracellular changes that are not accurately reflected by arterial blood chemistry.
- Excessive administration may cause hyperosmolality, hypernatraemia, hypokalaemia, and sodium overload.
- Bicarbonate may decrease tissue oxygen availability by a left shift of the oxyhaemoglobin dissociation curve.
- Sodium bicarbonate does have a place in the management of acid retention or alkali loss, e.g. chronic renal failure, renal tubular acidosis, fistulae, diarrhoea. Fluid and potassium deficit should be corrected first.

Ion content of sodium bicarbonate (mmol/L)

	Na$^+$	K$^+$	HCO$_3$$^-$	Cl$^-$	Ca^{2+}
1.26% sodium bicarbonate	150		150		
8.4% sodium bicarbonate	1000		1000		

See also:

Blood gas analysis, p154; Electrolytes (Na$^+$, K$^+$, Cl$^-$, HCO$_3$$^-$), p212; Electrolyte management, p482; Hypernatraemia, p484; Hypokalaemia, p490; Metabolic acidosis, p502.

Colloids

Types

- Albumin: e.g. 4.5–5%, 20–25% human albumin solution.
- Dextran: e.g. 6% Dextran 70.
- Gelatin: e.g. 3.5% polygeline, 4% succinylated gelatin.
- Hydroxyethyl starch: e.g. 6% hetastarch, 6% hexastarch, 6 and 10% pentastarch, 6% and 10% tetrastarch.

Uses

Replacement of plasma volume deficit.
- Short-term volume expansion (gelatin, dextran).
- Medium-term volume expansion (albumin, pentastarch, tetrastarch).
- Long-term volume expansion (hetastarch, hexastarch).

Routes

- IV.

Side effects

- Dilution coagulopathy.
- Anaphylaxis.
- Interference with blood crossmatching (Dextran 70).
- Nephropathy (high dose hydroxyethyl starches).

Notes

- Smaller volumes of colloid are required for resuscitation with less contribution to oedema. Maintenance of plasma colloid osmotic pressure (COP) is a useful effect not seen with crystalloids, but colloids contain no clotting factors or other plasma enzyme systems.
- Albumin is the main provider of COP in the plasma and has a number of other functions. There is no evidence that maintenance of plasma albumin levels, as opposed to maintenance of plasma COP with artificial plasma substitutes, is advantageous.
- Hyperoncotic colloids can be used where salt restriction is necessary. This is rarely necessary as plasma volume expansion relates to weight of colloid infused rather than concentration. Artificial colloids used with ultrafiltration or diuresis are just as effective in oedema states.
- Polygeline is a 3.5% solution and contains calcium (6.25mmol/L). The calcium content prevents the use of the same administration set for blood transfusions. Succinylated gelatin is a 4% solution and does not contain calcium.
- Hydroxyethyl starch solutions are protected from metabolism due to a high degree of substitution (proportion of glucose units substituted with hydroxyethyl groups—DS) or a high C2:C6 ratio of carbon atoms substituted. Prolonged itching related to intradermal deposition, coagulopathy, and nephropathy are complications if excessive doses of higher molecular weight hydroxyethyl starches are used.
- Pentastarch and tetrastarch provide only a short-term volume expanding effects.
- Hydroxyethyl starches in balanced electrolyte solutions are available. These avoid the problem of hyperchloraemic acidosis in higher doses. There is also some evidence of less coagulation disturbance.

Unique features of albumin

- Transport of various molecules.
- Free radical scavenging.
- Binding of toxins.
- Inhibition of platelet aggregation.

Relative persistence of colloid effect

Albumin	+++
Dextran 70	++
Succinylated gelatin	++
Polygeline	+
Hetastarch (high MW, high DS, low C2:C6 ratio)	++++
Hexastarch (medium MW, high DS, high C2:C6 ratio)	++++
Pentastarch (medium MW, low DS, low C2:C6 ratio)	++
Tetrastarch (low MW, low DS, high C2:C6 ratio)	++

- Persistence is dependent on molecular size and protection from metabolism.
- High DS and high C2:C6 ratio protect hydroxyethyl starch from metabolism.
- All artificial colloids are polydisperse (i.e. there is a range of molecular sizes).

Key papers

The SAFE Study Investigators. (2004) A comparison of albumin and saline for fluid resuscitation in the intensive care unit. *N Engl J Med* **350**: 2247–56.

Brunkhorst F, Engel C, Bloos F, et al. (2008) Intensive insulin therapy and pentastarch resuscitation in severe sepsis. *N Engl J Med* **358**: 125–39.

See also:

Colloid osmotic pressure, p238; Crystalloids, p242; Basic resuscitation, p338; Fluid challenge, p342; Anaphylactoid reactions, p578.

Blood transfusion

Blood storage

Blood cells are eventually destroyed by oxidant damage during storage of whole blood. Since white cells and plasma enzyme systems are important in this cellular destruction, effects are correspondingly less severe for packed red cells. Blood used for transfusion in most of Europe is now routinely leukodepleted to prevent acute non-haemolytic transfusion reactions. Microaggregate formation is associated with platelets, white cells, and fibrin, and range in size from 20–170μm. The risk of microaggregate damage is reduced with packed cells. In addition to spherocytosis and haemolysis, prolonged storage depletes ATP and 2,3-DPG levels, thus increasing the O_2 affinity of the red cells. If whole blood is to be used in critically ill patients, it should be as fresh as possible.

Compatibility

In an emergency with massive blood loss that threatens life, it is permissible to transfuse O-negative packed cells, but a sample must be taken for grouping prior to transfusion. With modern laboratory procedures, it is possible to obtain ABO compatibility for group specific transfusion within 5–10min and a full crossmatch in 30min.

Hazards of blood transfusion

- Citrate toxicity—hypocalcaemia is rarely a problem. The prophylactic use of calcium supplementation is not recommended.
- Potassium load—potassium returns to cells rapidly, but hyperkalaemia may be a problem if blood is stored at room temperature.
- Jaundice—haemolysis of incompatible or old blood.
- Pyrexia—immunological transfusion reactions to incompatible red or white cells or platelets or blood products
- DIC—partial activation of clotting factors and destruction of stored cells, either in old blood or when transfusion is incompatible.
- Anaphylactoid reaction—urticaria is common and probably due to a reaction to transfused plasma proteins; if severe, it may be treated by slowing the transfusion and giving chlorpheniramine 10mg IV/IM. In severe anaphylaxis, in addition to standard treatment, the transfusion should be stopped and saved for later analysis. A sample should be taken for further crossmatching.
- Transmission of disease—including viruses, parasites (malaria), prions.
- Transfusion-related acute lung injury (TRALI) and other immune reactions.
- A multicentre trial suggested liberal transfusion in the critically ill produced less favourable outcomes, particularly in younger, less sick patients, than using a trigger haemoglobin of 7g/dL. This was performed with non-leukodepleted blood; the validity with leukodepleted blood now in common use is uncertain.

Key paper

Hebert P, Wells G, Blajchman M, et al. for the Tranfusion Requirements in Critical Care Investigators. (1999) A multicentre, randomised, controlled clinical trial of transfusion requirements in critical care. *N Engl J Med* **340**: 409–17.

See also:

Basic resuscitation, p338; Upper gastrointestinal haemorrhage, p412; Bleeding varices, p414; Lower intestinal bleeding and colitis, p420; Jaundice, p428; Anaemia, p472; Sickle cell disease, p474; Haemolysis, p476; Hyperkalaemia, p488; Anaphylactoid reactions, p578.

Blood products

Types
- Plasma, e.g. fresh frozen plasma.
- Platelets.
- Concentrates of coagulation factors, e.g. cryoprecipitate, factor VIII concentrate, factor IX complex, Octaplex.
- Recombinant technologies, e.g. factor VIIa, factor VIII.

Uses
- Vitamin K deficiency (fresh frozen plasma, factor IX complex, Octaplex).
- Haemophilia (cryoprecipitate, factor VIII, recombinant factor VIIa).
- von Willebrand's disease (cryoprecipitate).
- Fibrinogen deficiency (cryoprecipitate).
- Christmas disease (factor IX complex).

Routes
- IV.

Notes
- A unit (150mL) of fresh frozen plasma is usually collected from one donor and contains all coagulation factors, including 200U factor VIII, 200U factor IX, and 400mg fibrinogen. It is stored at −30°C and should be infused within 2h once defrosted.
- Platelet concentrates are viable for three days when stored at room temperature. Viability decreases if they are refrigerated. They must be infused quickly via a short giving set with no filter.
- Indications for platelet concentrates include platelet count $<10 \times 10^9$ or $<50 \times 10^9$ with spontaneous bleeding or to cover invasive procedures and spontaneous bleeding with platelet dysfunction. They are less useful in conditions associated with immune platelet destruction (e.g. ITP).
- A 15mL vial of cryoprecipitate contains 100U factor VIII, 250mg fibrinogen, factor XIII, and von Willebrand factor and is stored at −30°C.
- In haemophilia, cryoprecipitate is given to achieve a factor VIII level >30% of normal.
- Factor VIII concentrate contains 300U factor VIII per vial. In severe haemorrhage due to haemophilia, 10–15U/kg are given 12-hourly.
- Recombinant factor VIIa is indicated for control of bleeding in patients with haemophilia with inhibitors to factors VIII or IX, or congenital factor VII deficiency. It forms complexes with exposed tissue factor and is not dependent on the presence of factors VIII or IX. It has been shown to reduce blood transfusion requirements in major blunt trauma. Success has been reported in cases of uncontrollable intra-operative bleeding (90mcg/kg repeated every 2–3h until bleeding stops).
- Octaplex is a prothrombin complex concentrate for the substitution of factors II, VII, IX, and X in treatment or prophylaxis of hereditary and acquired coagulation factor disorders, e.g. warfarin overdose.

Key paper

Boffard KD, for the NovoSeven Trauma Study Group. (2005) Recombinant factor VIIa as adjunctive therapy for bleeding control in severely injured trauma patients: two parallel randomised, placebo-controlled, double-blind clinical trials. *J Trauma* **59**: 8–15.

See also:

Plasma exchange, p114; Full blood count, p220; Coagulation monitoring, p222; Colloids, p246; Blood transfusion, p248; Anticoagulants, p318; Bleeding disorders, p468; Clotting disorders, p470; Platelet disorders, p478.

Respiratory drugs

Bronchodilators

Types

- β_2 agonists, e.g. salbutamol, epinephrine, terbutaline.
- Anticholinergics, e.g. ipratropium.
- Theophyllines, e.g. aminophylline.
- Others, e.g. magnesium, ketamine, isoflurane.

Uses

- Relief of bronchospasm.

Routes

- Inhaled (salbutamol, epinephrine, terbutaline, ipratropium, isoflurane).
- Nebulised (salbutamol, epinephrine, terbutaline, ipratropium).
- IV (salbutamol, epinephrine, terbutaline, ipratropium, aminophylline, magnesium, ketamine).
- PO (aminophylline).

Side effects

- CNS stimulation (salbutamol, epinephrine, terbutaline, aminophylline).
- Tachycardia (salbutamol, epinephrine, terbutaline, aminophylline, ketamine).
- Hypotension (salbutamol, terbutaline, aminophylline, isoflurane).
- Hyperglycaemia (hydrocortisone, prednisolone, epinephrine).
- Hypokalaemia (salbutamol, epinephrine, terbutaline).
- Lactic acidosis (salbutamol)—rare.

Notes

- Selective β_2 agonists are usually given by inhalation via a pressurised aerosol or a nebuliser. Inhalation often gives rapid relief of bronchospasm. The aerosol is of less benefit in severe asthma unless used with a spacer device. They can be given by IV infusion.
- Nebulised drugs require a minimum volume of 4mL and a driving gas flow of 6–8L/min (higher or lower flow creates the wrong particle size for drug delivery).
- *In extremis*, epinephrine may be used IV, SC, or injected down the endotracheal tube. As epinephrine is not selective, arrhythmias are more likely. However, the α agonist effect may reduce mucosal swelling by vasoconstriction, further improving airflow.
- Ipratropium bromide does not depress mucociliary clearance, but may thicken sputum due to its anticholinergic effect. It is synergistic with β_2 agonists, but has a slower onset of action. Its use in critical care is poorly studied.
- Aminophylline is synergistic with β_2 agonists. Dosages must be adjusted according to plasma levels (range 10–20mg/L) since toxic effects may be severe. Dose requirements are lower with heart failure, liver disease, chronic airflow limitation, fever, erythromycin, and higher in children, smokers, and those with a moderate to high alcohol intake.
- Magnesium is a useful adjunctive therapy for severe asthma.
- Ketamine or isoflurane may be useful for sedation and bronchodilatation in the ventilated asthmatic.

Drug dosages

	Aerosol*	Nebuliser*	IV bolus	IV infusion
Salbutamol	100–200mcg	2.5–5mg		3–20mcg/min
Terbutaline	250–500mcg	5–10mg	1.5–5mcg/min	
Epinephrine		0.5mg		
Ipratropium		250mcg		
Aminophylline			5mg/kg over 20min	0.5mg/kg/h
Magnesium			1.2–2g over 20min	
Ketamine			1–2mg/kg	<0.75mg/kg/h

* Aerosols and nebulisers are usually given four to six times daily, but may be given more frequently if necessary.

In extremis, epinephrine may be given as 0.1–0.5mg subcutaneously, injected down the endotracheal tube or by IV infusion.

See also:

Chest physiotherapy, p90; Pulmonary function tests, p148; Corticosteroids, p328; Chronic airflow limitation, p354; Acute chest infection (1), p356; Asthma—general management, p364.

Respiratory stimulants

Types
- Drug antagonists, e.g. naloxone, flumazenil.
- CNS stimulants, e.g. doxapram.

Uses
- Acute respiratory failure due to failure of ventilatory drive.
- Drug-induced ventilatory failure, e.g. as a result of excessive sedation or post-operatively.

Routes
- IV.

Modes of action
- Naloxone—short-acting opiate antagonist.
- Flumazenil—short-acting benzodiazepine antagonist.
- Doxapram—generalised central nervous system stimulant with predominant respiratory stimulation at lower doses. Stimulation of carotid chemoreceptors at very low doses with increased tidal volumes.

Side effects
- Seizures (flumazenil, doxapram).
- Tachyarrhythmias (naloxone, flumazenil).
- Hallucinations (doxapram).

Notes
- Respiratory stimulants are mainly used in patients with chronic airflow limitation who develop acute hypercapnic respiratory failure.
- Effects of doxapram are short-lived so infusion is necessary. After about 12h infusion, the effects on ventilatory drive are reduced.
- Naloxone may be used in respiratory depression due to opiate drugs. Since it reverses all opiate effects, it may be better to reverse respiratory depression with non-specific respiratory stimulants, e.g. doxapram leaving pain relief intact. It may need to be repeated where long-acting opiates are involved.
- Most benzodiazepines are long-acting compared to flumazenil so repeated doses may be necessary.
- Flumazenil should not be used in mixed overdose.

Drug dosages

	IV bolus	IV infusion
Naloxone	0.1–0.4mg	
Flumazenil	0.2mg over 15min (0.1mg/min to max 2mg)	
Doxapram	1–1.5mg/kg over 30s	2–3mg/min

Key paper

Greenstone M, Lasserson TJ. (2003) Doxapram for ventilatory failure due to exacerbations of chronic obstructive pulmonary disease. *Cochrane Database Syst Rev* CD000223. Review.

See also:

Respiratory failure, p350; Chronic airflow limitation, p354; Sedative poisoning, p526; Post-operative critical care, p620.

Nitric oxide

Nitric oxide (NO) is a fundamental mediator in many physiological processes. One of the most important effects is smooth muscle relaxation; NO is a major local controller of vascular tone via effects on cyclic GMP.

Inhaled NO

NO is provided for inhalation from cylinders and is added to the inspiratory limb of the ventilator circuit by a servo control device to achieve a concentration of 1–40ppm. Most patients require less than 20ppm. Inhalation produces vasodilatation at the site of gas exchange, and may improve ventilation-perfusion matching and reduce pulmonary artery pressures. However, randomised multicentre studies in patients with acute lung injury revealed no long-term benefit nor outcome improvement.

Side effects

NO is immediately bound to haemoglobin ensuring local effects only. There is no tolerance, but patients can become dependent on continued inhalation with rebound pulmonary hypertension and hypoxaemia on withdrawal. For this reason, withdrawal must be gradual. Excessive humidification of inspired gases may form nitric acid with NO; the use of heat-moisture exchangers rather than water baths is recommended.

Monitoring

NO and nitrogen dioxide concentrations can be monitored in the inspiratory limb of the ventilator circuit with fuel cell analysers or by chemiluminescence. It is extremely rare to see toxic nitrogen dioxide concentrations (>5ppm). Methaemoglobin is formed when NO binds to haemoglobin. Prolonged inhalation at higher doses may rarely produce significant methaemoglobinaemia (>5%) so this should be monitored daily.

Achieving the correct dose

Approximately 50% of patients with severe respiratory failure show short-term improvement in PaO_2 with NO. However, the most effective dose varies. It is usual to start at 1ppm for 10min and monitor the change in PaO_2/FIO_2 ratio. An increase should be followed by an increase in nitric oxide concentration to 5ppm for a further 10min. Thereafter, the dose is adjusted according to response at 10min intervals until the most effective dose is found. It is important to assess the dose response at daily intervals, aiming to keep the dose at the lowest effective level.

Scavenging

Since the concentrations used are so small, dilution of exhaled gases into the atmosphere is unlikely to produce important environmental concentrations. In the air-conditioned intensive care environment, air changes are so frequent as to make scavenging unnecessary.

Key papers

Dellinger RP, Zimmerman JL, Taylor RW, et al, for the Inhaled Nitric Oxide in ARDS Study Group. (1998) Effects of inhaled nitric oxide in patients with acute respiratory distress syndrome: results of a randomised phase II trial. *Crit Care Med* **26**: 15–23.

Lundin S, Mang H, Smithies M, et al, for the The European Study Group of Inhaled Nitric Oxide. (1999) Inhalation of nitric oxide in acute lung injury: results of a European multicentre study. *Intensive Care Med* **25**: 911–9.

See also:

Acute respiratory distress syndrome (2), p362.

Surfactant

In ARDS, there is decreased surfactant production, biochemical abnormality of the surfactant produced, and inhibition of surfactant function. The net result is alveolar and small airway collapse. Surfactant also contributes to host defence against microorganisms. Surfactant replacement would be expected to exert therapeutic effects on lung mechanics, gas exchange, and host defence.

Instillation of surfactant (either as a liquid or nebulised) via the ET tube into the lungs is associated with improved outcome in neonatal respiratory distress syndrome. Potential indications in adults include ARDS, pneumonia, chronic airflow limitation, and asthma. Multiple studies in ARDS have yet to demonstrate mortality benefit though this may be related to the type of surfactant, the volume, or the delivery system used.

Studies have demonstrated improved oxygenation with recombinant surfactant protein C but no improvement in survival in patients with ARDS.

Complications of surfactant treatment have included increased cough, sputum production, bronchospasm, increased peak airway pressure, and adverse effects on pulmonary function. These can be minimised by adequate sedation and neuromuscular blockade before instilling surfactant.

Key paper

Spragg RG, Lewis JF, Walmrath HD. et al. (2004) Effect of Recombinant Surfactant Protein C–Based Surfactant on the Acute Respiratory Distress Syndrome. *N Engl J Med* **351**: 884–92.

See also:

Acute respiratory distress syndrome (2), p362.

Cardiovascular drugs

Inotropes

Types

- Catecholamines, e.g. epinephrine, norepinephrine, dobutamine, dopamine.
- Phosphodiesterase (PDE) inhibitors, e.g. milrinone, enoximone.
- Dopexamine.
- Calcium sensitisers, e.g. levosimendan.
- Cardiac glycosides, e.g. digoxin (weak).

Modes of action

- Increase force of myocardial contraction, either by stimulating cardiac β_1 adrenoreceptors (catecholamines), decreasing cAMP breakdown (PDE inhibitors), increasing calcium sensitivity (Ca sensitizers), directly increasing contractility (digoxin), or inhibiting neuronal reuptake of noradrenaline (dopexamine). All agents, except digoxin, have, to greater or lesser degrees, associated dilator or constrictor properties via α_1 and β_1 adrenoreceptors, dopaminergic receptors, or K_{ATP} channels.
- Digoxin may cause splanchnic vasoconstriction and, for an inotropic effect, usually requires higher plasma levels.
- The increase in cardiac work is partially offset in those drugs possessing associated dilator effects.
- Other than epinephrine (when used for its vasoconstrictor effect in cardiopulmonary resuscitation) or digoxin (for long-term use in chronic heart failure), inotropes are usually given by continuous IV infusion titrated for effect.

Uses

- Myocardial failure, e.g. post-myocardial infarction, cardiomyopathy.
- Myocardial depression, e.g. sepsis.
- Augmentation of oxygen delivery in high-risk surgical patients.

Side effects

- Arrhythmias (usually associated with concurrent hypovolaemia).
- Tachycardia (usually associated with concurrent hypovolaemia).
- Hypotension (related to dilator properties ± concurrent hypovolaemia).
- Hypertension (related to constrictor properties).
- Anginal chest pain, or ST segment and T wave changes on ECG.
- Catecholamines decrease metabolic efficiency, enhance β-oxidation of fat, and are prothrombotic. They are used to create models of myocardial ischaemia/necrosis. *In vitro,* they cause immune suppression and enhance bacterial growth.

Notes

- Epinephrine, norepinephrine, dobutamine, and dopamine should be given via a central vein as tissue necrosis may occur secondary to peripheral extravasation.

Drug dosages

Epinephrine	Infusion starting from 0.05mcg/kg/min
Norepinephrine	Infusion starting from 0.05mcg/kg/min
Dobutamine	Infusion from 2.5–25mcg/kg/min
Dopamine	Infusion from 2.5–30mcg/kg/min
Dopexamine	Infusion from 0.5–6mcg/kg/min
Milrinone	Loading dose of 50mcg/kg over 10min, followed by infusion from 0.375–0.75mcg/kg/min
Enoximone	Loading dose of 0.5–1mg/kg over 10min, followed by infusion from 5–20mcg/kg/min
Digoxin	0.5mg given PO or IV over 10–20min. Repeat at 4–8h intervals until loading achieved (assessed by clinical response). Maintenance dose thereafter is 0.0625–0.25mg/d, depending on plasma levels and clinical response.
Levosimendan	12–24mcg/kg over 10min (avoid if hypotensive), followed by 0.1mcg/kg/min for 24h

Haemodynamic effects

	BP	HR	Cardiac output	SVR
Epinephrine	+	+	+/++	+
Norepinephrine	++	–	–	++
Dobutamine	0/–	+	++	–
Dopamine	+/++	–	+	+/++
Dopexamine	0/–	+	++	–
Milrinone	–	+	++	–
Enoximone	–	+	++	–
Digoxin	0/–	–	+	+
Levosimendan	0/–	+	++	–

BP blood pressure; HR heart rate, SVR systemic vascular resistance.

See also:

Intra-aortic balloon counterpulsation, p102; Cardiac output—central thermodilution, p178; Cardiac output—peripheral thermodilution, p180; Cardiac output—indicator dilution, p182; Cardiac output—Doppler ultrasound, p184; Cardiac output—pulse contour analysis, p186; Cardiac output—other techniques, p188; Basic resuscitation, p358; Cardiac arrest, p340; Hypotension, p380; Tachyarrhythmias, p384; Acute coronary syndrome (1), p388; Acute coronary syndrome (2), p390; Heart failure—management, p394; Multiresistant infection, p562; Care of the potential organ/tissue donor, p656.

Vasodilators

Types
- Nitrates, e.g. glyceryl trinitrate, isosorbide dinitrate.
- Angiotensin-converting enzyme (ACE) inhibitors, e.g. captopril.
- Smooth muscle relaxants, e.g. sodium nitroprusside, hydralazine.
- α-adrenergic antagonists, e.g. phentolamine.
- β_2-adrenergic agonists, e.g. salbutamol.
- Calcium antagonists, e.g. nifedipine, diltiazem.
- Dopaminergic agonists, e.g. dopexamine.
- Phosphodiesterase inhibitors, e.g. enoximone, milrinone.
- Prostaglandins, e.g. epoprostenol (prostacyclin, PGI_2), alprostadil (PGE_1).
- Brain natriuretic peptide analogues, e.g. nesiritide.

Modes of action
- Increase cGMP concentration (by nitric oxide donation or by inhibiting cGMP breakdown) or acts directly on dopaminergic receptors leading to vasodilatation.
- Reduce (to varying degrees) ventricular preload and/or afterload.
- Reduce cardiac work.

Uses
- Myocardial failure, e.g. post-myocardial infarction, cardiomyopathy.
- Angina/ischaemic heart disease.
- Systemic hypertension (specific causes, e.g. phaeochromocytoma).
- Peripheral vascular disease/hypoperfusion.
- Splanchnic perfusion (dopexamine, dopamine).
- Pulmonary hypertension (inhaled NO or prostaglandins).

Side effects/complications
- Hypotension (often associated with concurrent hypovolaemia).
- Tachycardia (often associated with concurrent hypovolaemia).
- Symptoms include headache, flushing, postural hypotension.
- Renal failure (ACE inhibitors)—especially with renal artery stenosis, hypovolaemia, non-steroidals.

Notes
- Glyceryl trinitrate and isosorbide dinitrate reduce both preload and afterload. At higher doses, the afterload effect is more prominent.
- Tolerance to nitrates usually commences within 24–36h. unless intermittent oral dosing is used. Progressive increases in dose are required to achieve the same effect.
- Prolonged (>24–36h) dose-related administration of sodium nitroprusside can rarely produce a metabolic acidosis related to cyanide accumulation.
- ACE inhibitor tablets can be crushed and given either sub-lingually or by naso-gastric tube.
- Dopaminergic drugs improve splanchnic blood flow though clinical benefits are unproved.
- Hydralazine has an unpredictable effect on blood pressure and, if given IV, should be used with caution.

Drug dosages

Nitrates	Glyceryl trinitrate 2–40mg/h
	Isosorbide dinitrate 2–40mg/h
Sodium nitroprusside	20–400mcg/min
Hydralazine	5–10mg by slow IV bolus, repeat after 20–30min.
	Alternatively, give by infusion starting at 200–300mcg/min and reducing to 50–150mcg/min.
ACE inhibitors	Captopril: 6.25mg test dose increasing slowly to 50–100mg tds
	Enalapril: 2.5mg test dose increasing to 40mg od or 20mg bd
	Lisinopril: 2.5mg test dose increasing to 40mg od
Nifedipine	5–20mg PO. Capsule fluid can be injected down nasogastric tube or given sublingually
Phentolamine	2–5mg IV slow bolus. Repeat as necessary.
Dopexamine	Infusion from 0.5–6mcg/kg/min
Milrinone	Loading dose of 50mcg/kg over 10min, followed by infusion from 0.375–0.75mcg/kg/min
Enoximone	Loading dose of 0.5–1 mg/kg over 10 min followed by infusion from 5–20mcg/kg/min
Epoprostenol, alprostadil	Infusion from 2–30ng/kg/min
Nitric oxide	Inhalation: 2–40ppm
Nesiritide	2mcg/kg bolus, followed by infusion of 0.01–0.03mcg/kg/min

See also:

Blood pressure monitoring, p164; Cardiac output—central thermodilution, p178; Cardiac output—peripheral thermodilution, p180; Cardiac output—indicator dilution, p182; Cardiac output—Doppler ultrasound, p184; Cardiac output—pulse contour analysis, p186; Cardiac output—other techniques, p188; Anti-anginal agents, p276; Hypertension, p382; Acute coronary syndrome (1), p388; Acute coronary syndrome (2), p390; Heart failure—management, p394.

Vasopressors

Types

- α-adrenergic, e.g. norepinephrine, epinephrine, dopamine, ephedrine, phenylephrine, methoxamine.
- Drugs reducing production of cyclic GMP (in septic shock), e.g. methylthioninium chloride (methylene blue).
- Vasopressin or synthetic analogues, e.g. terlipressin.

Modes of action

- Acting on peripheral α-adrenergic or vasopressin V1 receptors.
- Blocking cGMP and NO production (methylene blue).

Arteriolar vasoconstriction and venoconstriction increases SVR and CVP.

Uses

- To increase organ perfusion pressures, particularly in high output, low peripheral resistance states, e.g. sepsis, anaphylaxis, to maintain adequate cerebral perfusion pressure or following neurological injury.
- To raise coronary perfusion pressures in cardiopulmonary resuscitation (epinephrine, vasopressin).

Side effects/complications

- Increased cardiac work.
- Decreased cardiac output.
- Myocardial and splanchnic ischaemia.
- Increased myocardial irritability, arrhythmias, and tachycardia, especially with concurrent hypovolaemia.
- Decreased peripheral perfusion and distal ischaemia/necrosis.

Notes

- Pressor agents should be avoided, if possible, in low cardiac output states as they may further compromise the circulation.
- Methoxamine and phenylephrine are the 'purest' pressor agents; other α-adrenergic agents have some inotropic properties. Ephedrine is similar to epinephrine, but its effects are more prolonged.
- Effects of pressor agents on splanchnic, renal, and cerebral circulations are variable and unpredictable.
- Pulmonary vascular resistance is also raised by these agents.
- Methylthioninium chloride (methylene blue) inhibits the NO-cGMP pathway. Its use has only been reported in a few small case series. A multicentre study of a NO synthase inhibitor (L-NMMA) was prematurely discontinued due to adverse outcomes.
- Vasopressin (short half-life, infusion needed) and terlipressin (longer half-life, can be given by bolus) may be effective in treating catecholamine-resistant vasodilatory shock. Paradoxically, such patients respond to small doses that have no pressor effect in healthy people.
- Large RCTs in septic shock show no outcome difference between types of catecholamine, but improved outcomes from low-dose vasopressin (over norepinephrine) in the less severe shock subgroup.
- Excessive dosing of any pressor agent may lead to regional ischaemia, e.g. cardiac, splanchnic. Digital ischaemia may respond to prompt administration of intravenous prostanoids (e.g. PGE_1, PGI_2).

Drug dosages

Norepinephine	Infusion starting from 0.05mcg/kg/min
Epinephrine	Infusion starting from 0.05mcg/kg/min
Dopamine	Infusion from 5–50mcg/kg/min
Methoxamine	3–10 mg by slow IV bolus (rate of 1mg/min)
Ephedrine	3–30mg by slow IV bolus
Methylthioninium chloride (methylene blue)	1–2mg/kg over 15–30min
Vasopressin	0.01–0.04U/min for sepsis
Terlipressin	0.25–0.5mg bolus, repeated at 30min intervals as necessary to maximum 2mg

Key papers

López A, Lorente JA, Steingrub J, et al. (2004) Multiple-centre, randomised, placebo-controlled, double-blind study of the nitric oxide synthase inhibitor 546C88: effect on survival in patients with septic shock. *Crit Care Med* **32**: 21–30.

Annane D, Vignon P, Renault A, et al. for the CATS Study Group. (2007) Norepinephrine plus dobutamine versus epinephrine alone for management of septic shock: a randomised trial. *Lancet* **370**: 676–84.

Russell JA, Walley KR, Singer J, et al for the VASST Investigators. (2008) Vasopressin versus nore-pinephrine infusion in patients with septic shock. *N Engl J Med* **358**: 877–87.

See also:

Blood pressure monitoring, p164; Cardiac output—central thermodilution, p178; Cardiac output—peripheral thermodilution, p180; Cardiac output—indicator dilution, p182; Cardiac output—Doppler ultrasound, p184; Cardiac output—pulse contour analysis, p186; Cardiac output—other techniques, p188; Tissue perfusion monitoring, p194; Intracranial pressure monitoring, p200; Jugular venous bulb saturation, p202; Other neurological monitoring, p206; Basic resuscitation, p338; Cardiac arrest, p340; Hypotension, p380; Sepsis and septic shock—treatment, p560; Anaphylactoid reactions, p578; Head injury (2), p588; Spinal cord injury, p590; Care of the potential organ/tissue donor, p656.

Hypotensive agents

Types

- Vasodilators.
- β-blockers.

β-blockers are being used more often in critical care practice for their beneficial effects in heart failure, and for arrhythmia and blood pressure control. Care needs to be taken with regard to their negative inotropic and chronotropic effects so, if in doubt, use small doses to begin with or shorter-acting agents such as esmolol or labetalol given by infusion. Despite their promise in reducing post-operative cardiovascular mortality and morbidity, a recent large trial assessing peri-operative metoprolol showed reduction in cardiovascular complications, but an increased incidence of stroke.

Modes of action

- Vasodilators reduce preload and afterload to variable degrees, depending on type and dose. In addition, nitrates, sodium nitroprusside (acts more on arterial vessels), and ACE inhibitors will often increase cardiac output in heart failure states.
- β-blockers reduce the force of myocardial contractility.
- α-blockers reduce vascular tone and can increase cardiac output.

Uses

- Hypertension—systemic and pulmonary.
- Heart failure—to reduce afterload ± preload (caution with β-blockers).
- Control of blood pressure, e.g. dissecting aortic aneurysm.

Side effects/complications

- Excessive hypotension.
- Heart failure (with β-blockers).
- Peripheral hypoperfusion (with β-blockers).
- Bronchospasm (with β-blockers).
- Decreased sympathetic response to hypoglycaemia (with β-blockers).
- Tachyphylaxis (with nitrates).
- Cyanide toxicity (with sodium nitroprusside).
- Unpredictable blood pressure lowering with nifedipine. Exercise caution when treating a hypertensive emergency.
- Exercise caution when using β-blockers and calcium channel blockers together.

Drug dosages

Nitrates	Glyceryl trinitrate 2–40mg/h
	Isosorbide dinitrate 2–40mg/h
Sodium nitroprusside	20–400mcg/min
ACE inhibitors	Ramipril: 1.25mg test dose rising to 10mg od
	Captopril: 6.25mg test dose rising to 25mg tds
	Enalapril: 2.5mg test dose rising to 40mg od
	Lisinopril: 2.5mg test dose rising to 40mg od
Nifedipine	5–10mg PO. Capsule fluid can be injected down nasogastric tube or given sublingually.
Phentolamine	2–5mg IV slow bolus. Repeat as necessary.
Esmolol	A titrated loading dose regimen is commenced followed by infusion (50–200mcg/kg/min).
Propranolol	Initially given as slow IV 1mg boluses, repeated at 2min intervals until effect is seen (to maximum 5mg).
Labetalol	0.25–2mg/min

Key paper

POISE Study Group. (2008) Effects of extended-release metoprolol succinate in patients undergoing non-cardiac surgery (POISE trial): a randomised controlled trial. *Lancet* **371**: 1839–47.

See also:

Blood pressure monitoring, p164; Vasodilators, p266; Hypertension, p382.

Anti-arrhythmics

Only anti-arrhythmics commonly used in the ICU setting are described.
For supraventricular tachyarrhythmias:

- Adenosine, verapamil, amiodarone, digoxin, β-blockers, magnesium.

For ventricular tachyarrhythmias:

- Amiodarone, lidocaine, flecainide, bretylium, β-blockers, magnesium.

Uses

- Correction of supraventricular and ventricular tachyarrhythmias which either compromise the circulation or could potentially do so.
- Differentiation between supraventricular and ventricular arrhythmias using adenosine.

Side effects/complications

- All anti-arrhythmic agents have side effects; they are negatively inotropic to greater or lesser degrees and may induce profound hypotension (e.g. verapamil, β-blockers) or bradycardia (e.g. β-blockers, amiodarone, digoxin, lidocaine). β blockers, in particular, should be used with caution because of these effects.
- All A–V blockers are contraindicated in re-entry tachycardia (e.g. Wolff–Parkinson–White syndrome).

Notes

- Adenosine: very short-acting; may revert paroxysmal SVT (other than atrial flutter and fibrillation) to sinus rhythm. Ineffective for VT. Contraindicated in 2° and 3° heart block, sick sinus syndrome, asthma. May cause flushing, bronchospasm, and occasional severe bradycardia, especially in patients taking dipyridamole.
- Amiodarone: effective against all types of tachyarrhythmia. Usually given by IV infusion but requires initial loading dose. When converting from IV to oral dosing, initial high oral dosing (200mg tds) is still required. Contraindicated in patients with thyroid dysfunction. Has low acute toxicity though may cause severe bradycardia and both chronic and acute pulmonary fibrosis. Avoid with other class III agents (e.g. sotalol). Must be given via central vein as causes peripheral phlebitis. Can also cause pulmonary fibrosis and abnormal thyroid function.
- β-blockers: for SVT. Caution when using β-blockers with verapamil.
- Bretylium: may take 15–20min to take effect; now used predominantly for resistant VF/VT. CPR should be continued for at least 20min.
- Digoxin: slow-acting, requires loading (1–1.5mg) to achieve therapeutic plasma levels over 12–24h (can be done over 4–6h). Contraindicated in 2° and 3° heart block. May cause severe bradycardia. Low K^+ and Mg^{2+}, and markedly raised Ca^{2+} increase myocardial sensitivity to digoxin. Amiodarone raises digoxin levels.
- Lidocaine: 10mL of 1% solution contains 100mg. No effect on SVT. Contraindicated in 2° and 3° heart block. May cause bradycardia and CNS side effects, e.g. drowsiness, seizures.
- Verapamil: should generally not be given with β-blockers as profound hypotension and bradyarrhythmias may result. Pre-treatment with 3–5mL 10% calcium gluconate by slow IV bolus prevents the hypotensive effects of verapamil without affecting its anti-arrhythmic properties.

Modes of action (Vaughan–Williams classification)

Class	Action	Examples
I	Reduces rate of rise of action potential: Ia: Increases action potential duration Ib: Shortens duration Ic: Little effect	Ia: disopyramide Ib: lidocaine Ic: flecainide
II	Reduces rate of pacemaker discharge	β-blockers
III	Prolongs duration of action potential and hence length of refractory period	Amiodarone Sotalol
IV	Antagonises transport of calcium across cell membrane	Verapamil Diltiazem

Drug dosages

Adenosine	6mg rapid IV bolus. If no response after 1min, give 12mg. If no response after 1min, repeat 12mg.
Amiodarone	5mg/kg over 20min (or 150–300mg over 3min in emergency), then IV infusion of 15mg/kg/24h in 5% glucose via central vein. Reduce thereafter to 10mg/kg/24h (approx. 600mg/d) for 3–7d, then maintain at 5mg/kg/24h (300–400mg/d).
β-blockers	Esmolol: A titrated loading dose regimen is commenced followed by an infusion rate of 50–200mcg/kg/min. Propranolol: Initially given as slow IV boluses of 1mg, repeated at 2min intervals to a maximum of 5mg. Labetalol: 0.25–2mg/min Sotalol: Dosage range is 20–120mg IV (0.5–1.5mg/kg) administered over 10min. Repeat 6-hourly, if necessary. Metoprolol: 2.5–5 mg injected IV at rate of 1–2mg/min, repeated at 5min intervals until satisfactory response is seen or total dose of 10–15mg given. Atenolol: 2.5mg IV over 2.5min, repeated at 5min intervals until response is seen or maximum of 10mg
Bretylium	In emergency, 5mg/kg by rapid IV bolus. If no response after 5min, repeat or increase to 10mg/kg.
Digoxin	0.5mg given IV over 10–20min. Repeat at 4–8h intervals until loading achieved (assessed by clinical response). Maintenance dose thereafter is 0.0625–0.25mg/d, depending on plasma levels and clinical response.
Lidocaine	1mg/kg slow IV bolus for loading, then 2–4mg/min infusion. Should be weaned slowly over 24h.
$MgSO_4$	10–20mmol over 1–2h (over 5min in emergency).
Verapamil	2.5mg slow IV. If no response, repeat to a maximum of 20mg. An IV infusion of 1–10mg/h may be tried. 10% calcium gluconate solution should be readily available.

See also:

Electrical cardioversion, p94; ECG monitoring, p162; Cardiac arrest, p340; Tachyarrhythmias, p384.

Chronotropes

Types

- Anticholinergic, e.g. atropine, glycopyrronium bromide.

Modes of action

- The anticholinergic drugs act by competitive antagonism of acetylcholine at peripheral muscarinic receptors and decreases atrioventricular conduction time.

Uses

- All types of bradycardia including 3° heart block.
- High dose atropine is used in cardiopulmonary resuscitation protocols for treatment of asystole.

Side effects/complications

- Anticholinergic drugs produce dry mouth, reduction and thickening of bronchial secretions, and inhibition of sweating. Urinary retention may occur, but parenteral administration does not lead to glaucoma.

Notes

- The anticholinergic agents are usually given by IV bolus, repeated as necessary.
- They are frequently used as a bridge to temporary pacing, but should not be considered a substitute. External or internal pacing should be readily accessible.
- Atropine nebulisers have been used successfully in patients developing symptomatic bradycardia during endotracheal suction.
- Neurological effects may be seen with atropine but not glycopyrronium bromide.

Drug dosages

Atropine	0.3–0.6mg IV bolus. 3mg is needed for complete vagal blockade or cardiopulmonary resuscitation.
Glycopyrronium bromide	0.2–0.4mg IV bolus

See also:
Temporary pacing (1), p96; Temporary pacing (2), p98; ECG monitoring, p162; Cardiac arrest, p340; Bradyarrhythmias, p386.

Anti-anginal agents

Types
- Vasodilators, e.g. nitrates, calcium antagonists.
- β-blockers.
- Potassium channel openers, e.g. nicorandil.
- Antiplatelet/anticoagulant agents: aspirin, heparin, clopidogrel.

Modes of action
- Calcium channel blockers cause competitive blockade of cell membrane, slow calcium channels leading to decreased influx of calcium ions into cells. This leads to inhibition of contraction and relaxation of cardiac and smooth muscle fibres, resulting in coronary and systemic vasodilatation.
- Nitrates may cause efflux of calcium ions from smooth muscle and cardiac cells, and also increases cGMP synthesis resulting in coronary and systemic vasodilatation.
- β-blockers inhibit β-adrenoreceptor stimulation, reducing myocardial work and oxygen consumption. This effect is somewhat offset by compensatory peripheral vasoconstriction.
- Potassium channel openers vasodilate by relaxation of vascular smooth muscle. The potassium channel opening action works on the arterial circulation while a nitrate-type action provides some venodilatation.
- Though aspirin, heparin, and clopidogrel have no direct anti-anginal effect, patients with unstable angina benefit from the reduction in platelet aggregation and thrombus formation.

Uses
- Angina pectoris.

Side effects/complications
- See Dilators, Hypotensive agents.
- Nicorandil is contraindicated in hypotension and cardiogenic shock. It should be avoided in hypovolaemia. Headache and flushing are the major reported side effects. Rapid and severe hyperkalaemia has been reported after cardiac surgery.

Notes
- Combination therapy involving nitrates, β-blockade, aspirin, clopidogrel ± heparin ± calcium antagonists ± glycoprotein IIb/IIIa antagonists are used in acute coronary syndromes; thrombolytic therapy confers no added advantage. Local guidelines should be consulted.
- Potassium channel openers belong to a new class of drug yet to be extensively evaluated in critically ill patients and should be thus used with caution, especially when hyperkalaemia is a concern.
- Angina may occasionally be worsened by a 'coronary steal' phenomenon where blood flow is diverted away from stenosed coronary vessels. This does not occur with nicorandil.

Drug dosages

Glyceryl trinitrate	0.3mg sublingually, 0.4–0.8mg by buccal spray, 2–40mg/h by IV infusion
Isosorbide dinitrate	10–20mg tds orally, 2–40mg/h by IV infusion
Nifedipine	5–20mg PO. The capsule fluid can be aspirated then injected down nasogastric tube or given sublingually.
Propranolol	Given either orally at doses of 10–100mg tds or IV as slow boluses of 1mg, repeated at 2min intervals to a maximum of 5mg until effect is seen. This can be repeated 2–4 hourly as necessary.
Nicorandil	10–20mg PO bd
Clopidogrel	300mg PO loading dose, then 75mg PO od
Aspirin	75–150mg PO od

See also:

Coronary revascularisation techniques, p104; Echocardiography, p192; Vasodilators, p266; Acute coronary syndrome (2), p390.

Renal drugs

Diuretics

Types

- Loop diuretics, e.g. furosemide, bumetanide.
- Osmotic diuretics, e.g. mannitol.
- Thiazides, e.g. metolazone.
- Potassium-sparing diuretics, e.g. amiloride, spironolactone, potassium canrenoate.

Uses

- To increase urine volume.
- Control of chronic oedema (thiazides, loop diuretics).
- Control of hypertension (thiazides).
- To promote renal excretion (e.g. forced diuresis, hypercalcaemia).

Routes

- IV (mannitol, furosemide, bumetanide, potassium canrenoate).
- PO (metolazone, furosemide, bumetanide, amiloride, spironolactone).

Modes of action

- Osmotic diuretics—reduce distal tubular water reabsorption.
- Thiazides—inhibit distal tubular Na^+ loss and carbonic anhydrase, and increase Na^+ and K^+ exchange. This reduces the supply of H^+ ions for exchange with Na^+ ions, producing an alkaline natriuresis with potassium loss.
- Loop diuretics—inhibit Na^+ and Cl^- reabsorption in the ascending loop of Henlé.
- Potassium-sparing diuretics—inhibit distal tubular Na^+ and K^+ exchange.

Side effects

- Hypovolaemia.
- Hyponatraemia or hypernatraemia.
- Hypokalaemia.
- Hyperkalaemia with potassium-sparing diuretics.
- Oedema formation (mannitol).
- Reduced catecholamine effect (thiazides).
- Hyperglycaemia (thiazides).
- Metabolic alkalosis (loop diuretics).
- Hypomagnesaemia (loop diuretics).
- Pancreatitis (furosemide).

Notes

- It is important to correct pre-renal causes of oliguria before resorting to diuretic use.
- Diuretics do not prevent renal failure, but may convert oliguric to polyuric renal failure.
- If there is inadequate glomerular filtration, mannitol is retained and passes to the extracellular fluid to promote oedema formation.
- Potassium-sparing diuretics should be avoided with ACE inhibitors as there is an increased risk of hyperkalaemia.

Drug dosages

	Oral	IV	Infusion
Mannitol		100g over 20min 6-hourly	
Metolazone	5–10mg od		
Furosemide	20–40mg 6–24 hourly	5–80mg 6–24 hourly	1–10mg/h
Bumetanide	0.5–1mg 6-24 hourly	0.5–2mg 6–24 hourly	1–5mg/h
Amiloride	5–10mg 12–24 hourly		
Spironolactone	100–400mg od		
K$^+$ canrenoate		200–400mg od	

See also:

Electrolytes (Na$^+$, K$^+$, Cl$^-$, HCO$_3^-$), p212; Fluid challenge, p342; Hypertension, p382; Oliguria, p398; Pancreatitis, p424; Hyponatraemia, p484; Hypokalaemia, p488; Metabolic alkalosis, p504.

Dopamine

The effects of dopamine are dependent on the dose infused. Dopamine was used widely at low doses in an attempt to secure preferential DA_1 stimulation and increase renal perfusion. However, a large, multicentre, randomised, controlled study comparing 'renal dose' dopamine and diuretics showed no difference in the incidence of renal failure. The previous widespread use of low dose dopamine (<3mcg/kg/min) has thus diminished considerably. Higher doses increase cardiac contractility via β_1 stimulation and produce vasoconstriction via α stimulation. Where vasoconstriction is inappropriate, this will reduce renal perfusion. However, there is evidence of natriuresis and diuresis by enhanced Na^+ transport in the ascending loop of Henlé. This effect is similar to that of a loop diuretic. In addition to the renal effects of DA_1 stimulation, there may be preferential perfusion of the splanchnic bed though any benefits to patients have yet to be shown.

Key paper

Bellomo R for the Australian and New Zealand Intensive Care Society (ANZICS) Clinical Trials Group. (2000) Low-dose dopamine in patients with early renal dysfunction: a placebo-controlled randomised trial. *Lancet* **356**: 2139–43.

Gastrointestinal drugs

H₂ blockers and proton pump inhibitors

Types
- H₂-antagonists, e.g. ranitidine, cimetidine.
- Proton pump inhibitors, e.g. omeprazole, pantoprazole.

Modes of action

These agents inhibit secretion of gastric acid, reducing both volume and acid content, either by antagonism of the histamine H_2 receptor or by inhibiting H^+K^+-ATPase which fuels the parietal cell proton pump on which acid secretion depends.

Uses
- Peptic ulceration, gastritis, duodenitis.
- Reflux oesophagitis.
- Prophylaxis against stress ulceration.
- Upper gastrointestinal haemorrhage of peptic/stress ulcer origin.
- With non-steroidal anti-inflammatory agents in patients with dyspepsia.

Side effects/complications
- The major concern voiced against these agents is the increased risk of nosocomial pneumonia by removal of the acid barrier. However, a multicentre randomised controlled trial (RCT) comparing ranitidine with sucralfate showed no difference in pneumonia rate and a lower incidence of GI bleeding.
- H₂-antagonists: rare but include arrhythmias, altered liver function tests, confusion (in the elderly).
- Proton pump inhibitors: altered liver function tests.

Notes
- Although licensed and frequently used for stress ulcer prophylaxis, overwhelming supportive evidence is scanty. Enteral nutrition has been shown to be as effective. No adequately powered study of proton pump inhibitors has yet been performed in ICU patients.
- Some studies have shown efficacy in upper gastrointestinal haemorrhage secondary to stress ulceration or peptic ulceration.
- Dosages should be modified in renal failure.
- Cimetidine can affect metabolism of other drugs, in particular, warfarin, phenytoin, theophylline, and lidocaine (related to hepatic cytochrome P450-linked enzyme systems). This does not occur with ranitidine.
- Omeprazole can delay elimination of diazepam, phenytoin, and warfarin.

Drug dosages

Ranitidine	50mg tds by slow IV bolus, 150mg bd PO
Cimetidine	200–400mg qds by slow IV bolus, 400mg bd PO
Omeprazole	40mg od IV(over 20–30min) or 20–40mg od PO
Pantoprazole	40mg od PO or slow IV

Key paper

Cook D, Guyatt G, Marshall J, et al. (1998) A comparison of sucralfate and ranitidine for the prevention of upper gastrointestinal bleeding in patients requiring mechanical ventilation. Canadian Critical Care Trials Group. *N Engl J Med* **338**: 791–7.

See also:

Upper gastrointestinal haemorrhage, p412.

Sucralfate

Modes of action

- Sucralfate is a basic aluminium salt of sucrose octasulphate and is probably not absorbed from the gastrointestinal tract.
- Exerts a cytoprotective effect by preventing mucosal injury. A protective barrier is formed both over normal mucosa and any ulcer lesion providing protection against penetration of gastric acid, bile, and pepsin as well as irritants such as aspirin and alcohol.
- Directly inhibits pepsin activity and absorbs bile salts.
- Weak antacid activity.

Uses

- Peptic ulceration, gastritis, duodenitis.
- Reflux oesophagitis.
- Prophylaxis against stress ulceration.

Side effects/complications

- Constipation.
- Reduced bioavailability of some drugs given orally, e.g. digoxin, phenytoin. Can be overcome by giving agents at least 2h apart.
- Use with caution in renal failure due to risk of increased aluminium absorption.

Notes

- Although licensed and frequently used for stress ulcer prophylaxis, overwhelming supportive evidence is scanty. Enteral nutrition and gastric acid blockers have been shown to be as effective.
- Evidence for a reduced incidence of nosocomial pneumonia compared to H_2 blocker therapy is also conflicting. Significant reduction in nosocomial pneumonia has been shown compared to a combination of H_2 blocker plus antacid, but not against H_2 blocker alone. Indeed, a large multicentre RCT comparing ranitidine with sucralfate showed no difference in pneumonia rate and a lower incidence of GI bleeding with ranitidine.
- Antacids should not be given for 30min before and after sucralfate.

Drug dosage

Sucralfate	1g six times a day PO or via NG tube.

Key paper

Cook D, Guyatt G, Marshall J, et al. (1998) A comparison of sucralfate and ranitidine for the prevention of upper gastrointestinal bleeding in patients requiring mechanical ventilation. Canadian Critical Care Trials Group. *N Engl J Med* **338**: 791–7.

See also:

Upper gastrointestinal haemorrhage, p412

Antacids

Types
- Sodium bicarbonate.
- Magnesium-based antacids, e.g. magnesium trisilicate.
- Aluminium-based antacids, e.g. aluminium hydroxide.
- Proprietary combinations, e.g. Gaviscon®.

Modes of action
- Neutralises gastric acid.
- Provides protective coating on upper gastrointestinal mucosa.

Uses
- Symptomatic relief of gastritis, duodenitis, oesophagitis.
- Stress ulcer prophylaxis (contentious).

Side effects/complications
- Possible increased risk of nosocomial pneumonia.
- Aluminium toxicity (if aluminium-containing antacids are used long-term in patients with renal dysfunction).
- Diarrhoea (magnesium-based antacids).
- Constipation (aluminium-based antacids).
- Metabolic alkalosis if large amounts are administered.
- Milk-alkali syndrome resulting in hypercalcaemia, metabolic alkalosis, and renal failure is very rare.

Notes
- As their main use is for symptomatic relief, antacids are rarely needed in mechanically ventilated patients.
- Continual nasogastric infusion of a weak sodium bicarbonate solution has been used successfully in treating stress ulcer-related haemorrhage.

Drug dosages

Magnesium trisilicate	10–20mL qds
Aluminium hydroxide	10–20mL qds
Gaviscon®	10–20mL qds

See also:
Upper gastrointestinal haemorrhage, p412.

Anti-emetics

Types
- Phenothiazines, e.g. prochlorperazine, chlorpromazine.
- Dopamine receptor blocker, e.g. metoclopramide, domperidone.
- Anti-histamines, e.g. cyclizine.
- $5HT_3$ receptor antagonists, e.g. ondansetron, granisetron.

Modes of action
- Phenothiazines increase the threshold for vomiting at the chemo-receptor trigger zone via central DA_2 dopaminergic blockade; at higher doses, there may also be some effect on the vomiting centre.
- Metoclopramide acts centrally and by increasing gastric motility.
- Cyclizine increases lower oesophageal sphincter tone and may inhibit the midbrain emetic centre.
- Ondansetron is a highly selective $5HT_3$ receptor antagonist; its precise mode of action is unknown, but may act both centrally and peripherally.

Uses
- Nausea.
- Vomiting.

Side effects/complications
- Dystonic or dyskinetic reactions, oculogyric crises (prochlorperazine, metoclopramide).
- Arrhythmias (metoclopramide, prochlorperazine).
- Headaches, flushing (ondansetron).
- Urticaria, drowsiness, dry mouth, blurred vision, urinary retention (cyclizine).
- Postural hypotension (prochlorperazine, cyclizine).
- Rarely neuroleptic malignant syndrome (prochlorperazine, metoclopramide).

Notes
- The initial choice should fall between prochlorperazine, metoclopramide, or cyclizine. Prochlorperazine and cyclizine are preferable when vomiting is related to drugs and metabolic disturbances acting at the chemoreceptor trigger zone while metoclopramide or domperidone should be tried first if a gastrointestinal cause is implicated.
- Metoclopramide and prochlorperazine dosage should be reduced in renal and hepatic failure.
- Ondansetron dosage should be reduced in hepatic failure.

Drug dosages

Prochlorperazine	5–10mg tds PO, 12.5mg qds IM or by slow IV bolus (note: not licensed for IV use)
Metoclopramide	10mg tds by slow IV bolus, IM, or PO
Cyclizine	50mg tds slow IV bolus, IM, or PO
Ondansetron	4–8mg tds by slow IV bolus, IM, or PO
Granisetron	1–3mg by slow IV bolus up to max 9mg/24h

See also:

Enteral nutrition, p128; Vomiting/gastric stasis, p406.

Gut motility agents

Types
- Metoclopramide.
- Domperidone.
- Erythromycin.

Modes of action
- Metoclopramide and domperidone probably act by blocking peripheral DA$_2$ dopaminergic receptors.
- Erythromycin is a motilin agonist acting on antral enteric neurons.

Uses
- Ileus, large nasogastric aspirates.
- Vomiting.

Side effects/complications
- Dystonic or dyskinetic reactions, oculogyric crises (metoclopramide).
- Arrhythmias (metoclopramide and erythromycin).
- Cholestatic jaundice (erythromycin).

Notes
- Metoclopramide dosing should be reduced in renal failure and hepatic failure, while erythromycin dosing should be reduced in hepatic failure.

Drug dosages

Metoclopramide	10mg tds by slow IV bolus, IM, or PO
Erythromycin	250mg qds PO or IV

See also:
Enteral nutrition, p128; Vomiting/gastric stasis, p406.

Anti-diarrhoeals

Types
- Loperamide.
- Codeine phosphate.

Modes of action
Loperamide and codeine phosphate bind to gut wall opiate receptors, reducing propulsive peristalsis and increasing anal sphincter tone.

Side effects/complications
- Abdominal cramps, bloating.
- Constipation (if excessive amounts given).

Notes
- Should not be used when abdominal distension develops, particularly with ulcerative colitis or pseudomembranous colitis.
- Avoid in infective diarrhoea as may prolong illness.
- Caution with loperamide in liver failure and codeine in renal failure.

Drug dosages

Loperamide	2 capsules (20mL) initially, then 1 capsule (10mL) after every loose stool for up to 5 days
Codeine phosphate	30–60mg 4–6 hourly PO, IM, or by slow IV bolus

See also:
Enteral nutrition, p128; Diarrhoea, p406.

Anti-constipation agents

Types
- Laxatives, e.g. lactulose, propantheline, mebeverine.
- Bulking agents, e.g. dietary fibre (bran), hemicelluloses (methylcellulose, ispaghula husk).
- Suppositories, e.g. glycerin.
- Enemata, e.g. warmed normal saline, olive oil, or arachis oil retention enemata.

Modes of action
- Laxatives include:
  - Anti-spasmodic agents such as anticholinergics (e.g. propantheline) and mebeverine (a phenylethylamine derivative of reserpine).
  - Non-absorbable disaccharides (e.g. lactulose) which soften the stool by an osmotic effect and by lactic acid production from a bacterial fermenting effect.
  - Irritants, such as castor oil, which is hydrolysed in the small intestine, releasing ricinoleic acid.
- Bulking agents are hydrophilic and thus increase water content of the stool.

Side effects/complications
- Bloating and abdominal distension.
- Diarrhoea if excessive amounts given.

Notes
- Surgical causes presenting as constipation such as bowel obstruction must be excluded. Other measures should be taken if possible to improve bowel function e.g. reducing concurrent opiate dosage, starting enteral nutrition.
- The agent of choice is lactulose.
- Larger doses of lactulose are used in hepatic failure as the pH of the colonic contents is reduced; this lowers formation and absorption of ammonium ions and other nitrogenous products into the portal circulation. Benefit in patients has not been shown.
- Anthraquinone glycosides (e.g. senna) and liquid paraffin are no longer recommended for routine use.

Drug dosage

Lactulose	15–50mL tds PO

See also:
Failure to open bowels, p410.

Neurological drugs

Non-opioid analgesics

Types

- Paracetamol.
- Non-steroidal anti-inflammatory drugs (NSAIDs): e.g. aspirin, ibuprofen, indometacin, diclofenac, ketorolac, sulindac.
- Ketamine.
- Nitrous oxide.
- Local anaesthetics, e.g. lidocaine, bupivacaine.
- α_2 agonists—clonidine, dexmedetomidine (see under sedatives).

Uses

- Pain associated with inflammatory conditions (aspirin, NSAIDs).
- Post-operative pain and musculoskeletal pain (aspirin, NSAIDs, paracetamol, ketamine, nitrous oxide, lidocaine, bupivicaine).
- Opiate-sparing effect (aspirin, paracetamol, NSAIDs).
- Antipyretic (aspirin, paracetamol, NSAIDs).

Routes

- IV (paracetamol, ketamine).
- IM (diclofenac, ketamine).
- PO (aspirin, NSAIDs, paracetamol).
- PR (aspirin, diclofenac, paracetamol).
- Local/regional (lidocaine, bupivacaine).
- Inhaled (nitrous oxide).

Side effects

- Gastrointestinal bleeding (aspirin, indometacin, diclofenac).
- Renal dysfunction (indometacin, diclofenac if any hypovolaemia).
- Reduced platelet aggregation (aspirin, indometacin, diclofenac).
- Reduced prothrombin formation (aspirin, indometacin, diclofenac).
- Myocardial depression (lidocaine, bupivacaine).
- Hypertension and tachycardia (ketamine).
- Seizures (lidocaine, bupivacaine).
- Hallucinations and psychotic tendencies (ketamine—prevented by concurrent use of benzodiazepines or droperidol).

Notes

- The WHO analgesia ladder concept requires mild to moderate pain to be managed with simple analgesics, progressing to opioids if pain relief is not adequate.
- Non-steroidal anti-inflammatory agents should be generally avoided in patients with renal dysfunction, GI bleeding, or coagulopathy.
- In sub-anaesthetic doses, ketamine is a powerful analgesic. It is associated with good airway maintenance, allows spontaneous respiration, and provides cardiovascular stimulation. It is also a bronchodilator.
- Nitrous oxide is a powerful, short-acting analgesic used with 50% oxygen (Entonox) to cover short, painful procedures. Do not use in cases of undrained pneumothorax since it may diffuse into the pneumothorax, resulting in tension.
- Cox-2 inhibitors are not currently recommended by the authors due to emerging evidence of cardiovascular side effects.
- Clonidine and dexmedetomidine have intrinsic analgesic properties.

Drug dosages

Aspirin	600mg PO/PR 4-hourly
Ibuprofen	400mg PO 4–8 hourly
Indometacin	50–100mg PO/PR 12-hourly
Diclofenac	25–50mg PO 8-hourly, 100mg PR 12–24 hourly, 75mg IM 12-hourly
Ketorolac	10mg PO 4–6 hourly, 10–30mg IV/IM 4–6 hourly
Sulindac	200mg PO 12-hourly
Paracetamol	0.5–1g PO/PR/IV 4–6 hourly
Ketamine	5–25mcg/kg/min IV or 0.5–1.0mg/kg IM
Clonidine	100–150mcg/min
Dexmedetomidine	1mcg/kg over 10min, followed by a maintenance infusion of 0.2 to 0.7mcg/kg/h
Lidocaine	Maximum 200mg
Bupivacaine	Maximum 150mg*

*Local anaesthetic doses vary according to area to be anaesthetised. Maximum doses may be increased if epinephrine is used locally.

See also:

Opioid analgesics, p304; Rheumatic disorders, p572; Pyrexia—management, p604; Pain, p618; Post-operative critical care, p620; Pain and comfort, p624.

Opioid analgesics

Types

- Natural opiates, e.g. morphine, codeine.
- Semi-synthetic, e.g. diamorphine, dihydrocodeine.
- Synthetic, e.g. pethidine, fentanyl, alfentanil, remifentanil, tramadol.

Uses

- Analgesia: Strong analgesics are extracts from opium or synthetic substances with similar properties. They are more useful for continuous pain rather than sharp, intermittent pain.
- Sedation.
- Anxiolysis in heart failure (diamorphine, morphine).
- Anti-diarrhoeal (codeine).

Routes

- IV (morphine, diamorphine, papaveretum, pethidine, fentanyl, alfentanil, remifentanil, tramadol).
- IM/SC (morphine, codeine, diamorphine, dihydrocodeine, pethidine, tramadol).
- PO (morphine, codeine, diamorphine, dihydrocodeine, pethidine, tramadol).
- Percutaneous (fentanyl).

Side effects

- Respiratory depression.
- Central nervous system depression.
- Stimulation of the vomiting centre.
- Decreased gastric emptying and gut motility, constipation.
- Histamine release and itching.
- Dry mouth.
- Increased muscular tone.
- Appetite loss.
- Withdrawal syndrome (withdraw slowly).
- Addiction (rare in the critically ill).

Notes

- Mild to moderate pain requiring opioids is usually treated with less potent drugs such as codeine, dihydrocodeine, or tramadol.
- Morphine is poorly absorbed from the gastrointestinal tract, and therefore, is usually administered parenterally. It is metabolised to morphine-6-glucuronide in the liver which is six times more potent than morphine and accumulates in renal failure.
- Pethidine has local anaesthetic properties associated with cardiac depression and vasodilatation. It is metabolised to norpethidine which may lead to seizures on accumulation. Respiratory depression occurs despite maintenance of respiratory rate.
- Fentanyl and alfentanil are good, short-acting analgesics with poor sedative quality. However, long-term infusion leads to accumulation. They cause severe respiratory depression and muscular rigidity.
- Remifentanil is ultra short-acting, and the patient may suffer from rebound pain if the infusion is stopped temporarily.

Drug dosages
Intravenous

	Bolus	Infusion
Morphine	0.1–0.2mg/kg	0.05–0.07mg/kg/h
Diamorphine	0.05–0.1mg/kg	0.03–0.06mg/kg/h
Pethidine	0.5mg/kg	0.1–0.3mg/kg/h
Fentanyl	5–7.5mcg/kg	5–20mcg/kg/h
Alfentanil	15–30mcg/kg	20–120mcg/kg/h
Remifentanil	1mcg/kg	0.05–2mcg/kg/min
Tramadol	50–100mg 4–6 hourly	

Other routes

Morphine	10mg IM/SC 4-hourly	5–20mg PO 4-hourly
Codeine	30–60mg IM 4-hourly	30–60mg PO 4-hourly
Diamorphine	5mg IM/SC 4-hourly	5–10mg PO 4-hourly
Dihydrocodeine	50mg IM/SC 4–6 hourly	30mg PO 4–6 hourly
Pethidine	25–100mg IM/SC 4-hourly	50–150mg PO 4-hourly
Tramadol	50–100mg IM 4–6 hourly	50–100mg PO 4–6 hourly
Fentanyl	12–100mcg/h percutaneous	

Note the above doses are a guide only and may need to be altered widely according to individual circumstances. The correct dose of an opiate analgesic is generally enough to ablate pain.

See also:
Non-opioid analgesics, p302; Pain, p618; Post-operative critical care, p620; Pain and comfort, p624.

Epidural analgesia

Types
- Opioid analgesics (morphine, diamorphine, fentanyl, alfentanil).
- Local anaesthetics (bupivacaine).
- Adjuvants (clonidine).

Uses
- Post-operative analgesia.
- Regional anaesthesia.

Side effects
- As lower doses of opioids are required to achieve effective analgesia, there is a lower incidence of opioid-related side effects.
- Hypotension (local anaesthetics, clonidine).
- Bradycardia (local anaesthetic with a high block above T4).
- Central nervous system and respiratory depression (opioids).
- Stimulation of the vomiting centre (opioids).
- Appetite loss (opioids).
- Dry mouth (opioids).
- Decreased gastric emptying and gut motility (opioids).
- Histamine release and itching (opioids).
- Increased muscular tone (opioids).
- Motor blockade (local anaesthetics).
- Urinary retention (opioids, local anaesthetics).
- Headache (dural puncture).
- Abscess or haematoma (catheter-related).
- Total spinal block (profound hypotension, apnoea, unconsciousness and dilated pupils due to inadvertent spinal injection of epidural dose).

Notes
- The epidural catheter should typically be placed in the mid-dermatome range of the site of the pain.
- Fentanyl is more lipid-soluble than non-synthetic opioids so gains faster access to opioid receptors.
- Low bupivacaine concentrations are less likely to block larger diameter motor fibres allowing the patient to mobilise.
- It is usual to infuse combinations of drugs in lower doses to maximise the analgesic effect while minimising side effects.
- Higher volume infusions block a greater range of nerve routes. A bolus of 1–2mL of local anaesthetic will typically block one dermatome. Age reduces the volume required.
- Inadequate block may respond to a bolus dose or increasing the infusion rate.
- Clonidine may enhance analgesia provided by epidural opioids and local anaesthetics.
- Coagulation should be checked before removing an epidural catheter to avoid haematoma. At least 12 hours should be left after the last dose of low molecular weight heparin.

Drug dosages

	Concentration	Dose
Fentanyl	2–4mcg/mL	0–40mcg/h
Morphine	50mcg/mL	0–0.5mg/h
Diamorphine	20mcg/mL	0–0.2mg/h
Bupivacaine	0.1–0.125%	12.5mg/h
Clonidine	2mcg/mL	15–20mcg/h

See also:
Non-opioid analgesics, p302; Opioid analgesics, p304; Respiratory failure, p350; Hypotension, p380;
Bradyarrhythmias, p386.

Sedatives and tranquilisers

Types

- Benzodiazepines, e.g. diazepam, midazolam, lorazepam.
- Major tranquillisers, e.g. chlorpromazine, haloperidol.
- Anaesthetic agents, e.g. propofol, isoflurane.
- α_2 agonists, e.g. clonidine, dexmedetomidine.

Uses

- Sedation and anxiolysis.

Routes

- IV (benzodiazepines, haloperidol, propofol, clonidine, dexmedetomidine).
- IM (benzodiazepines, chlorpromazine, haloperidol).
- PO (diazepam, lorazepam, chlorpromazine, haloperidol, clonidine).
- Inhaled (isoflurane).

Side effects

- Hypotension (benzodiazepines, chlorpromazine, haloperidol, propofol, clonidine, dexmedetomidine).
- Respiratory depression (benzodiazepines, chlorpromazine, haloperidol, propofol).
- Arrhythmias (chlorpromazine, haloperidol).
- Dry mouth (clonidine, dexmedetomidine).
- Extrapyramidal disorder (chlorpromazine, haloperidol).
- Fluoride toxicity (isoflurane).
- Rebound agitation on drug withdrawal (benzodiazepines).

Notes

- Sedative drugs have cardiovascular and respiratory side effects. Objective assessment of the depth of sedation is necessary to ensure comfort does not give way to excessive sedation.
- All sedatives are cumulative so doses must be kept to a minimum. Stopping sedation daily has been shown to reduce critical care stay.
- Benzodiazepines have an advantage of being amnesic.
- Midazolam is slowly metabolised in 10% of patients.
- All benzodiazepines accumulate in renal failure; care must be taken to avoid excessive dosage by regular reassessment of need.
- Propofol in sub-anaesthetic doses is short-acting, but effects are cumulative with prolonged infusion or with coexisting hepatic/renal failure.
- Large dose propofol may contribute significantly to calorie intake via the fat emulsion.
- As chlorpromazine and haloperidol antagonise catecholamines, they may cause vasodilatation and hypotension. Dystonic reactions and arrhythmias (e.g. torsade de pointes) are also occasionally seen.
- α_2 antagonists offer both analgesia and sedation, and are synergistic with opiates.
- Dexmedetomidine causes minimal respiratory depression and the patient is easily rousable. Bradycardia and hypotension may occur, especially with the loading dose.
- Isoflurane is short-acting although cumulative effects have been recorded with prolonged use that also carries the theoretical risk of fluoride toxicity. Exhaled isoflurane should be adequately scavenged.

Drug dosages

	Bolus	Infusion
Diazepam	0.05–0.15mg/kg IV/IM	Too long-acting
Midazolam	50mcg/kg IV/IM	10–50mcg/kg/h
Lorazepam	1mg IV	Too long-acting
Propofol	0.5–2mg/kg IV	1–3mg/kg/h
Chlorpromazine	25–50mg IM	Too long-acting
Haloperidol	2–10mg IV/IM	Too long-acting
Clonidine		100–150mcg/h
Dexmedetomidine	Loading infusion of 6.0mcg/kg/h over 10min, followed by maintenance infusion of 0.2–0.7mcg/kg/h.	

Note that the above doses are a guide only and may need to be altered widely according to individual circumstances.

Key papers

Kress JP, Pohlman AS, O'Connor MF, et al. (2000) Daily interruption of sedative infusions in critically ill patients undergoing mechanical ventilation. *N Engl J Med* **342**: 1471–7.

Pandharipande PP, Pun BT, Herr DL, et al. (2007) Effect of sedation with dexmedetomidine vs lorazepam on acute brain dysfunction in mechanically ventilated patients: the MENDS randomized controlled trial. *JAMA* **298**: 2644–53.

Girard TD, Kress JP, Fuchs BD, et al. (2008) Efficacy and safety of a paired sedation and ventilator weaning protocol for mechanically ventilated patients in intensive care (Awakening and Breathing Controlled trial): a randomised controlled trial. *Lancet* **371**: 126–34.

Monitoring sedation

Frequent, objective reassessment of sedation depth and degree of agitation with corresponding adjustment of infusion doses is necessary to avoid severe cardiovascular and respiratory depression. Simple sedation scores are available to aid assessment, e.g. Riker Score, CAM-ICU.

UCL Hospitals Sedation Score

Agitated and restless	+3
Awake and uncomfortable	+2
Aware but calm	+1
Roused by voice, remains calm	0
Roused by movement	−1
Roused by painful or noxious stimuli	−2
Unrousable	−3
Natural sleep	A

Sedation doses are adjusted to achieve a score as close as possible to. Positive scores require increased sedation doses and negative scores require reduced sedation doses.

See also:

IPPV—failure to tolerate ventilation, p52; IPPV—assessment of weaning, p60; EEG/CFM monitoring, p204; Respiratory stimulants, p256; Delirium, p442.

Muscle relaxants

Types
- Depolarising, e.g. suxamethonium.
- Non-depolarising, e.g. pancuronium, atracurium, cisatracurium, vecuronium, rocuronium.

Mode of action
- Suxamethonium is structurally related to acetylcholine and causes initial stimulation of muscular contraction seen clinically as fasciculation. During this process, continued stimulation leads to desensitisation of the post-synaptic membrane of the neuromuscular junction with efflux of K^+ ions. Subsequent flaccid paralysis is short-acting (2–3min) and cannot be reversed (is actually potentiated) by anticholinesterase drugs. Prolonged effects occur with congenital or acquired pseudo-cholinesterase deficiency.
- Non-depolarising muscle relaxants prevent acetylcholine from depolarising the post-synaptic membrane of the neuromuscular junction by competitive blockade. Reversal of paralysis is achieved by anticholinesterase drugs such as neostigmine. They have a slower onset and longer duration of action than the depolarising agents.

Uses
- To facilitate endotracheal intubation.
- To facilitate mechanical ventilation where optimal sedation does not prevent patient interference with the function of the ventilator.

Routes
- IV.

Side effects
- Hypertension (suxamethonium, pancuronium).
- Bradycardia (suxamethonium).
- Tachycardia (pancuronium).
- Hyperkalaemia (suxamethonium).

Notes
- Modern practice and developments in ventilator technology have rendered use of muscle relaxants less common. It is now rarely necessary to fully paralyse muscles to facilitate mechanical ventilation.
- Frequently reassess requirements for muscle relaxants. Ideally, relaxants should be stopped intermittently to allow depth of sedation to be assessed. If mechanical ventilation proceeds smoothly when relaxants have been stopped, they probably should not be restarted.
- Suxamethonium is contraindicated in spinal neurological disease, hepatic disease, and for 5–50 days after burns.
- Atracurium and cisatracurium are non-cumulative and popular choices for infusion. Non-enzymatic (Hoffman) degradation allows clearance independent of renal or hepatic function, although effects are prolonged in hypothermia.
- Rocuronium has the most rapid onset of the non-depolarising muscle relaxants.

Drug dosages

	Bolus	Infusion
Suxamethonium	50–100mg	2–5mg/min
Pancuronium	4mg	1–4mg/h
Atracurium	25–50mg	25–50mg/h
Cisatracurium	10mg	2–4mg/h
Vecuronium	5–7mg	Excessive half life
Rocuronium	40–50mg	20–40mg/h

See also:

Endotracheal intubation, p42; IPPV—failure to tolerate ventilation, p52; IPPV—failure to deliver ventilation, p54; Sedatives and tranquilisers, p308; Critical care neuromuscular disorders, p460; Post-operative critical care, p620.

Anticonvulsants

Types

- Benzodiazepines, e.g. lorazepam, diazepam, clonazepam.
- Phenytoin.
- Carbamazepine.
- Sodium valproate.
- Magnesium sulphate.
- Thiopental.

Uses

- Control of status epilepticus.
- Intermittent seizure control.
- Myoclonic seizures (clonazepam, sodium valproate).

Routes

- IV (lorazepam, diazepam, clonazepam, phenytoin, sodium valproate, magnesium sulphate, thiopental).
- PO (diazepam, clonazepam, phenytoin, carbamazepine, sodium valproate).
- PR (diazepam).

Side effects

- Sedation (benzodiazepines, thiopental).
- Respiratory depression (benzodiazepines, thiopental).
- Nausea and vomiting (phenytoin, sodium valproate).
- Ataxia (phenytoin, carbamazepine).
- Visual disturbance (phenytoin, carbamazepine).
- Hypotension (diazepam, thiopental)).
- Arrhythmias (phenytoin, carbamazepine).
- Pancreatitis (thiopental).
- Hepatic failure (sodium valproate).

Notes

- Common insults causing seizures include cerebral ischaemic damage, space-occupying lesions, drugs or drug/alcohol withdrawal, metabolic encephalopathy (including hypoglycaemia), and neurosurgery.
- Anticonvulsants provide control of seizures but do not replace removal of the cause where this is possible.
- Onset of seizure control may be delayed by up to 24h with phenytoin, but a loading dose is usually given during the acute phase of seizures.
- Magnesium sulphate is especially useful in eclamptic seizures (and in their prevention).
- Phenytoin has a narrow therapeutic range and a non-linear relationship between dose and plasma levels. Therefore, it is essential to monitor plasma levels.
- Enteral feeding should be stopped temporarily while oral phenytoin is administered.
- Carbamazepine has a wider therapeutic range than phenytoin and there is a linear relationship between dose and plasma levels. Therefore, it is not critical to monitor plasma levels.
- Plasma concentrations of sodium valproate are not related to effects so monitoring of plasma levels is not useful.

Intravenous drug dosages

	Bolus	**Infusion**
Lorazepam	4mg	
Diazepam	2.5mg repeated to 20mg	
Phenytoin	18mg/kg at <50mg/min	100mg 8-hourly
Magnesium sulphate	20mmol over 10–20min	5–10mmol/h
Sodium valproate	400–800mg	
Clonazepam	1mg	1–2mg/h
Thiopental	1–3mg/kg	Lowest possible dose

Key papers

Treiman VA for the Veterans Affairs Status Epilepticus Cooperative Study Group. (1998) A comparison of four treatments for generalized convulsive status epilepticus. *N Engl J Med* **339**: 792–8.

Magpie Trial Collaboration Group. (2002) Do women with pre-eclampsia, and their babies, benefit from magnesium sulphate? The Magpie Trial: a randomised placebo-controlled trial. *Lancet* **359**: 1877–90.

The Collaborative Eclampsia Trial. (1995) Which anticonvulsant for women with eclampsia? Evidence from the Collaborative Eclampsia Trial. *Lancet* **345**: 1455–63.

See also:

EEG/CFM monitoring, p204; Generalised seizures, p444.

Neuroprotective agents

Types
- Diuretics, e.g. mannitol, furosemide.
- Corticosteroids, e.g. dexamethasone.
- Calcium antagonists, e.g. nimodipine.
- Barbiturates, e.g. thiopental.

Uses
- Reduction of cerebral oedema (mannitol, furosemide, dexamethasone).
- Prevention of cerebral vasospasm (nimodipine).
- Reduction of cerebral metabolic rate (thiopental).

Routes
- IV.

Notes
- Cerebral protection requires generalised sedation and abolition of seizures to reduce cerebral metabolic rate, cerebral oedema, and neuronal damage during ischaemia and reperfusion.
- Mannitol reduces cerebral interstitial water as a result of its osmotic load. The effect is transient and best where the blood brain barrier is intact. Interstitial water is mainly reduced in normal areas of brain and this may accentuate cerebral shift. Repeated doses accumulate in the interstitium and may eventually increase oedema formation; mannitol should only be given 4–5 times in 48h. In addition to its osmotic effect, there is some evidence of cerebral vasoconstriction due to a reduction in blood viscosity and free radical scavenging.
- The loop diuretic effect of furosemide encourages salt and water loss. There may also be a reduction of CSF chloride transport, reducing the formation of CSF.
- Dexamethasone reduces oedema around space-occupying lesions such as tumours. Corticosteroids are not currently considered useful in head injury or after a cerebrovascular accident, but benefit has been shown if given early after spinal injury. Corticosteroids encourage salt and water retention and must be withdrawn slowly to avoid rebound oedema.
- Nimodipine is used to prevent cerebral vasospasm during recovery from cerebrovascular insults. As a calcium channel blocker, it also prevents calcium ingress during neuronal injury. This calcium ingress is associated with cell death. It is commonly used in the management of subarachnoid haemorrhage for 5–14 days.
- Thiopental reduces cerebral metabolism, thus prolonging the time that the brain may sustain an ischaemic insult. However, it also reduces cerebral blood flow although blood flow is redistributed preferentially to ischaemic areas. Thiopental acutely reduces intracranial pressure and this is probably the main cerebroprotective effect. Seizure control is a further benefit. Despite these effects, barbiturate coma has not been shown to improve outcome in cerebral insults of various causes.

Drug dosages

	Bolus	Infusion
Mannitol	20–40g 6-hourly	
Furosemide		1–5mg/h
Dexamethasone	4mg 6-hourly or 8–16mg od	
Nimodipine		0.5–2.0mg/h
Thiopental	1–3mg/kg	Lowest possible dose

Key papers

Edwards P, Arango M, Balica L, et al and the CRASH trial collaborators. (2005) Final results of MRC CRASH, a randomised placebo-controlled trial of intravenous corticosteroid in adults with head injury-outcomes at 6 months. *Lancet* **365**: 1957–9.

Allen GS, Ahn HS, Preziosi TJ, et al. (1983) Cerebral arterial spasm—a controlled trial of nimodipine in patients with subarachnoid haemorrhage. *N Engl J Med* **308**: 619–24.

Bracken MB, Shepard MJ, Holford TR, et al. (1997) Administration of methylprednisolone for 24 or 48 hours or tirilazad mesylate for 48 hours in the treatment of acute spinal cord injury. Results of the Third National Acute Spinal Cord Injury Randomised Controlled Trial. National Acute Spinal Cord Injury Study. *JAMA* **277**: 1597–604.

See also:

Intracranial pressure monitoring, p200; Jugular venous bulb saturation, p202; EEG/CFM monitoring, p204; Other neurological monitoring, p206; Anticonvulsants, p312; Coma, p438; Generalised seizures, p444; Intracranial haemorrhage, p448; Subarachnoid haemorrhage, p450; Stroke, p452; Raised intracranial pressure, p454; Head injury (1), p594; Head injury (2), p596.

Haematological drugs

Anticoagulants

Types

- Heparin.
- Low molecular weight (LMW) heparin, e.g. dalteparin, enoxaparin, tinzaparin, fondaparinux.
- Heparinoids, e.g. danaparoid.
- Direct thrombin inhibitors, e.g. lepirudin, dabigatran, rivaroxaban.
- Anticoagulant prostanoids, e.g. epoprostenol, alprostadil.
- Sodium citrate.
- Warfarin.

Modes of action

- Heparin potentiates naturally occurring antithrombin, reduces platelet adhesion to injured vessels, and promotes *in vitro* aggregation.
- LMW heparin appears to influence factor Xa activity specifically; simpler pharmacokinetics allow a smaller dose to be effective.
- Heparanoids are similar to heparin, with 10–20% risk of cross-reactivity. Use is mainly restricted to treating heparin-induced thrombocytopaenia syndrome (HITS) and DVT prophylaxis. No antidote is available.
- Lepirudin is a recombinant form of hirudin that forms an irreversible complex with thrombin. It is unrelated to heparin so can be used to treat HITS. Antibody formation occurs in 40% of patients treated with lepirudin >6 days. Half-life is long and there is no antidote.
- Dabigatran and rivaroxaban are being developed for oral thromboprophylaxis or treatment of thromboembolism without monitoring. There are no antidotes, but half-lives are short.
- Prostanoids affect the balance between native TXA_2 and PGI_2.
- Sodium citrate chelates ionised calcium.
- Warfarin produces a controlled deficiency of vitamin K-dependent coagulation factors (II, VII, IX, and X). Effects develop in 48–72h.

Uses

- Maintenance of an extracorporeal circulation.
- Prevention or treatment of thromboembolism.

Routes

- IV (heparins, heparinoids, prostanoids, sodium citrate).
- SC (heparins).
- PO (warfarin).

Side effects

- Bleeding.
- Hypotension (anticoagulant prostanoids).
- Heparin-induced thrombocytopaenia.
- Hypocalcaemia and hypernatraemia (sodium citrate).

Notes

- Alprostadil is less potent than epoprostenol. As it is metabolised in the lungs, systemic vasodilatation effects are usually minimal.
- For extracorporeal use, citrate has advantages over heparin as it has no antiplatelet activity and is readily haemofiltered.

Drug Dosages

Unfractionated heparin
Dose is titrated to produce an APTT of 1.5–3 times control. This usually requires 500–2000IU/h with an initial loading dose of 3000–5000IU.

Low molecular weight heparin
For DVT prophylaxis, give 2500–5000IU dalteparin or 20–40mg enoxaparin SC daily.

For anticoagulation of an extracorporeal circuit, an IV bolus of 35IU/kg dalteparin or 0.25mg/kg enoxaparin is followed by an infusion of 13IU/kg dalteparin or 0.1mg/kg enoxaparin. Adjust dose to maintain anti-factor Xa activity at 0.5–1IU/mL (or 0.2–0.4IU/mL if high risk of haemorrhage).

For DVT or pulmonary embolism, give 200IU/kg dalteparin or 1.5mg/kg enoxaparin SC daily (or 100IU/kg dalteparin bd if at risk of bleeding).

Heparinoids
Caution in patients with renal insufficiency.

For DVT, prophylaxis give 750 anti-Xa units danaparoid SC bd.

For DVT or pulmonary embolism with history of HITS, give a loading dose of 2500 anti-Xa units danaparoid IV, then infusion of 400U/h for 2h, 300U/h for 2h, then maintenance of 200U/h for five days. Target a therapeutic anti-Xa level during the infusion of 0.5–0.7 anti-Xa units/mL.

For anticoagulation of an extracorporeal circuit, a loading dose of 3,500 anti-Xa units danaparoid IV is followed by continuous infusion of 100 anti-Xa units/h.

Direct thrombin inhibitors
Lepirudin: 0.1–0.4mg/kg bolus followed by 0.1–0.15mg/kg/h infusion. Caution in patients with renal insufficiency.

Anticoagulant prostaglandins
Usual dose range is 2.5–10ng/kg/min. If used for an extracorporeal circulation, infusion should be started 30min prior to commencement.

Sodium citrate
Infused at 5mmol/L of extracorporeal blood flow. Monitor Ca^{2+} (ideally ionised levels and treat as needed).

Warfarin
Start at 10mg/day orally for two days, then 1–6mg/day according to INR. For DVT prophylaxis, pulmonary embolus, mitral stenosis, atrial fibrillation, and tissue valve replacements, maintain INR between 2–3. For recurrent DVT or pulmonary embolus, and mechanical valve replacements, the INR should be kept between 3–4.5

See also:
Extracorporeal respiratory support, p78; Electrical cardioversion, p94; Intra-aortic balloon counterpulsation, p102; Coronary revascularisation techniques, p104; Haemo(dia)filtration (2), p110; Plasma exchange, p114; Coagulation monitoring, p222; Blood products, p250; Coagulants and antifibrinolytics, p322; Pulmonary embolus, p376; Acute coronary syndrome (1), p388; Clotting disorders, p470.

Thrombolytics

Types
- More fibrin-specific, e.g. alteplase (rtPA), tenecteplase, reteplase.
- Older agents, e.g. streptokinase, urokinase.

Modes of action
Activate plasminogen to form plasmin which degrades fibrin.

Uses
- Life-threatening thrombosis or embolus.
- Acute myocardial infarction.
- Acute ischaemic stroke (alteplase).
- To unblock indwelling vascular access catheters.

Routes
- IV.

Side effects
- Bleeding—treat with tranexamic acid 1g IV tds.
- Hypotension and arrhythmias.
- Embolisation from pre-existing clot as it is broken down.
- Anaphylactoid reactions (anistreplase, streptokinase, urokinase).

Contraindications (absolute)—ESC guidelines
- Previous intracranial hemorrhage or stroke of unknown origin.
- Structural cerebrovascular lesion or malignant intracranial neoplasm.
- Ischaemic stroke within six months (not acute stroke within 3h).
- Recent major trauma/surgery/head injury (<3wk).
- Gastrointestinal bleeding within last month.
- Aortic dissection.
- Active bleeding or bleeding diathesis.

Contraindications (relative)—ESC guidelines
- Transient ischaemic attack in preceding six months.
- Oral anticoagulant therapy.
- Pregnancy within one week post-partum.
- Non-compressible vascular puncture.
- Traumatic CPR.
- Poorly controlled hypertension (systolic blood pressure >180mmHg).
- Advanced liver disease.
- Infective endocarditis.
- Active peptic ulcer.

Notes
- In acute myocardial infarction, they are of most value when used within 12h of onset. They may require adjuvant therapy (e.g. aspirin with streptokinase or heparin with rtPA) to maximise the effect.
- In acute ischaemic stroke, alteplase may be beneficial within three hours of onset. Exclude haemorrhage and diffuse swelling by CT scan.
- Anaphylactoid reactions to streptokinase are not uncommon, particularly in those who have had streptococcal infections. Do not expose patients twice between five days and one year of the last dose.

Drug dosages

Alteplase (rtPA)	Dose schedule for acute myocardial infarction is 15mg IV bolus, then 0.75mg/kg over 30min, then 0.5mg/kg over 1h to a maximal dose of 100mg. This is then followed by heparin for 24–48h.
	For pulmonary embolism: 10mg over 1–2min, then 90mg over 2h, followed by heparin.
	For acute ischaemic stroke: 0.1mg/kg over 1–2min, then 0.8mg/kg over 60min. Avoid heparin for 24h.
Tenecteplase	For acute MI: IV bolus of 0.5mg/kg over 10s followed by heparin for 24–48h.
Reteplase	For acute MI: two IV boluses of 10 units given 30min apart followed by heparin for 24–48h.
Streptokinase	For acute MI: 1.5 million units over 60min. Heparin for 24–48h optional.
	For severe venous thrombosis: 250,000 units over 30min followed by 100,000 units/h for 24–72h).
	For pulmonary embolism: 1.5 million units over 2h.
Urokinase	For unblocking indwelling vascular catheters: 5000 IU are instilled.
	For thromboembolic disease: 4400IU/kg is given over 10min followed by 4400IU/kg/h for 12–24h

Key papers

Task Force on management of acute myocardial infarction of the European Society of Cardiology. (2003) Management of acute myocardial infarction in patients with ST-segment elevation. *Eur Heart J* **24**: 28–66.

Task Force Report of the European Society of Cardiology. (2000) Guidelines on diagnosis and management of acute pulmonary embolism. *Eur Heart J* **21**: 1301–66.

British Thoracic Society guidelines for the management of suspected acute pulmonary embolism. (2003) *Thorax* **58**: 470–84.

See also:

Coagulation monitoring, p222; Coagulants and antifibrinolytics, p322; Pulmonary embolus, p376; Acute coronary syndrome (1), p388.

Coagulants and antifibrinolytics

Types
- Vitamin K.
- Prothrombin complex concentrate, e.g. Octaplex®, Beriplex®.
- Protamine.
- Tranexamic acid.
- Activated factor VII (FVIIa).
- Fresh frozen plasma.

Uses
- To reverse a prolonged prothrombin time, e.g. malabsorption, oral anticoagulant therapy, β-lactam antibiotics or critical illness (vitamin K, Octaplex®, Beriplex®).
- To reverse the effects of heparin (protamine).
- Bleeding from raw surfaces, e.g. prostatectomy, dental extraction (tranexamic acid).
- Bleeding from thrombolytics (tranexamic acid).
- Bleeding from major trauma or haemophilia (FVIIa).

Routes
- IV (vitamin K, protamine, tranexamic acid, FVIIa).
- PO (vitamin K, tranexamic acid).

Notes
- The effects of vitamin K are prolonged so avoid where patients are dependent on oral anticoagulant therapy. A dose of 10mg is given PO or by slow IV injection daily. In life-threatening haemorrhage due to warfarin excess, 5–10mg is given by slow IV injection with other coagulation factor concentrates (Octaplex®, Beriplex®). If INR >7 or in less severe haemorrhage, 0.5–2mg may be given by slow IV injection with minimum lasting effect on oral anticoagulant therapy.
- Protamine has an anticoagulant effect of its own in high doses. Protamine 1mg neutralises 100IU unfractionated heparin if given within 15min. Less is required if given later since heparin is excreted rapidly. Protamine should be given by slow IV injection according to the APTT. Total dose should not exceed 50mg. Protamine injection may cause severe hypotension.
- Tranexamic acid has an antifibrinolytic effect by antagonising plasminogen.
- Recombinant factor VIIa is licensed for use in haemophilia, but a number of case series in major trauma, orthopaedic and cardiac surgery report benefit in severe, intractable bleeding that had not responded to standard measures.

Drug dosages

Vitamin K	5–10mg IV
Octaplex®	30–50IU/kg IV
Beriplex®	30IU/kg IV
Protamine	25–50mg slow IV
Tranexamic acid	1–1.5g IV 6–12 hourly
Factor VIIa	90mcg/kg slow IV, repeated as necessary 1.5–2 hourly

See also:

Coagulation monitoring, p222; Blood products, p250; Anticoagulants, p318; Thrombolytics, p320; Bleeding disorders, p468; Clotting disorders, p470.

Miscellaneous drugs

Antimicrobials

Types

- Penicillins, e.g. benzylpenicillin, flucloxacillin, piperacillin, ampicillin.
- Cephalosporins, e.g. cefotaxime, ceftazidime, cefuroxime.
- Carbapenems, e.g. imipenem, meropenem.
- Aminoglycosides, e.g. gentamicin, amikacin, tobramycin.
- Quinolones, e.g. ciprofloxacin.
- Glycopeptides, e.g. teicoplanin, vancomycin.
- Macrolides, e.g. erythromycin, clarithromycin.
- Tetracyclines, e.g. tigecycline.
- Other, e.g. clindamycin, metronidazole, linezolid, co-trimoxazole, rifampicin.
- Antifungals, e.g. amphotericin, fluconazole, caspofungin, voriconazole, itraconazole.
- Antivirals, e.g. aciclovir, ganciclovir.

Uses

- Treatment of infection.
- Prophylaxis against infection, e.g. peri-operatively.
- Local choice of antimicrobial varies. As a guide, the following choices are common:
  - Pneumonia (hospital-acquired Gram-negative)—ceftazidime, ciprofloxacin, meropenem or piperacillin/tazobactam (piptazobactam).
  - Pneumonia (community acquired)—cefuroxime + clarithromycin.
- Systemic sepsis—cefuroxime ± gentamicin (+ metronidazole if anaerobes likely).

Routes

- Generally given IV in critically ill patients.

Side effects

- Hypersensitivity reactions (all).
- Seizures (high dose penicillins, high dose metronidazole, ciprofloxacin).
- Gastrointestinal disturbance (cephalosporins, erythromycin, clindamycin, teicoplanin, vancomycin, co-trimoxazole, rifampicin, metronidazole, ciprofloxacin, amphotericin, flucytosine).
- Vestibular damage (aminoglycosides).
- Renal failure (aminoglycosides, teicoplanin, vancomycin, ciprofloxacin, rifampicin, amphotericin, aciclovir).
- Erythema multiforme (co-trimoxazole).
- Leucopaenia (co-trimoxazole, metronidazole, teicoplanin, ciprofloxacin, flucytosine, aciclovir).
- Thrombocytopaenia (linezolid).
- Peripheral neuropathy (metronidazole).

Notes

- Antimicrobials should be chosen according to microbial sensitivities, usually based on advice from the microbiology laboratory.
- Appropriate empiric therapy for serious infections should be determined by likely organisms, taking into account known community and hospital infection, and resistance patterns.
- Up to 10% of penicillin-allergic patients are also cephalosporin-allergic.
- Optimal duration of therapy is unknown.

Drug dosages (intravenous)

Benzylpenicillin	1.2g 6-hourly (2-hourly for pneumococcal pneumonia)
Flucloxacillin	500mg–2g 6-hourly
Ampicillin	500mg–1g 6-hourly
Piptazobactam	4.5g 6–8 hourly
Ceftazidime	2g 8-hourly
Ceftriaxone	1–4g daily
Cefuroxime	750mg–1.5g 8-hourly
Gentamicin	1.5mg/kg stat, then by levels (usually 80mg 8-hourly)
Amikacin	7.5mg/kg stat, then by levels (usually 500mg 12-hourly)
Tobramycin	5mg/kg stat, then by levels (usually 100mg 8-hourly)
Erythromycin	500mg–1g 6–12hourly
Metronidazole	500mg 8-hourly or 1g 12-hourly PR
Clindamycin	300–600mg 6-hourly
Ciprofloxacin	200–400mg 12-hourly
Co-trimoxazole	960mg 12-hourly in *Pneumocystis carinii* pneumonia
Tigecycline	100mg initially, then 50mg 12-hourly
Imipenem	1–2g 6–8 hourly
Meropenem	500mg–1g 8-hourly
Rifampicin	600mg daily
Teicoplanin	400mg 12-hourly for 3 doses, then 400mg daily
Vancomycin	500mg 6-hourly (monitor levels)
Linezolid	600mg 12-hourly
Chloramphenicol	1–2g 6-hourly
Amphotericin	250mcg–1mg/kg daily
Flucytosine	25–50mg/kg 6-hourly
Fluconazole	200–400mg daily
Caspofungin	70mg stat, then 50–70mg daily
Voriconazole	400mg 12-hourly on first day, then 200–300mg 12-hourly
Itraconazole	200mg 12-hourly for 2 days, then 200mg daily
Aciclovir	10mg/kg 8-hourly
Ganciclovir	5mg/kg 12-hourly

Most antimicrobials need dose adjustment for renal or hepatic failure.

Common choices for specific organisms

S. aureus	Flucloxacillin
MRSA	Teicoplanin, vancomycin, linezolid
S. pneumoniae	Cefuroxime, benzylpenicillin
N. meningitidis	Ceftriaxone, cefotaxime, benzylpenicillin
H. influenzae	Cefuroxime, cefotaxime
E. coli	Ampicillin, ceftazidime, ciprofloxacin, gentamicin, imipenem, meropenem
Klebsiella spp.	Ceftazidime, ciprofloxacin, gentamicin, imipenem, meropenem
P. aeruginosa	Ceftazidime, ciprofloxacin, gentamicin, imipenem, meropenem, piptazobactam

See also:
Virology, serology and assays, p226; Infection—treatment, p554; Multi-resistant infection, p562.

Corticosteroids

Uses

- Anti-inflammatory—corticosteroids are often given in high dose for their anti-inflammatory effect, e.g. asthma, allergic and anaphylactoid reactions, vasculitic disorders, rheumatoid arthritis, inflammatory bowel disease, neoplasm-related cerebral oedema, ARDS, laryngeal oedema (e.g. after intubation), and after spinal cord injury. Benefit is unproven in cerebral oedema following head injury or cardiac arrest.
- Infection—though their immunosuppressive actions may increase susceptibility to infection, corticosteroids are often used with antibiotics as first-line therapy to reduce the inflammatory response of microbial killing, e.g. miliary TB, bacterial meningitis, pneumocystis pneumonia. Only in cerebral malaria has specific detriment been shown. In septic shock, high dose, short-course corticosteroids were ineffective/detrimental. However, more recent trials found improved survival with 'low dose' hydrocortisone (50mg qds) ± fludrocortisone (50mcg), although only in the severe 'vasopressor-unresponsive' subset. Pressor requirements fell faster with corticosteroid therapy. The short corticotropin (ACTH) test is not reliable in determining adrenal responders from non-responders. Free cortisol levels should ideally be assayed, but this is not routinely offered by hospitals.
- Replacement therapy—for patients with Addison's disease and post-adrenalectomy or pituitary surgery. Fludrocortisone is also usually required long-term for its mineralocorticoid Na^+ retaining effect. Higher replacement doses are needed in chronic corticosteroid takers undergoing stress, e.g. surgery, infection.
- Immunosuppressive—after organ transplantation.

Side effects/complications

- Sodium and water retention (especially with mineralocorticoids).
- Hypoadrenal crisis if stopped abruptly after prolonged treatment.
- Immunosuppressive: increased infection risk.
- Neutrophilia.
- Impaired glucose tolerance/diabetes mellitus.
- Hypokalaemic alkalosis.
- Osteoporosis, proximal myopathy (long-term use).
- Increased susceptibility to peptic ulcer disease and GI bleeding.

Notes

- Oral fungal infection is relatively common with inhaled corticosteroids, but systemic and pulmonary fungal infection is predominantly seen in the severely immunocompromised (e.g. AIDS, post-chemotherapy) and not those taking high-dose corticosteroids alone.
- Choice of corticosteroid for short-term anti-inflammatory effect is probably irrelevant, provided the dose is sufficient. Chronic hydrocortisone should be avoided for anti-inflammatory use because of its mineralocorticoid effect, but is appropriate for adrenal replacement.
- Prednisone and cortisone are inactive until metabolised by the liver to prednisolone and hydrocortisone, respectively. Glucocorticoids antagonise the effects of anticholinesterase drugs.
- Corticosteroids probably do not cause critical illness myopathy.

Relative potency and activity

Drug	Glucocorticoid activity	Mineralocorticoid activity	Equivalent anti-inflammatory dose (mg)
Cortisone	++	++	25
Dexamethasone	++++	–	0.75
Hydrocortisone	++	++	20
Methylprednisolone	+++	+	4
Prednisolone	+++	+	5
Prednisone	+++	+	5
Fludrocortisone	+	++++	–

Drug dosages

Drug	Replacement dose	Anti-inflammatory dose
Dexamethasone	–	4–20mg tds IV
Hydrocortisone	20–30mg daily	100–200mg qds IV
Methylprednisolone	–	500mg–1g IV daily
Prednisolone	2.5–15mg mane	40–60mg od PO
Fludrocortisone	0.05–0.3mg daily	–

Weaning

Acute use (<3–4 days):   can stop immediately.
Short-term use (≥3–4 days):   wean over 2–5 days.
Medium-term use (weeks):   wean over 1–2 weeks.
Long-term use (months/years):   wean slowly (months to years).

Key papers

Bracken MB, Shepard MJ, Holford RT, et al. (1997) Administration of methylprednisolone for 24 or 48 hours or tirilazad mesylate for 48 hours in the treatment of acute spinal cord injury. Results of the Third National Acute Spinal Cord Injury Randomised Controlled Trial. National Acute Spinal Cord Injury Study. *JAMA* **277**: 1597–604.

Prasad K, Garner P. (2000) Steroids for treating cerebral malaria. *Cochrane Database Syst Rev.* (2): CD000972. Review.

de Gans J, van de Beek D; European Dexamethasone in Adulthood Bacterial Meningitis Study Investigators. (2002) Dexamethasone in adults with bacterial meningitis. *N Engl J Med* **347**: 1549–56.

Annane D, Sébille V, Charpentier C, et al. (2002) Effect of treatment with low doses of hydrocortisone and fludrocortisone on mortality in patients with septic shock. *JAMA* **288**: 862–71.

Sprung C, Annane D, Keh D, et al for the CORTICUS study group. (2008) Hydrocortisone therapy for patients with septic shock. *N Engl J Med* **358**: 111–24.

See also:

Electrolytes (Na⁺, K⁺, Cl⁻, HCO₃⁻), p212; Full blood count, p220; Immunomodulatory therapies in sepsis, p332; Airway obstruction, p348; Acute respiratory distress syndrome (2), p364; Asthma—general management, p364; Meningitis, p446; Raised intracranial pressure, p454; Myasthenia gravis, p458; Platelet disorders, p478; Hypercalcaemia, p494; Hypoadrenal crisis, p524; Sepsis and septic shock—treatment, p560; HIV related disease, p566; Rheumatic disorders, p572; Vasculitis, p574; Anaphylactoid reactions, p578; Spinal cord injury, p590.

Prostaglandins

Types
- Epoprostenol (prostacyclin, PGI_2).
- Alprostadil (PGE_1).

Modes of action
- Stimulate adenyl cyclase, thus increasing platelet cAMP concentration; this inhibits phospholipase and cycloxygenase, and thus reduces platelet aggregation (epoprostenol is the most potent inhibitor known).
- Reduces platelet procoagulant activity and release of heparin neutralising factor.
- May have a fibrinolytic effect.
- Pulmonary and systemic vasodilator by relaxation of vascular smooth muscle.

Uses
- Anticoagulation, particularly for extracorporeal circuits, either as a substitute or in addition to heparin.
- Pulmonary hypertension.
- Microvascular hypoperfusion (including digital vasculitis).
- Haemolytic uraemic syndrome.
- Acute respiratory failure (by inhalation).

Side effect and complications
- Hypotension.
- Bleeding (particularly at cannula sites).
- Flushing, headache.

Notes
- Epoprostenol is active on both pulmonary and systemic circulations. Although alprostadil is claimed to be metabolised in the lung and have only pulmonary vasodilating effects, falls in systemic blood pressure are not uncommonly seen, especially if metabolism is incomplete.
- Avoid extravasation into peripheral tissues as solution has high pH.
- Effects last up to 30min following discontinuation of the drug.
- Prostaglandins may potentiate the effect of heparin.
- Recent studies have shown improvement in gas exchange by selective pulmonary vasodilatation following inhalation of epoprostenol at doses of 10–15ng/kg/min. The efficacy appears similar to that of nitric oxide inhalation, but is not as rapid.

Drug dosages

Epoprostenol	2–20ng/kg/min
Alprostadil	2–20ng/kg/min

See also:
Haemo(dia)diltration (2), p110; Vasodilators, p266; Anticoagulants, p318; Vasculiitis, p574.

Immunomodulatory therapies in sepsis

Agents modulating different components of the inflammatory response have been studied. These target triggers (e.g. endotoxin), cytokines (e.g. tumour necrosis factor, interleukin-1, and effector cells and their products (e.g. neutrophils, free oxygen radicals, NO)), aim to replace or boost often depleted endogenous anti-inflammatory response systems, e.g. corticosteroids, activated protein C, antithrombin, immunoglobulin.

However, there is a variable degree of disruption and imbalance between pro- and anti-inflammatory systems. Outside small research studies, current monitoring capability precludes the ability to determine which patient would benefit from either boosting or suppressing their inflammatory response, and to what degree, at a precise point of time. This issue has likely affected identification of subgroups who could have benefited from a large number of immunomodulatory drug trials that have failed to show outcome benefit. Only corticosteroids in severe septic shock, and activated protein C (also in a more severe subset) have demonstrated mortality reduction in reasonably sized multicentre trials. For the others, promising results from post hoc subgroup analysis and from tightly controlled small patient studies have not been reproduced.

Activated protein C

Drotrecogin alfa (activated) is a recombinant form of activated protein C and has anti-inflammatory, anticoagulant and fibrinolytic properties. Its beneficial role in adult sepsis is most likely related to anti-inflammatory effects. The pivotal PROWESS study demonstrated overall outcome benefit for patients with severe sepsis treated within 48h of presentation with a 96h infusion of 24mcg/kg/h. However, subset analysis showed benefit was restricted to those with a higher risk of death. Subsequent studies have failed to show benefit in lower risk adults (APACHE score <25) or in children. The major side effect is bleeding so caution should be exercised in those at high risk of potentially catastrophic bleeding, e.g. concurrent coagulopathy or a recent history of surgery, major trauma, head injury and/or peptic ulcer disease. Ongoing trials are attempting to reproduce the PROWESS findings and to use plasma protein C levels as a biomarker against which treatment will be titrated.

Corticosteroids

Hydrocortisone (50mg qds) ± fludrocortisone (50mcg) improves survival in severe 'vasopressor-unresponsive' sepsis.

Immunoglobulin (IV Ig)

Intravenous immunoglobulin (IV Ig) has been studied in both general sepsis and in specific toxin-related conditions. Meta-analyses suggest benefit in general sepsis though no single large study has shown significant overall benefit. A single dose of 2g/kg should be given, and repeated only if the patient relapses after initial response. If an anaphylactoid reaction occurs, slow down/stop infusion and consider corticosteroids.

Uses

- Severe invasive group A streptococcal disease (e.g. necrotising fasciitis).
- Staphylococcal toxic shock syndrome or necrotising (Panton-Valentine Leukocidin (PVL)-associated) staphylococcal sepsis.
- Severe or recurrent *Clostridium difficile* colitis.

Examples of drugs investigated in multi-centre studies

- Corticosteroids (methylprednisolone, hydrocortisone).
- Immunoglobulin.
- Anti-endotoxin antibody (HA-1A, E5).
- Anti-tumour necrosis factor antibody.
- Tumour necrosis factor soluble receptor antibody.
- Interleukin-1 receptor antagonist.
- Platelet activating factor antagonists, PAF-ase.
- Bradykinin antagonists.
- Naloxone.
- Ibuprofen.
- N-acetylcysteine, procysteine.
- L-N-mono-methyl-arginine (L-NMMA).
- Antithrombin.
- Tissue factor pathway inhibitor.
- Activated protein C.

Key papers

Bernard GR, for the PROWESS study group. (2001) Efficacy and safety of recombinant human activated protein C for severe sepsis. *N Engl J Med* **344**: 699–709.

Annane D, Sébille V, Charpentier C, et al. (2002) Effect of treatment with low doses of hydrocortisone and fludrocortisone on mortality in patients with septic shock. *JAMA* **288**: 862–71.

Sprung C, Annane D, Keh D, et al for the CORTICUS study group. (2008) Hydrocortisone therapy for patients with septic shock. *N Engl J Med* **358**: 111–24.

Turgeon AF, Hutton B, Fergusson DA, et al. (2007) Meta-analysis: intravenous immunoglobulin in critically ill adult patients with sepsis. *Ann Intern Med* **146**: 193–203.

See also:
Corticosteroids, p328; Sepsis and septic shock—treatment, p560.

Rituximab

This is an anti-CD20 antibody directed against B lymphocytes that is finding increasing use in a variety of haematological, immune, and rheumatological conditions. Many of its uses are still off-label, but it is increasingly popular.

Modes of action
- Anti-CD20 antibody directed against normal and malignant B cells.

Uses
- Non-Hodgkin's lymphoma.
- Other haematological malignancies, including Burkitt's lymphoma, CLL, Waldenstrom's macroglobulinaemia.
- Post-transplant lymphoproliferative disorder (PTLD) without evidence of allograft rejection.
- Acquired haemophilia.
- Thrombotic thrombocytopaenic purpura.
- Idiopathic thrombocytopaenic purpura.
- Rheumatoid arthritis not responding to anti-TNF therapy.
- Other autoimmune conditions, including SLE.
- Multifocal motor neuropathy.

Routes
- IV infusion.

Adverse effects
- Pulmonary events (hypoxaemia, pulmonary infiltrates, acute respiratory failure).
- Hepatitis B reactivation.
- Tumour lysis syndrome.
- Severe mucocutaneous reactions (e.g. Stevens–Johnson syndrome).
- Abdominal pain, bowel obstruction, and perforation.
- Neutropaenia and thrombocytopaenia.
- Reactivation of JC virus resulting in progressive multifocal leukoencephalopathy.
- Arrhythmias.
- Infusion-related syndrome with hypotension, rigors, pyrexia, urticaria, angioedema, and bronchospasm.

See also:
Clotting disorders, p470; Platelet disorders, p478; Rheumatic disorders, p572; Vasculitis, p574; Leukaemia/lymphoma, p630.

Resuscitation

Basic resuscitation

In any severe failure of the cardiorespiratory system, the order of priority should be to secure the airway, maintain respiration (manual ventilation if necessary), restore the circulation (with external cardiac massage if necessary), and consider mechanical ventilation. Initial assessment should include airway patency, palpation of pulses, measurement of blood pressure, presumptive diagnosis, and consideration of treatment of the cause.

Airway protection

The airway should be opened by tilting the head back with one hand on the forehead and lifting the chin with the fingers of the other hand. If there is a neck injury or an inadequate airway with the head tilt and chin lift, a jaw thrust should be performed. The fingers should be placed behind the angle of the mandible on both sides, and the mandible lifted forward and upward until the lower teeth (or gum) are in front of the upper teeth (or gum). The mouth and pharynx should be cleared by suction and loose fitting dentures removed. If necessary, an oropharyngeal (Guedel) airway may be inserted.

Manual ventilation

Once the airway is protected the patient who is not breathing requires manual ventilation with a self-inflating bag and mask (Ambu bag). Oxygen should be delivered in high concentration (FIO_2 1.0 for manual ventilation, FIO_2 0.6–1.0 for spontaneously breathing patients) to achieve adequate arterial oxygen saturation. Hyperoxia should not be allowed to persist as this can be detrimental. If the patient breathes inadequately (poor arterial saturation, hypercapnia, rapid shallow breathing), ventilatory support should continue.

Circulation

If pulses are impalpable or weak, or if the patient has a severe bradycardia, external cardiac massage is required and treatment should continue as for a cardiac arrest. Hypotension should be treated initially with a fluid challenge although life-threatening hypotension may require blind treatment with epinephrine 0.05–0.2mg IV increments at 1–2min intervals until a satisfactory blood pressure is restored. Such treatment should not be prolonged without circulatory monitoring to ensure the adequacy of cardiac output as well as correction of hypotension.

Venous access

Venous access must be secured early during basic resuscitation. Large-bore cannulae are necessary, e.g. 14G. In cases of haemorrhage, two cannulae are required. Small peripheral veins should be avoided; forearm flexure veins are appropriate if nowhere else is available. In very difficult patients, a Seldinger approach to the femoral vein or a central vein may be appropriate. The latter has the advantage of providing central venous monitoring.

See also:
Oxygen therapy, p38; Airway maintenance, p40; Endotracheal intubation, p42; Ventilatory support—indications, p44; Electrical cardioversion, p94; Central venous catheter—insertion, p168; Colloids, p246; Inotropes, p264; Vasopressors, p268; Cardiac arrest, p340; Fluid challenge, p342.

Cardiac arrest

As with basic resuscitation, the order of priority is airway, breathing, circulation, and drug treatment. Initial management of airway and breathing is as described for basic resuscitation. Only attempt intubation after adequate pre-oxygenation. Tube placement and return of circulation should ideally be confirmed with capnography. If intubation is difficult, maintain manual ventilation with an Ambu bag, mask, and 100% O_2.

Therapeutic hypothermia is useful to improve cerebral outcome, post-cardiac arrest (particularly out-of-hospital VF or pulseless VT).

Cardiac massage

External massage provides minimal circulatory support during cardiac arrest. A rate of 100/min with a compression depth of 5cm is recommended. Once an artificial airway is established, give manual breaths at a rate of 8–10/min. Compressions should not be paused for ventilation.

Cardioversion

Cardioversion is performed urgently if VT or VF cannot be excluded. Restart cardiac massage immediately without waiting to review the ECG. Cerebral damage continues while there is no blood flow.

Drugs

Few drugs are necessary for first-line cardiac arrest management. Drugs should be given via a large vein since vasoconstriction and poor flow delay peripheral injections reaching the central circulation. If early venous access cannot be secured, the intraosseous route may be used.

Epinephrine

The α constrictor effects predominate during cardiac arrest, helping to maintain diastolic blood pressure, and coronary and cerebral perfusion. Irrespective of rhythm give 1mg (10mL of 1:10000 solution) after every third shock and every 3–5min.

Vasopressin

A recent trial comparing vasopressin and epinephrine showed improved outcomes with vasopressin in asystole. The vasopressin dose is 40IU, and may be repeated after 3min if the first dose is ineffective.

Magnesium

A dose of 8mmol can be given in refractory VF, torsades de pointes, hypomagnesaemia, or if digoxin toxicity is suspected.

Amiodarone

In VF/VT give amiodarone 300mg IV bolus after every third shock.

Calcium chloride

Used in pulseless electrical activity if there is hyperkalaemia, hypocalcaemia, or calcium antagonist use. Give 10mL 10% solution.

Bicarbonate

Only used if cardiac arrest is due to hyperkalaemia or tricyclic poisoning. A dose of 50mL of 8.4% solution is given.

Key papers

The Hypothermia after Cardiac Arrest Study Group. (2002) Mild therapeutic hypothermia to improve the neurologic outcome after cardiac arrest. *N Engl J Med* **346**: 549–56.

Wenzel V for the European Resuscitation Council. (2004) Vasopressor during CPR study. A comparison of vasopressin and epinephrine for out-of-hospital cardiopulmonary resuscitation. *N Engl J Med* **350**: 105–13.

The European Resuscitation Council (ERC). (2005) Guidelines for Resuscitation 2005. *Resuscitation* **67S1**: S1–S189.

Resuscitation Council Guidelines (2010) http://www.resus.org.uk/pages/medimain.htm.

Fluid challenge

Treat hypovolaemia urgently to avoid the serious complication of multi-organ failure. Ensure an adequate circulating volume before considering other methods of circulatory support. Clinical signs of hypovolaemia (reduced skin turgor, low CVP, oliguria, tachycardia, and hypotension) are late indicators. Lifting the legs of a supine patient and watching for an improvement in the circulation is a useful indicator of hypovolaemia. A high index of suspicion must be maintained; normal heart rate, BP, and CVP do not exclude hypovolaemia. The CVP is particularly unreliable in pulmonary vascular disease, right ventricular disease, isolated left ventricular failure, and valvular heart disease. The absolute CVP or PAWP are also difficult to interpret since peripheral venoconstriction may maintain CVP despite hypovolaemia; indeed, CVP may fall in response to fluid. The response to a fluid challenge is the safest method of assessment.

Choice of fluid

The aim of a fluid challenge is to produce a significant (200mL) and rapid increase in plasma volume. Colloid fluids are ideal; a gelatin solution is recommended for short-term plasma volume expansion in simple hypovolaemia. Consider hydroxyethyl starch when there is a probability of capillary leak. Packed red cells have a high haematocrit and do not adequately expand the plasma volume. Crystalloid fluids are rapidly lost from the circulation and give a less reliable increase in plasma volume.

Assessing the response to a fluid challenge

Ideally, the response of CVP, PAWP or, preferably, stroke volume should be monitored during a fluid challenge. Fluid challenges should be repeated if the response suggests continuing hypovolaemia. However, if such monitoring is not available, it is reasonable to assess the clinical response to up to two fluid challenges (200mL each).

CVP (or PAWP) response

The change in CVP/PAWP after a 200mL fluid challenge depends on the starting blood volume (see figure opposite). A ≥3mmHg rise in CVP/PAWP represents a significant increase and suggests an adequate circulating volume. A positive response may sometimes occur in the vasoconstricted patient with a lower blood volume. It is also important to assess clinical response; if inadequate, it may be appropriate to monitor stroke volume before further fluid challenges or considering further circulatory support (see figure 21.1.).

Stroke volume response

In the inadequately filled left ventricle, a fluid challenge will increase stroke volume. Failure to increase stroke volume may be due to a well-filled ventricle (usually accompanied by a ≥3mmHg rise in filling pressure), ongoing rapid fluid loss (e.g. massive haemorrhage), right heart failure or obstruction (e.g. pericardial tamponade, massive PE, mitral stenosis). It is important to monitor stroke volume rather than cardiac output during a fluid challenge. If the heart rate falls appropriately in response to a fluid challenge, the cardiac output may not increase despite an increase in stroke volume (see figure 21.1).

CVP/PAWP

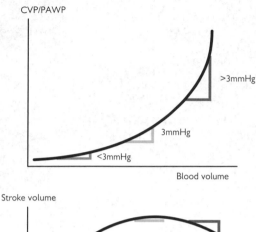

>3mmHg

3mmHg

<3mmHg

Blood volume

Stroke volume

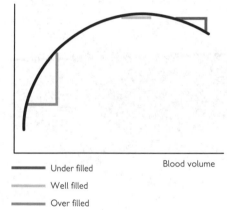

Blood volume

— Under filled

— Well filled

— Over filled

Fig. 21.1. CVP and stroke volume response to fluid challenge.

See also:
Central venous catheter—insertion, p168; Central venous catheter—use, p170; Cardiac output—central thermodilution, p178; Cardiac output—peripheral thermodilution, p180; Cardiac output—indicator dilution, p182; Cardiac output—Doppler ultrasound, p184; Cardiac output—pulse contour analysis, p186; Cardiac output—other techniques, p188; Pressure and stroke volume variation, p190; Echocardiography, p192; Colloids, p246; Basic resuscitation, p338.

Respiratory disorders

Dyspnoea

Defined as difficulty in breathing. The respiratory rate may be increased or decreased though the respiratory effort is usually increased with the use of accessory muscles. The patient may show signs of progressive fatigue and impaired gas exchange.

Common ICU causes

Respiratory	Respiratory failure
Circulatory	Heart failure, hypoperfusion, pulmonary embolism, severe anaemia
Metabolic	Acidosis
Central	Stimulants, e.g. aspirin
Anaphylactic	Upper airway obstruction, bronchospasm
Psychiatric	Hysterical

- A psychiatric cause of dyspnoea is only made after exclusion of other treatable causes.
- Dual coexisting pathologies should be considered, e.g. chest infection and hypovolaemia.

Principles of management

1. O_2 therapy to maintain SaO_2 (ideally 92–98%).
2. Correct abnormality where possible.
3. Support therapy until recovery.
   —Mechanical, e.g. positive pressure ventilation, CPAP.
   —Pharmacological treatment, e.g. bronchodilators, vasodilators.
4. Relieve anxiety.

Airway obstruction

Causes
- In the lumen, e.g. foreign body, blood clot, vomitus, sputum plug.
- In the wall, e.g. epiglottitis, laryngeal oedema, anaphylaxis, neoplasm.
- Outside the wall, e.g. trauma (facial, neck), thyroid mass.

Presentation
- In spontaneously breathing patient: stridor, dyspnoea, fatigue, cyanosis.
- In ventilated patient (e.g. due to intraluminal obstruction): raised airway pressures, decreased tidal volume, hypoxaemia, hypercapnia.

Diagnosis
- Chest and lateral neck X-ray.
- Fibreoptic laryngoscopy/bronchoscopy.
- CT scan.

Management
Presentation outside ICU/operating theatre
1. High FIO_2.
2. If collapsed or *in extremis*: perform immediate orotracheal intubation. If impossible, emergency cricothyroidotomy or tracheostomy.
3. If symptomatic but not *in extremis*: consider cause and treat as appropriate, e.g. removal of foreign body. Elective intubation or tracheostomy may be required.
4. With acute epiglottitis, the use of a tongue depressor or nasendoscopy may precipitate complete obstruction so this should be undertaken in an operating theatre ready to perform emergency tracheostomy. The responsible organism is usually *H. influenzae*. Treat early with chloramphenicol. Acute epiglottitis is recognised in adults.
5. Consider Heliox (79% He/21% O_2) alone or as a supplement to oxygen to reduce viscosity and improve airflow.

Presentation within ICU/operating theatre
If intubated:
- High FIO_2.
- Pass suction catheter down the ET tube, assess ease of passage and the contents suctioned. If ET tube is patent, attempt repeated suction interspersed with 5mL boluses of 0.9% saline. Urgent fibreoptic bronchoscopy may be necessary for diagnosis and, if possible, removal of a foreign body. If a foreign body cannot be removed by fibreoptic bronchoscopy, urgent rigid bronchoscopy should be performed by an experienced operator. If the ET tube is obstructed, remove the tube, oxygenate by face mask, then reintubate.

If not intubated:
- As for out-of-ICU presentation.
- If recently extubated, consider laryngeal oedema. Post-extubation laryngeal oedema is unpredictable though occurs more commonly after prolonged or repeated intubation; the incidence may be reduced by proper tethering of the endotracheal tube and prevention of excessive coughing. Diagnosed by nasendoscopy. Dexamethasone 4mg x3 doses over 24h may reduce the swelling though re-intubation is often necessary in the interim.

See also
Endotracheal intubation, p42; Continuous positive airway pressure, p70; Tracheotomy, p80;
Fibreoptic bronchoscopy, p88; Corticosteroids, p328.

Respiratory failure

Defined as impaired pulmonary gas exchange leading to hypoxaemia and/or hypercapnia.

Common ICU causes

Central	Cerebrovascular accident, drugs (e.g. opiates, sedatives), raised intracranial pressure, trauma
Brainstem/spinal cord	Trauma (at or above phrenic level), tetanus, Pickwickian syndrome, motor neurone disease
Neuropathy	Guillain–Barré, critical illness polyneuropathy
Neuromuscular	Muscle relaxants, organophosphorus poisoning, myasthenia gravis
Chest wall/muscular	Flail chest, heart failure, myopathy (including critical illness and disuse myopathy)
Airways	Upper airways obstruction, airway disruption, asthma, anaphylaxis
Parenchymal	Pneumonia, ARDS, fibrosis, pulmonary oedema
Extra-pulmonary	Pneumothorax, pleural effusion, haemothorax
Circulatory	Pulmonary embolus, heart failure, Eisenmenger intracardiac shunt

Types of respiratory failure

- Type I: hypoxaemic—often parenchymal in origin.
- Type II: hypoxaemic, hypercapnic—often mechanical in origin.

Principles of management

1. Ensure SaO_2 is compatible with survival (i.e. usually >80%, preferably >92–98%).
2. Correct abnormality where possible, e.g. drain pneumothorax, relieve/bypass obstruction.
3. Support therapy until recovery:
   —Positive pressure ventilation.
   —Non-invasive respiratory support.
   —Pharmacological treatment, e.g. bronchodilators, antibiotics.
   —Opiate antagonists, respiratory stimulants.
   —General measures, e.g. hydration, airway humidification.
   —Removal of secretions, physiotherapy, bronchoscopy.
4. Unless the patient is symptomatic (e.g. drowsy, dyspnoeic), the $PaCO_2$ may be left elevated to minimise ventilator trauma (permissive hypercapnia) or if chronically hypercapnic (type II respiratory failure).

Atelectasis and pulmonary collapse

A collapsed lobe or segment is usually visible on a chest X-ray. Macroatelectasis is also evident as volume loss. In microatelectasis, the chest X-ray may be normal, but the A–aDO$_2$ will be high. Atelectasis reduces lung compliance and PaO$_2$, and increases work of breathing. This may result in poor gas exchange, increased airway pressures, reduced tidal volume and, if severe, circulatory collapse.

Causes

- Collapsed lobe/segment—bronchial obstruction (e.g. sputum retention, foreign body, blood clot, vomitus, misplaced endotracheal tube).
- Macroatelectasis—air space compression by heavy, oedematous lung tissue, external compression (e.g. pleural effusion, haemothorax), sputum retention.
- Microatelectasis—inadequate depth of respiration, nitrogen washout by 100% oxygen with subsequent absorption of oxygen occurring at a rate greater than replenishment.

Sputum retention

Excess mucus (sputum) normally stimulates coughing. If ciliary clearance is reduced (e.g. smoking, sedatives) or mucus volume is excessive (e.g. asthma, bronchiectasis, cystic fibrosis, chronic bronchitis), sputum retention may occur. Sputum retention may also be the result of inadequate coughing (e.g. chronic obstructive pulmonary disease, pain, neuromuscular disease) or increased mucus viscosity (e.g. hypovolaemia, inadequate humidification of inspired gas).

Preventive measures

- Sputum hydration—maintenance of systemic hydration and humidification of inspired gases (e.g. nebulised saline/bronchodilators, heated water bath, heat-moisture exchanging filter).
- Cough—requires inspiration to near total lung capacity, glottic closure, contraction of abdominal muscles, and rapid opening of the glottis. Dynamic compression of the airways and high velocity expiration expels secretions. The process is limited if total lung capacity is reduced, abdominal muscles are weak, pain limits contraction, or small airways collapse on expiration. It is usual to flex the abdomen on coughing, and this should be simulated in supine patients by drawing the knees up. This also limits pain in patients with an upper abdominal wound.
- Physiotherapy—postural drainage, percussion and vibration, hyperinflation, intermittent positive pressure breathing, incentive spirometry, or manual hyperinflation.
- Maintenance of lung volumes—increased V$_T$, CPAP, PEEP, positioning to reduce compression of lung tissue by oedema.

Management

Specific management depends on the cause and should be corrective. All measures taken for prevention should continue. If there is lobar or segmental collapse with obstruction of proximal airways, bronchoscopy may be useful to allow directed suction, foreign body removal, and saline instillation. Patients with high FIO$_2$ may deteriorate due to the effects of excessive lavage or suction reducing minute ventilation.

See also:
Fibreoptic bronchoscopy, p88; Chest physiotherapy, p90; Bronchodilators, p254; Chronic airflow limitation, p354; Acute weakness, p440; Critical care neuromuscular disorders, p460; Pain, p618; Post-operative critical care, p620.

Chronic airflow limitation

Many patients requiring ICU admission for community-acquired pneumonia have chronic respiratory failure. An acute exacerbation (which may or may not be infection-related) results in decompensation and symptomatic deterioration. Such infections include viruses, *Haemophilus influenzae*, *Klebsiella*, and *Staphylococcus aureus*, in addition to *Streptococcus pneumoniae*, and rarely, *Mycoplasma pneumoniae* and *Legionella pneumophila*. Otherwise, patients are admitted with coincidental chronic airflow limitation (CAL) or as a prophylactic measure in view of their limited respiratory function, e.g. for elective post-operative ventilation.

Problems in managing CAL patients on the ICU

- Disability due to chronic ill health.
- Fatigue, muscle weakness, and decreased physiological reserve leading to earlier need for ventilatory support, increased difficulty in weaning, and greater physical dependency on support therapies.
- Psychological dependency on support therapies.
- More prone to pneumothorax.
- Usually have greater levels of sputum production.
- Right ventricular dysfunction (cor pulmonale).

Notes

- Trials of non-invasive ventilatory support ± respiratory stimulants such as doxepram have shown considerable success in avoiding intubation and mechanical ventilation.
- Decisions on whether or not to intubate should be made in consultation with the patient (if possible), the family, and a respiratory physician or GP with knowledge of the patient. The patient should be given the benefit of the doubt, and intubated in an acute situation where a precise history and quality of life are not known.
- Accept lower target levels of PaO_2 or SpO_2 (e.g. 88–92%).
- Accept higher target levels of $PaCO_2$ if patient is known or suspected to have chronic CO_2 retention (e.g. elevated plasma bicarbonate levels on admission to hospital).

Weaning the patient with CAL

- An early trial of extubation may be worthwhile.
- Weaning may be a lengthy procedure. Daily trials of spontaneous breathing may reveal faster-than-anticipated progress.
- Provide plentiful encouragement and psychological support. Setting daily targets and early mobilisation may be advantageous.
- Do not tire by prolonged spontaneous breathing. Consider gradually increasing periods of spontaneous breathing interspersed by periods of rest. Ensure a good night's sleep, ideally by natural means.
- Use patient appearance and lack of symptoms (e.g. tachypnoea or fatigue) rather than specific blood gas values to judge duration of spontaneous breathing.
- Early tracheostomy may benefit when difficulty in weaning is expected.
- The patient may cope better with a tracheostomy mask than CPAP.
- Extrinsic PEEP or CPAP may prevent early airway closure reducing the work of breathing. However, there is a risk of air trapping.
- Consider heart failure as a cause of difficulty in weaning.

Key papers

Brochard L, Mancebo J, Wysocki M, et al. (1995) Non-invasive ventilation for acute exacerbations of chronic obstructive pulmonary disease. *N Engl J Med* **333**: 817–22.

Antonelli M, Conti G, Rocco M, et al. (1998) A comparison of non-invasive positive-pressure ventilation and conventional mechanical ventilation in patients with acute respiratory failure. *N Engl J Med* **339**: 429–35.

Epstein SK, Ciubotaru RL. (1998) Independent effects of aetiology of failure and time to reintubation on outcome for patients failing extubation. *Am J Respir Crit Care Med* **158**: 489–93.

See also:

Oxygen therapy, p38; Positive end expiratory pressure (1), p66; Continuous positive airway pressure, p70; Non-invasive respiratory support, p76; Chest physiotherapy, p90; Blood gas analysis, p156; Bronchodilators, p254; Respiratory stimulants, p256; Antimicrobials, p326; Acute chest infection (1), p356; Pneumothorax, p368.

Acute chest infection (1)

Patients may present with or may develop infection as a complication of critical care management. Typical features include fever, cough, purulent sputum production, breathlessness, pleuritic pain, and bronchial breathing. Urgent investigation includes arterial gases, chest X-ray, blood count, cultures of blood and sputum. In community-acquired pneumonia, acute phase antibody titres and urinary antigen (e.g. *S. pneumoniae*, *L. pneumophilia*) should be measured. If Panton-Valentine Leukocidin (PVL) producing *S. aureus* is suspected (necrotising pneumonia, especially in younger patients), perform PCR testing

Diagnosis and initial antimicrobial treatment

Basic resuscitation is required if there is cardiorespiratory compromise. Appropriate treatment of the infection depends on chest X-ray and microbiology findings, and although empiric, 'best guess' antibiotic treatment may be started before culture results are available. Treatment includes physiotherapy and methods to aid sputum clearance.

Clear chest X-ray

Acute bronchitis is associated with cough, mucoid sputum, and wheeze. In the previously healthy, a viral aetiology is most likely, often with an upper respiratory prodrome. Symptomatic relief is often all that is needed. Likely organisms in acute-on-chronic bronchitis include *S. pneumoniae*, *H. influenzae* or *S. aureus*. Use appropriate antibiotics, e.g. cefuroxime or ampicillin ± flucloxacillin. Bacteria in sputum may confuse viral pneumonia although secondary bacterial infection is common.

Consolidation on chest X-ray

Recent history is important for deciding the cause of pneumonia (see figure 22.1):

- Hospital-acquired pneumonia—enteric (Gram-negative) organisms treated with ceftazidime and gentamicin, or carbapenems if extended spectrum beta-lactamase (ESBL) producing; *S. aureus* is treated with flucloxacillin (or teicoplanin/vancomycin/linezolid if resistant).
- Recent aspiration—anaerobic or Gram-negative infection treated with clindamycin or cefuroxime and metronidazole.
- Community-acquired pneumonia in a previously healthy individual—for *S. pneumoniae* (often lobar, acute onset) or atypical pneumonia (insidious onset, known community outbreaks, renal failure, and electrolyte disturbance in Legionnaire's disease), treat with cefuroxime and clarithromycin. Treat PVL-positive *S. aureus* pneumonia with clindamycin and linezolid. Both *S. aureus* and *H. influenzae* are common in those debilitated by chronic disease (e.g. alcoholism, diabetes, chronic airflow limitation, or the elderly). *S. aureus* pneumonia complicates influenza.
- Immunosuppressed—opportunistic infections (e.g. tuberculosis, *Pneumocystis carinii*, Herpes viruses, CMV, or fungi).

Pulmonary cavitation on chest X-ray

Cavitation should alert to the possibility of anaerobic infection (sputum is often foul-smelling) (see figure 22.2). *S. aureus*, *K. pneumoniae* or tuberculosis are also associated with cavitation. Appropriate antibiotics include metronidazole or clindamycin for anaerobic infection, flucloxacillin for *S. aureus*, and ceftazidime and gentamicin for *K. pneumoniae*. A foreign body or pulmonary infarct should also be considered where there is a single abscess.

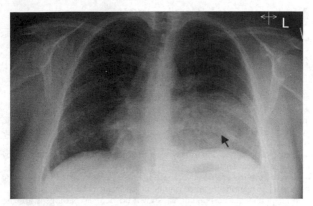

Fig 22.1. X-ray showing left (L) basal consolidation (arrow).

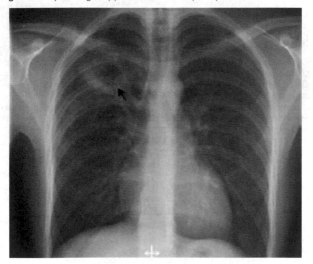

Fig 22.2. X-ray showing right upper zone cavitation (arrow).

See also:

Blood gas analysis, p154; Respiratory imaging, p158; Full blood count, p220; Bacteriology, p224; Virology, serology and assays, p226; Antimicrobials, p326; Respiratory failure, p350; Chronic airflow limitation, p354; Acute chest infection (2), p358; Infection—diagnosis, p552; HIV-related disease, p566; SARS, VHF, and H5N1, p570.

Acute chest infection (2)

Laboratory diagnosis

The following samples are required for laboratory diagnosis:

- Sputum (e.g. cough specimen, endotracheal tube aspirate, protected brush specimen, bronchoalveolar lavage specimen).
- Blood cultures.
- Serology and PCR (in community-acquired pneumonia).
- Urine for antigen (if *Legionella*, *Pneumococcus*, or *Candida* suspected).

In severe pneumonia, blind antibiotic therapy should not be withheld while awaiting results. However, specimens should be taken before starting antibiotics.

Microbiological yield is usually very low, especially if antibiotic therapy has started before sampling.

Where cultures are positive, there is often multiple growth. Separating pathogenic organisms from colonising organisms may be difficult.

In hospital-acquired pneumonia, known nosocomial pathogens are the likely source, e.g. local Gram-negative flora, MRSA.

Continuing treatment

Antibiotics should be adjusted according to sensitivities once available. Failure to respond to treatment in 72h should prompt consideration of infections more common in the immunocompromised.

Hospital-acquired pneumonia requires treatment with appropriate antibiotics for 24h after symptoms subside (usually 3–5 days). Some Critical Care Units use longer courses, but a multicentre study showed no difference in outcome between 7 and 14 days' treatment.

In atypical or pneumococcal pneumonia, 10–14 days antibiotic treatment is usual (though no evidence base exists to indicate optimal duration of therapy).

Antimicrobial treatment

Drug	Dose	Organism
Aciclovir	10mg/kg 8-hourly IV	Herpes viruses
Amphotericin B	250mg–1g 6-hourly IV	Fungi
Ampicillin	500mg–1g 6-hourly IV	H. influenzae Gram-negative spp.
Benzylpenicillin	1.2g 2–6 hourly IV	S. pneumoniae
Ceftazidime	2g 8-hourly IV	K. pneumoniae P. aeruginosa Gram-negative spp.
Cefuroxime	750mg–1.5g 8-hourly IV	S. pneumoniae H. influenzae Gram-negative spp.
Clarithromycin	500mg 12-hourly IV (250–500mg 12-hourly PO if less severe)	Atypical pneumonia S. pneumoniae
Erythromycin	1g 6–12 hourly (500mg 6-hourly PO if less severe)	Atypical pneumonia S. pneumoniae
Clindamycin	300–600mg 6-hourly IV	Anaerobes Gram-negative spp.
Cotrimoxazole	120mg/kg/d IV	Pneumocystis carinii
Flucloxacillin	2g 6-hourly IV (500mg–1g 6-hourly PO if less severe)	S. aureus
Ganciclovir	5mg/kg 12-hourly IV (over 1h)	CMV
Gentamicin	1.5mg/kg stat IV (thereafter by levels, usually 80mg 8-hourly)	K. pneumoniae, P. aeruginosa Gram-negative spp.
Metronidazole	500mg 8-hourly IV or 1g 12-hourly PR	Anaerobes
Teicoplanin	400mg 12-hourly for 3 doses, then 400mg daily	Methicillin-resistant S. aureus
Vancomycin	500mg 6-hourly (monitor levels)	Methicillin-resistant S. aureus
Linezolid	600mg 12-hourly IV or PO	Methicillin-resistant S. aureus

Key papers

Iregui M, Ward S, Sherman G, et al. (2002) Clinical importance of delays in the initiation of appropriate antibiotic treatment for ventilator-associated pneumonia. *Chest* **122**: 262–8.

Chastre J, for the PneumA Trial Group. (2003) Comparison of 8 vs 15 days of antibiotic therapy for ventilator-associated pneumonia in adults: a randomised trial. *JAMA* **290**: 2588–98.

See also

Bacteriology, p224; Virology, serology and assays, p226; Antimicrobials, p326; Acute chest infection (1), p356; HIV related disease, p566; SARS, VHF, and H5N1, p570.

Acute respiratory distress syndrome (1)

Acute respiratory distress syndrome (ARDS) is the respiratory component of multiple organ dysfunction. It may predominate the clinical picture or be of lesser importance in relation to dysfunction of other organ systems.

Aetiology

As part of the exaggerated inflammatory response following a major exogenous insult which may be either direct (e.g. chest trauma, inhalation injury) or distant (e.g. peritonitis, major haemorrhage, burns). Histology reveals aggregation and activation of neutrophils and platelets, patchy endothelial and alveolar disruption, interstitial oedema, and fibrosis. Classically, the acute phase is characterised by increased capillary permeability and the fibroproliferative phase (after seven days) by a predominant fibrotic reaction. However, recent data suggest such distinctions are not so clear-cut; evidence of markers of fibrosis is present as early as day 1.

Definitions

Acute lung injury (ALI):
- PaO_2/FIO_2 ≤300mmHg (40kPa).
- RegardLess of level of PEEP.
- With bilateral infiltrates on chest X-ray.
- With pulmonary artery wedge pressure <18mmHg.

Acute respiratory distress syndrome (ARDS):
- As above but PaO_2/FIO_2 ≤200 mmHg (26.7kPa).

Prognosis

Prognosis depends in part on the underlying insult, the presence of other organ dysfunctions, and the age and chronic health of the patient. Predominant single-organ ARDS carries a mortality of 30–50%; there has been outcome improvement over the last decade.

Some deterioration on lung function testing is usually detectable in survivors of ARDS, even in those who are relatively asymptomatic. Recent studies indicate that a significant proportion of survivors of ARDS have physical and/or psychological sequelae at one year.

Key papers

Bernard GR for the American-European Consensus Conference on ARDS. (1994) Definitions, mechanisms, relevant outcomes, and clinical trial coordination. *Am J Respir Crit Care Med* **149**: 818–24.

Marshall RP, Bellingan G, Webb S, et al. (2000) Fibroproliferation occurs early in the acute respiratory distress syndrome and impacts on outcome. *Am J Respir Crit Care Med* **162**: 1783–8.

Herridge MS, Cheung AM for the Canadian Critical Care Trials Group. (2003) One-year outcomes in survivors of the acute respiratory distress syndrome. *N Engl J Med* **348**: 683–93.

Cheung AM, Tansey CM, Tomlinson G, et al. (2006) Two-year outcomes, health care use, and costs of survivors of acute respiratory distress syndrome. *Am J Respir Crit Care Med* **174**: 538–44.

See also:

Acute respiratory distress syndrome (2), p362; Inhalation injury, p374; Systemic inflammation/ multi-organ failure—causes, p556; Multiple trauma (1), p582; Multiple trauma (2), p584; Burns— fluid management, p592; Burns—general management, p594; Blast injury, p596.

Acute respiratory distress syndrome (2)

General management

1. Remove the cause whenever possible, e.g. drain pus, antibiotics, fix long bone fracture.
2. Sedate with an opiate-benzodiazepine combination as mechanical ventilation is likely to be prolonged. Doses should be kept to the lowest possible but consistent with adequate sedation.
3. Muscle relaxation can be used in severe ARDS to improve chest wall compliance and gas exchange.
4. Haemodynamic manipulation with either fluid, dilators, pressors, diuretics and/or inotropes may improve oxygenation. This may be achieved by either increasing cardiac output and thus mixed venous saturation in low output states, or by decreasing cardiac output thereby lengthening pulmonary transit times in high output states. Care should be taken not to compromise the circulation.

Respiratory management

1. Maintain adequate gas exchange with increased FIO_2, and depending on severity, either non-invasive respiratory support (e.g. CPAP, BiPAP) or positive pressure ventilation. Specific modes may be utilised such as pressure-controlled ventilation. V_T should be targeted at 6–7mL/kg and plateau inspiratory pressures ≤30cmH₂O, if possible. However, there is no consensus regarding the upper desired levels of FIO_2 and PEEP. Greater emphasis is currently placed on higher levels of PEEP (up to 20cmH₂O). While the European view generally favours use of high FIO_2 (up to 1.0), a common US approach is to keep FIO_2 ≤0.60, yet maintaining SaO_2 with high PEEP. Recent studies assessing high and low levels of PEEP found no mortality benefit.
2. Non-ventilatory respiratory support techniques such as $ECCO_2R$ can be used in severe ARDS, but have yet to show convincing benefit over conventional ventilatory techniques.
3. Blood gas values should be aimed at maintaining survival without striving to necessarily achieve normality. Permissive hypercapnia, where $PaCO_2$ values are allowed to rise, sometimes >10kPa, is controversial; in general, values 93–98% are targeted, but in severe ARDS, this may be progressively relaxed to 80–85% or even lower, provided organ function remains adequate.
4. Patient positioning may improve gas exchange. This includes kinetic therapy using special rotational beds, and prone positioning with the patient turned frequently through 180°. Care must be taken during turning to prevent tube displacement and shoulder injuries.
5. Inhaled nitric oxide or epoprostenol improves gas exchange in some 50% of patients though no outcome benefit has been shown.
6. High-dose corticosteroids are beneficial in 50–60% of patients, at least in terms of improving gas exchange.
7. Surfactant therapy is currently not indicated for ARDS.
8. Neutral fluid balance (after initial resuscitation) improves outcomes.
9. Ventilator trauma is ubiquitous. Multiple pneumothoraces may occur and may require multiple chest drains. They may be difficult to diagnose by X-ray and, despite the attendant risks, CT scanning may reveal undiagnosed pneumothoraces and aid drain placement.

Key papers

Hickling KG, Walsh J, Henderson S, et al. (1994) Low mortality rate in adult respiratory distress syndrome using low-volume, pressure-limited ventilation with permissive hypercapnia: a prospective study. *Crit Care Med* **22**: 1568–78.

Meduri GU, HeadLey AS, Golden E, et al. (1998) Effect of prolonged methylprednisolone therapy in unresolving acute respiratory distress syndrome: a randomised controlled trial. *JAMA* **280**: 159–65.

Acute Respiratory Distress Syndrome Network. (2000) Ventilation with lower tidal volumes compared with traditional tidal volumes for acute lung injury and the acute respiratory distress syndrome. *N Engl J Med* **342**: 1301–8.

Gattinoni L, for the Prone-Supine Study Group. (2001) Effect of prone positioning on the survival of patients with acute respiratory failure. *N Engl J Med* **345**: 568–73.

NHLBI Acute Respiratory Distress Syndrome (ARDS) Clinical Trials Network. (2006) Comparison of two fluid-management strategies in acute lung injury. *N Engl J Med* **354**: 2564–75.

Meade MO, for the Lung Open Ventilation Study Investigators. (2008) Ventilation strategy using low tidal volumes, recruitment manoeuvres, and high positive end-expiratory pressure for acute lung injury and acute respiratory distress syndrome: a randomised controlled trial. *JAMA* **299**: 637–45.

Mercat A, Richard J-C, Vielle B, et al. (2008) Positive end-expiratory pressure setting in adults with acute lung injury and adult respiratory distress syndrome. *JAMA* **299**: 646–55.

See also:

Oxygen therapy, p38; Ventilatory support—Indications, p44; IPPV—adjusting the ventilator, p50; IPPV—complications of ventilation, p56; High frequency oscillatory ventilation, p64; Positive end expiratory pressure (1), p66; Positive end expiratory pressure (2), p68; Lung recruitment, p72; Prone positioning, p74; Extracorporeal respiratory support, p78; Blood gas analysis, p154; Extravascular lung water measurement, p156; Nitric oxide, p258; Surfactant, p260; Corticosteroids, p328; Acute respiratory distress syndrome (1), p360; Pneumothorax, p368.

Asthma—general management

Pathophysiology

Acute bronchospasm and mucus plugging are often secondary to an insult such as infection. The patient may progress to fatigue, respiratory failure, and collapse. The onset may develop slowly over days or occur rapidly within minutes to hours.

Clinical features

- Dyspnoea, wheeze (expiratory ± inspiratory), difficulty in talking, use of accessory respiratory muscles, fatigue, agitation, cyanosis, coma, collapse.
- Pulsus paradoxus is a poor indication of severity; a fatiguing patient cannot generate significant respiratory swings in intrathoracic pressure.
- A 'silent' chest is also a late sign suggesting severely limited airflow.
- Pneumothorax and lung/lobar collapse.

Management of asthma

Asthmatics must be managed in a well-monitored area. If clinical features are severe, they should be admitted to an intensive care unit where rapid institution of mechanical ventilation is available. Monitoring should comprise, as a minimum, pulse oximetry, continuous ECG, regular blood pressure measurement, and blood gas analysis. If severe, an intra-arterial cannula ± central venous access should be inserted.

1. FIO_2 to maintain SpO_2 92–98%.
2. Nebulised β_2-agonist (e.g. salbutamol)—may be repeated every 2–4h or, in severe attacks, administered continuously.
3. IV corticosteroids for 24h, then oral prednisolone. Nebulised ipratropium bromide rarely gives additional benefit and may thicken sputum.
4. IV bronchodilators, e.g. salbutamol, magnesium sulphate.
5. Exclude pneumothorax and lung/lobar collapse.
6. Ensure adequate hydration and fluid replacement.
7. Commence antibiotics (e.g. cefuroxime ± clarithromycin) if strong evidence of bacterial chest infection. Green sputum does not necessarily indicate a bacterial infection.
8. If no response to above measures or *in extremis*, consider:
- IV salbutamol infusion.
- Epinephrine SC or by nebuliser.
- Mechanical ventilation.
- Anecdotal success has been reported with sub-anaesthetic doses of a volatile anaesthetic agent such as isoflurane or sevoflurane which both calm/sedate and bronchodilate.

Indications for mechanical ventilation

- Increasing fatigue.
- Respiratory failure—rising $PaCO_2$, falling PaO_2.
- Cardiovascular collapse.

Facilitating endotracheal intubation

Summon senior assistance. Pre-oxygenate with 100% O_2. Perform rapid sequence induction. 'Breathing down' with an inhalational anaesthetic (e.g. isoflurane) pre-intubation should only be attempted by an experienced clinician. To minimise barotrauma, care should be taken to avoid excess air trapping, high airway pressures, and high tidal volumes.

Drug dosages

Epinephrine	0.5mL 1:1000 solution SC or 2mL 1:10000 solution by nebuliser
Hydrocortisone	100–200mg qds
Ipratropium bromide	250–500mcg qds by nebuliser
Prednisolone	40–60mg od initially
Salbutamol	2.5–5mg by nebuliser 5–20mcg/min by IV infusion
Magnesium sulphate	1.2–2.0g IV over 20min

Key paper

British Thoracic Society Scottish Intercollegiate Guidelines Network. (2008) British Guideline on the Management of Asthma. *Thorax* **63** (Suppl 4): 1–121.

See also:

Oxygen therapy, p38; Endotracheal intubation, p42; Ventilatory support—indications, p44; Pulmonary function tests, p148; Blood gas analysis, p154; Bronchodilators, p254; Antimicrobials, p326; Corticosteroids, p328; Asthma—ventilatory management, p366; Pneumothorax, p368.

Asthma—ventilatory management

1. Initially give low V_T (5mL/kg) breaths at low rate (5–10/min) to assess degree of bronchospasm and air trapping. Slowly increase V_T (to 6–7mL/kg) ± increase rate, taking care to avoid significant air trapping and high inspiratory pressures. Low rates with prolonged I:E ratio (e.g. 1:1) may be advantageous. Avoid very short expiratory times. Do not strive to achieve normocapnia.

2. Administer muscle relaxants for a minimum 2–4h until severe bronchospasm has abated and gas exchange improved. Although atracurium may cause histamine release, it does not appear clinically to worsen bronchospasm.

3. Sedate with either standard medication or with agents such as ketamine or isoflurane that have bronchodilating properties. Ketamine given alone may cause hallucinations while isoflurane carries a theoretical risk of fluoride toxicity and can excessively vasodilate.

4. If significant air trapping remains, consider ventilator disconnection and forced manual chest compressions every 10–15min.

5. If severe bronchospasm persists, consider injecting 1–2mL of 1:10000 epinephrine down ET tube. Repeat at 5min intervals as necessary.

Maintenance

1. Ensure adequate rehydration.

2. Generous humidification should be given to loosen mucus plugs. Use a heat-moisture exchanger plus either hourly 0.9% saline nebulisers or instillation of 5mL 0.9% saline down the endotracheal tube or a hot water bath humidifier.

3. Physiotherapy assists mobilisation of secretions and removal of mucus plugs. Hyperventilation should be avoided.

4. With improvement, gradually normalise ventilator settings (VT, rate, I:E ratio) to achieve normocapnia before allowing patient to waken and breathe spontaneously.

5. If acute deterioration, consider pneumothorax or lung/lobar collapse.

6. If mucus plugging constitutes a major problem, instillation of a mucolytic (N-acetylcysteine) may be considered though this may induce further bronchospasm. Bronchoscopic removal of plugs should only be performed by an experienced operator.

Assessment of air trapping (intrinsic PEEP, PEEPi)

- Measure PEEPi by pressing end-expiratory hold button of ventilator.
- No pause between expiratory and inspiratory sounds.
- Disconnection of ventilator and timing of audible expiratory wheeze.
- An increasing $PaCO_2$ may respond to reductions in minute volume which will lower the level of intrinsic PEEP.

Weaning

- Bronchospasm may increase on lightening sedation due to awareness of ET tube and increased coughing.
- May need trial of extubation while still on high FIO_2.
- Consider extubation under inhalational or short-acting IV sedation.
- Space out intervals between β$_2$-agonist nebulisers. Convert other anti-asthmatic drugs to oral medication. Theophylline dose (if used) should be adjusted to ensure therapeutic levels.

See also:

Ventilatory support—indications, p44; IPPV—modes of ventilation, p48; IPPV—adjusting the ventilator, p50; IPPV—failure to deliver ventilation, p54; IPPV—complications of ventilation, p56; IPPV—weaning techniques, p58; Positive end expiratory pressure (1), p66; Positive end expiratory pressure (2), p68; Chest physiotherapy, p90; Sedatives and tranquilisers, p308; Muscle relaxants, p310.

Pneumothorax

Significant collection of air in the pleural space that may occur spontane-ously or following trauma (including iatrogenic), asthma, and chronic lung disease. It is a common result of ventilator trauma.

Clinical features

- May be asymptomatic.
- Dyspnoea, pain.
- Decreased breath sounds, hyper-resonant, asymmetric chest expansion—may be difficult to assess in a ventilated patient.
- Respiratory failure and deterioration in gas exchange.
- Increasing airway pressures and difficulty to ventilate.
- Cardiovascular deterioration with mediastinal shift (tension).

Diagnosis

Chest X-ray—most easily seen on erect views where absent lung mark-ings are seen lateral to a well-defined lung border. Tension pneumo-thorax results in marked mediastinal shift away from the affected side. Pneumothorax must be distinguished from bullae, especially with long-standing emphysema; inadvertent drainage of a bulla may cause a bron-chopleural fistula. Advice should be sought from a radiologist.

Since ventilated patients are often imaged in a supine position, pneu-mothorax may be missed as it may be anterior to normal lung, giving lung markings on the radiograph. A lateral chest X-ray may help. Supine pneu-mothorax should be considered if the following are seen (see figure 22.3):
- Hyperlucent lung field compared to the contralateral side.
- Loss of clarity of the diaphragm outline.
- 'Deep sulcus' sign, giving the appearance of an inverted diaphragm.
- A particularly clear part of the cardiac contour.

Ultrasound—may be helpful but is operator-dependent.

CT scan—very sensitive and may be useful in difficult situations, e.g. ARDS, and to direct drainage of a localised pneumothorax.

Management

1. Increase FIO_2 if hypoxaemic.
2. If life-threatening with circulatory collapse, aspirate air on affected side with a needle, followed by formal chest drain insertion.
3. Repeated needle aspiration may be sufficient in spontaneously breath-ing patients without respiratory failure.
4. Chest drain insertion. This may need to be done under ultrasound or CT guidance if localised due to surrounding lung fibrosis.

A small pneumothorax (<10% hemithorax) may be left undrained, but prompt action should be instituted if cardiorespiratory deterioration occurs. Patients should not be transferred between hospitals, particularly by aeroplane, with an undrained pneumothorax. Drains may be removed if not swinging/bubbling for several days.

Bronchopleural fistula

Denoted by continual drainage of air. Usually responds to conservative treatment with continual application of 5kPa negative pressure; this may take weeks to resolve. For severe leak and/or compromised ventilation, high frequency jet ventilation and/or a double-lumen endobronchial tube may be considered. Surgical intervention is rarely necessary.

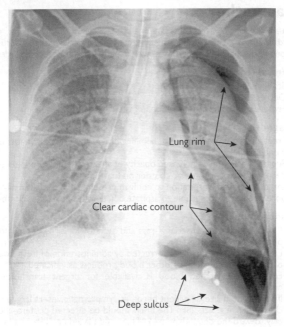

Fig 22.3. Chest X-ray appearance.

See also:
Chest drain insertion, p84; Respiratory imaging, p158; Dyspnoea, p346; Respiratory failure, p350.

Haemothorax

Usually secondary to chest trauma or following a procedure, e.g. cardiac surgery, chest drain insertion, central venous catheter insertion. Spontaneous haemothorax is rare, even in patients with clotting disorders.

Clinical features

- Stony dullness.
- Decreased breath sounds.
- Hypovolaemia and deterioration in gas exchange (if large).

Diagnosis

- Erect chest X-ray—blunting of hemidiaphragm and progressive loss of basal lung field.
- Supine chest X-ray—increased opacity of affected hemithorax plus decreased clarity of cardiac contour on that side.
- Large-bore needle aspiration to confirm presence of blood. A small-bore needle may be unable to aspirate a haemothorax if it has clotted.

Management

1. If small, observe with serial X-rays and monitor for signs of cardiorespiratory deterioration.
2. Ensure any coagulopathy is corrected by administration of fresh frozen plasma and/or platelets or other blood products as indicated.
3. Ensure crossmatched blood is available for urgent transfusion if necessary.
4. If significant in size or patient becomes symptomatic, insert large-bore chest drain, e.g. size 28Fr. The drain should be directed postero-inferiorly toward the dependent area of lung and placed on 5kPa suction.
5. If drainage exceeds 1000mL or >200mL/h for 3–4h despite correcting any coagulopathy, contact a thoracic surgeon.
6. Factor VIIa may be considered for intractable bleeding though only anecdotal reports of benefit exist.
7. Drains inserted for a haemothorax may be removed after 1–2 days if no further bleeding occurs.

Perforation of an intercostal vessel during chest drain insertion may cause considerable bleeding into the pleura. If deep tension sutures around the chest drain fail to stem blood loss, remove the chest drain and insert a Foley urethral catheter through the hole. Inflate the balloon and apply traction on the catheter to tamponade the bleeding vessel. If these measures fail, contact a thoracic surgeon.

See also:

Chest drain insertion, p84; Coagulants and antifibrinolytics, p322; Bleeding disorders, p468;
Multiple trauma (1), p582; Multiple trauma (2), p584.

Haemoptysis

- May range from a few specks of blood in expectorated sputum to massive pulmonary haemorrhage.
- Likely to disrupt gas exchange before hypovolaemia is life-threatening.
- May be a presenting feature of a patient admitted to intensive care or may result from critical illness and its treatment.

Causes

Massive haemoptysis

- Disruption of a bronchial artery by acute inflammation or invasion (e.g. pulmonary neoplasm, trauma, cavitating TB, bronchiectasis, lung abscess, and aspergilloma).
- Rupture of arterio-venous malformations and bronchovascular fistulae.
- Pulmonary infarction secondary to prolonged pulmonary artery catheter wedging or pulmonary artery rupture.

Minor haemoptysis

- Intrapulmonary inflammation or infarction (e.g. pulmonary embolus).
- Endotracheal tube trauma (e.g. mucosal erosion, balloon necrosis, trauma from the tube tip, trauma to a tracheostomy stoma, trauma from suction catheters).
- Tissue breakdown in critically ill patients (e.g. tissue hypoperfusion, coagulopathy, poor nutritional state, sepsis, and hypoxaemia).

Investigation and assessment

Assess cardiorespiratory function and monitor closely. Massive haemoptysis may require resuscitation and urgent intubation. The diagnosis may be suggested by the history and a chest X-ray may identify a cavitating lesion. Lower lobe shadowing on a chest X-ray may be the result of overspill of blood from elsewhere in the bronchial tree. Early surgical intervention should be prompted by a changing air-fluid level, persistent opacification of a previous cavity, or a mobile mass. Early bronchoscopy may identify the source of haemoptysis although only while bleeding is active. Blood in multiple bronchial orifices may be confusing but saline lavage may leave the source visible. Rigid bronchoscopy is useful in massive haemoptysis allowing oxygenation and wide bore suction.

Management

- Basic resuscitation (high FIO_2, endotracheal intubation, and blood transfusion) is needed for cardiorespiratory compromise.
- Correction of coagulopathy is a priority.
- Bronchoscopy allows direct instillation of 1 in 200,000 epinephrine if the source of haemorrhage can be found or, alternatively, endobronchial tamponade with a balloon catheter.
- In cases of severe haemorrhage from one lung, a double-lumen endotracheal tube may prevent some overspill to the other lung while definitive treatment is organised.
- Definitive treatment may include radiological bronchial artery embolisation or surgical resection.
- Induced hypotension may be useful in bronchial artery haemorrhage.
- In cases of pulmonary artery haemorrhage, PEEP may be used with mechanical ventilation to reduce pulmonary bleeding.

See also:

Positive end expiratory pressure (1), p66; Positive end expiratory pressure (2), p68; Continuous positive airway pressure, p70; Fibreoptic bronchoscopy, p88; Coagulation monitoring, p222.

Inhalation injury

Causes include smoke, steam, noxious gases, and aspiration of gastric contents.

Clinical features

- Dyspnoea, coughing.
- Stridor (if upper airway obstruction).
- Bronchospasm.
- Signs of lung/lobar collapse (especially with aspiration).
- Signs of respiratory failure.
- Cherry-red skin colour (carbon monoxide).
- Agitation, coma.
- ARDS (late).

General principles of management

1. High flow, high concentration O_2 targeting an SaO_2 of 92–98%.
2. Early intubation if upper airway is compromised or threatened.
3. Early bronchoscopy if inhalation of soot, debris, vomit suspected.

Specific conditions

Smoke inhalation

- Smoke rarely causes thermal injury beyond the major bronchi as it has a low specific heat content. However, soot is a major irritant to the upper airways and can produce very rapid and marked inflammation.
- Urgent laryngoscopy should be performed if soot is present in the nares, mouth, or pharynx.
- If soot is seen or the larynx appears inflamed, perform early endotracheal intubation. As the upper airway can obstruct within minutes, it is advisable to intubate as a prophylactic measure rather than as an emergency where it may prove impossible.
- After intubation, perform urgent bronchoscopy with bronchial toilet using warmed 0.9% saline to remove as much soot as possible.
- Commence benzylpenicillin 1.2gqds IV.
- Specific treatment for poisons contained within smoke (e.g. carbon monoxide, cyanide).

Steam inhalation

- Consider early/prophylactic intubation.
- Steam has a much higher heat content than smoke and can cause injury to the whole respiratory tract.
- Consider early bronchoscopy and lavage with cool 0.9% saline.

Aspiration of gastric contents

- Early bronchoscopy and physiotherapy to remove as much particulate and liquid matter as possible.
- Either cefuroxime plus metronidazole, or clindamycin for 3–5 days. Some authorities argue that antibiotics are unnecessary.
- Corticosteroid therapy has no proven benefit.

See also:
Fibreoptic bronchoscopy, p88; Antimicrobials, p326; Basic resuscitation, p338; Inhaled poisons, p534; Burns—fluid management, p592; Burns—general management, p594.

Pulmonary embolus

- Usually arises from a DVT in femoral or pelvic veins. Risk increases with prolonged immobility, polycythaemia, or hyperviscosity disorders.
- Amniotic fluid embolus.
- Fat embolus after pelvic or long bone trauma.
- Right heart source, e.g. mural thrombus.

Clinical features

- Pleuritic-type chest pain, dyspnoea ± haemoptysis.
- The patient with a major embolus often prefers to lie flat. Dyspnoea improves due to increased venous return and right heart loading.
- Deterioration in gas exchange: may find a low PaO_2, low or high $PaCO_2$, and a metabolic acidosis.
- Cardiovascular features, e.g. tachycardia, low/high BP, and collapse.
- Chest X-ray: may be normal but a massive embolus may produce fewer vascular markings (pulmonary oligaemia) in a hemithorax ± a bulging pulmonary hilum. A wedge-shaped peripheral pulmonary infarct may be seen after a few days following a smaller embolus.
- ECG: acute right ventricular strain, i.e. $S_1Q_3T_3$, tachycardia, right axis deviation, right bundle branch block, P pulmonale.
- Echocardiogram: may reveal evidence of pulmonary hypertension and acute right ventricular strain. A large embolus may be visualised.
- D-dimers: a normal value probably excludes a pulmonary embolus.

Definitive diagnosis

- CT scan with contrast: the investigation of choice for major embolus.
- Echocardiography: may identify embolus.
- Pulmonary angiography.
- Ventilation-perfusion scan: degree of certainty is reduced if area of non-perfused lung corresponds to any chest X-ray abnormality.
- Fat globules or fetal cells in pulmonary artery blood may be found in fat and amniotic fluid embolus, respectively.

General management

1. FIO_2 0.6–1.0 to maintain SaO_2 93–98%.
2. Lie patient flat to increase venous return.
3. Fluid challenge to optimise right heart filling.
4. Epinephrine infusion if circulation still compromised.
5. Mechanical ventilation may be needed. Gas exchange may worsen due to loss of preferential shunting and decreases in cardiac output.

Management of blood clot embolus

Start anticoagulation with low molecular weight heparin adjusted for weight. Consider thrombolysis if there is a major embolus and cardio-vascular compromise, and embolectomy if the patient remains moribund. Otherwise, at 24–48h, commence warfarinisation regimen but continue heparin for further 2–3 days after adequate oral dosing.

Management of fat embolus

Other than general measures including oxygenation, fluid resuscitation, and right heart loading, treatment remains controversial. Various authorities advocate corticosteroids, heparinisation, or no specific therapy.

Drug dosages

Low molecular weight heparin regimens

Subcutaneous low molecular weight heparin is given until oral anticoagulant therapy is fully established.

Dalteparin: 200 units/kg (max. 18,000 units) every 24h (or 100 units/kg twice daily if increased risk of haemorrhage)

Enoxaparin: 1mg/kg 12-hourly or 1.5mg/kg (150 units/kg) every 24h

Tinzaparin: 175 anti-Xa units/kg once daily

Unfractionated heparin regimen

IV heparin is given until oral anticoagulant therapy is fully established.

80 units/kg bolus (do not exceed 8,000 units initial bolus) followed by 18 unit/kg/h (not to exceed 1,800 units/h) titrated to achieve APTT 2–3x normal.

Thrombolytic regimens

rtPA: (100mg over 90min) should be given followed by a heparin infusion (24,000–36,000 units/d) to maintain the partial thromboplastin time at 2–3x normal. This is the treatment of choice if surgery or angiography is contemplated.

Streptokinase (500,000 units as a loading dose over 30min followed by 100,000 units/h for 24h).

NB. Central venous catheters should ideally be inserted pre-thrombolysis by an experienced operator to minimise the risk of bleeding/haematoma.

Key papers

Task Force Report of the European Society of Cardiology. (2000) Guidelines on diagnosis and management of acute pulmonary embolism. *Eur Heart J* **21**: 1301–66.

Konstantinides S, for the Management Strategies and Prognosis of Pulmonary Embolism-3 Trial Investigators. (2002) Heparin plus alteplase compared with heparin alone in patients with submassive pulmonary embolism. *N Engl J Med* **347**: 1143–50.

British Thoracic Society guidelines for the management of suspected acute pulmonary embolism. (2003) *Thorax* **58**: 470–84.

See also:

Ventilatory support—indications, p44; Blood gas analysis, p154; Coagulation monitoring, p222; Anticoagulants, p318; Thrombolytics, p320; Basic resuscitation, p338; Cardiac arrest, p340.

Cardiovascular disorders

Hypotension

The overall management aim is to maintain a minimum mean arterial pressure that will ensure adequate tissue perfusion. This will vary between patients so individual titration is necessary. A normal BP does not guarantee an adequate cardiac output; circulatory support should aim to achieve adequate blood flow as well as an adequate pressure. For patients *in extremis*, first-line treatment options should include external cardiac massage and epinephrine 0.05–0.2mg IV boluses (1mg in cardiac arrest). BP elevation should not be excessive as this may compromise tissue perfusion.

Assessment of hypotension

Hypotension requires treatment if there are signs of poor tissue perfusion (e.g. oliguria, confusion, altered consciousness, cool peripheries, metabolic acidosis). This will usually be at mean BP <60mmHg (higher if patient has a hypertension history) with xxx Specific treatment should be given for the underlying cause, e.g. haemorrhage, acute myocardial infarction, arrhythmias, pulmonary embolus, sepsis, and poisoning.

Initial treatment of hypotension

Most cases require fluid as first-line management to restore an adequate circulating volume. Exceptions may include acute heart failure, arrhythmias, cardiac tamponade, and pneumothorax. In cases of severe haemorrhage, blood should be used as soon as available; if life-threatening, group specific or O negative blood should be used considered.

Pharmacological treatment

If hypotension persists after restoring an adequate circulating volume, the appropriate choice of drug treatment depends on whether there is myocardial failure (signs of low cardiac output or known measured low stroke volume) or peripheral vascular failure (warm, vasodilated periphery, or measured normal/high stroke volume). A low stroke volume should be treated with an inotropic agent (e.g. epinephrine, dobutamine) and peripheral vascular failure with a vasopressor (e.g. norepinephrine).

Inotropic support

Most hypotensive patients requiring inotropes (epinephrine, dopamine, or dobutamine) should have flow monitoring. Titrating against BP alone carries the danger of inappropriate vasoconstriction and reduced cardiac output. The agent should be titrated against stroke volume as tachycardia may maintain output. Dobutamine and PDE inhibitors (e.g. milrinone) can cause excessive vasodilatation and hypotension.

Vasopressors

Once stroke volume has been corrected, norepinephrine (or high-dose dopamine) should be titrated against mean BP. In most patients, 60mmHg is an adequate target, but may need to be higher to ensure organ perfusion in the elderly and previous hypertensives. Pressors may reduce cardiac output. This effect should be monitored and corrected by adjustment of dose. Vasopressin (or its synthetic analogue, terlipressin) is increasingly used for high output, catecholamine-resistant, vasodilatory shock. Care should be taken to avoid excessive peripheral constriction or impairment of organ perfusion.

Drug dosages

Epinephrine	Infusion starting from 0.05mcg/kg/min
Dobutamine	Infusion from 2.5–25mcg/kg/min
Dopamine	Infusion from 2.5–30mcg/kg/min
Norepinephrine	Infusion starting from 0.05mcg/kg/min
Vasopressin	0.01–0.04U/min for sepsis
Terlipressin	0.25–0.5mg bolus, repeated at 30min intervals as necessary to maximum 2mg

Key papers

Russell JA, for the VASST Investigators. (2008) Vasopressin versus norepinephrine infusion in patients with septic shock. *N Engl J Med* **358**: 877–87.

Annane D, for the CATS Study Group. (2007) Norepinephrine plus dobutamine versus epinephrine alone for management of septic shock: a randomised trial. *Lancet* **370**: 676–84.

See also:

Intra-aortic balloon counterpulsation, p102; Blood pressure monitoring, p164; Arterial cannulation, p166; Colloids, p246; Inotropes, p264; Vasopressors, p268; Basic resuscitation, p338; Cardiac arrest, p340; Fluid challenge, p348; Pneumothorax, p368; Haemothorax, p370; Pulmonary embolus, p376; Acute coronary syndrome (1), p300; Acute coronary syndrome (2), p390; Heart failure—assessment, p392; Upper gastrointestinal haemorrhage, p412; Bleeding varices, p414; Intra-abdominal bowel perforation and obstruction, p418; Lower intestinal bleeding and colitis, p420; Abdominal sepsis, p422; Pancreatitis, p424; Sepsis and septic shock—treatment, p560; Multiple trauma (1), p582; Spinal cord injury, p590; Burns—fluid management, p592; Post-partum haemorrhage, p638; Amniotic fluid embolus, p640.

Hypertension

Often defined in adult patients as a diastolic pressure >95mmHg and a systolic pressure >180mmHg.

Common causes in intensive care

- Idiopathic/essential.
- Agitation/pain, especially where muscle relaxants are used.
- Excessive vasoconstriction, e.g. cold, vasopressor drugs.
- Head injury, cerebrovascular accidents.
- Drug-related.
- Dissecting aneurysm, aortic coarctation.
- Vasculitis, thrombotic thrombocytopaenic purpura.
- (Pre-)eclampsia.
- Aortic coarctation (may present acutely in adulthood).
- Endocrine, e.g. phaeochromocytoma (rare).
- Renal failure, renal artery stenosis (rare).
- Spurious—underdamped transducer system.

Indications for acute treatment

Hypertensive encephalopathy, heart failure, eclampsia, and acute dissecting aneurysm are the prime indications for rapid and aggressive, albeit controlled, reduction of blood pressure.

In other conditions, especially chronic hypertension and following acute neurological events, e.g. head injury, cerebrovascular accidents, a rapid reduction in BP may adversely affect perfusion. Hypertension after a cerebral event is not usually treated unless very high, e.g. mean BP >140–150mmHg, systolic BP >220–230mmHg. In this instance, controlled and partial reduction is mandatory, e.g. with sodium nitroprusside infusion with continuous invasive monitoring. In the presence of a raised ICP, a cerebral perfusion pressure ≥60–70mmHg is usually targeted.

Hypertensive crisis

Occurs when symptomatic (increasing drowsiness, seizures, papilloedema, retinopathy) in the presence of elevated systemic pressures. The diastolic BP usually exceeds 120–130mmHg and the mean BP >140–150mmHg, although encephalopathy can occur at lower pressures.

Principles of management

1. Adequate monitoring (invasive BP, ECG, CVP, cardiac output, urine output).
2. Consider pain, hypovolaemia, hypothermia, and agitation.
3. Consider specific treatment, e.g. phaeochromocytoma, thyroid crisis, aortic dissection, inflammatory vasculitis.
4. Slow intravenous infusion of nitrate or nitroprusside. Other options include labetalol or esmolol infusions, hydralazine (IV or IM). Sublingual nifedipine or IV hydralazine may sometimes produce precipitate falls in BP. Use cautiously and start with low doses.
5. Aim to reduce to mildly hypertensive levels unless dissecting aneurysm where systolic BP should be lowered <100–110mmHg. After certain types of surgery (e.g. cardiac, aortic), control of systolic BP <100–120mmHg may be requested to reduce risk of bleeding.
6. Longer-term oral treatment, e.g. calcium channel blocker, ACE inhibitor, should be instituted.

Drug dosages

GTN	0.5–20mg/h
Sodium nitroprusside	0.5–1.5mcg/kg/min, increased slowly to 0.5–8mcg/kg/min
Labetalol	50mg IV over 1min repeated every 5min to maximum 200mg
Metoprolol	5mg slow IV or 0–0.1mg/kg/h
Esmolol	50–200mcg/kg/min
Hydralazine	5–10mg slow IV, followed by 50–150mcg/min

See also:

Tachyarrhythmias

If pulses are not palpable or there is severe hypotension, a tachyarrhythmia requires cardiac massage and urgent DC cardioversion. Otherwise, the initial treatment prior to diagnosis includes correction of hypoxaemia, potassium (to ensure a plasma K^+ 4.5–5.8mmol/L) and magnesium (targeting plasma levels of 1.5–2mmol/L).

Causes of tachyarrhythmias

Where possible, the cause should be treated. Specific treatment should be given as appropriate, e.g. for hypovolaemia, hypotension (may also be due to the arrhythmia), acute myocardial infarction, pain, anaemia, hypercapnia, fever, anxiety, thyrotoxicosis, and digoxin toxicity.

Diagnosis

Broad complex tachycardia

Assumed to be ventricular tachycardia (VT) until proven otherwise (e.g. slows with adenosine). Regular complexes with AV dissociation (fusion beats, capture beats, QRS >140ms, axis <–30°, concordance) suggest VT. If there is no AV dissociation, the arrhythmia is probably supraventricular with aberrant conduction; adenosine may be used as a diagnostic test since SVT may respond and VT will not. Irregular broad complexes are probably atrial fibrillation with aberration. Torsades de pointes are a form of ventricular tachycardia with a variable axis.

Narrow complex tachycardia

The absence of P waves suggests atrial fibrillation. A P wave rate >150 suggests SVT, whereas slower rates may represent sinus tachycardia or atrial flutter with block. P waves are abnormal (flutter waves) in atrial flutter and QRS complexes may be irregular in variable block. Extremely fast SVT may be due to a re-entry pathway with retrograde conduction and premature ectopic atrial excitation. In Wolff Parkinson White syndrome, the re-entry pathway inserts below the His bundle allowing rapid AV conduction and re-entry tachyarrhythmias. Prior to onset of the arrhythmia, there may be a short PR interval and a delta wave.

Treatment

Ventricular tachycardia

Lidocaine, amiodarone, or magnesium is the mainstay of drug treatment. Overdrive pacing may be used if a pacing wire is *in situ*, capturing the ventricle at a pacing rate higher than the arrhythmia and gradually reducing the pacing rate. Torsades de pointes may be exacerbated by anti-arrhythmics so magnesium or overdrive pacing are safest.

Supraventricular tachycardia and atrial flutter

Carotid sinus massage may be used in patients with no risk of calcified atheromatous carotid deposits. Amiodarone, adenosine, or magnesium is usually the most useful drugs in the critically ill. Verapamil may be used if complexes are narrow (no risk of misdiagnosed ventricular tachycardia) although this drug and other AV node blockers should be avoided in re-entry tachycardias.

Atrial fibrillation

If onset <48 hours, cardiovert, especially if haemodynamic compromise. If rate control desired, β-blockers are first-line; digoxin has a secondary role.

Drug dosages and cautions

Adenosine	6mg IV as a rapid bolus. If no response in 1min give 12mg followed by a repeat 12mg.
Verapamil	2.5mg IV slowly. If no response, repeat to a maximum of 20mg. An IV infusion of 1–10mg may be used. 10mL $CaCl_2$ 10% should be available to treat hypotension associated with verapamil. Verapamil should be avoided in re-entry tachyarrhythmias since ventricular response may increase. Life-threatening hypotension may occur in misdiagnosed ventricular tachycardia and life-threatening bradycardia may occur if the patient has been β-blocked.
Lidocaine	1mg/kg IV as a bolus, followed by an infusion of 2–4mg/min.
Amiodarone	5mg/kg over 20min, then infused at up to 15mg/kg/24h in 5% glucose via a central vein. Avoid with other class III agents (e.g. sotalol) since QT interval may be severely prolonged.
Magnesium	20mmol $MgSO_4$ over 2–3h. In an emergency it may be given over 5min.

See also:

Electrical cardioversion, p94; ECG monitoring, p162; Electrolytes (Na^+, K^+, CT, HCO_3^-), p212; Antiarrhythmics, p272; Basic resuscitation, p338.

Bradyarrhythmias

If peripheral pulses are not palpable, a bradyarrhythmia requires external cardiac massage and treatment as for asystole. For asymptomatic brady-cardia, treatment may not be required other than close monitoring and correction of the cause. The exception to this is higher degrees of heart block occurring after an acute anterior myocardial infarction where pacing may be required prophylactically.

Causes

Where possible, treat the cause. Common causes for which specific treat-ment may be required include hypovolaemia, hyperkalaemia, hypotension (may also be due to the arrhythmia), acute myocardial infarction, digoxin toxicity, β-blocker toxicity, hyperkalaemia, hypothyroidism, hypopitui-tarism, and raised intracranial pressure. Digoxin toxicity may require treat-ment with anti-digoxin antibodies.

Diagnosis

Sinus bradycardia

Slow ventricular rate with normal P waves, normal PR interval, and 1:1 AV conduction.

Heart block

- Normal P waves, a prolonged PR interval, and 1:1 AV conduction suggest 1° heart block.
- In 2° heart block, the ventricles fail to respond to atrial contraction intermittently. This may be associated with regular P waves and an increasing PR interval until ventricular depolarisation fails (Mobitz I or Wenkebach) or a normal PR interval with regular failed ventricular depolarisation (Mobitz II). In the latter case, the AV conduction ratio may be 2:1 or more.
- In 3° heart block, there is complete AV dissociation with a slow, idioventricular rate.

Absent P wave bradycardia

Absent P waves may represent slow atrial fibrillation or sino-atrial dys-function. In the latter case, there will be a slow, idioventricular rate.

Treatment

Hypoxaemia must be corrected in all symptomatic bradycardias. First-line drug treatment is usually atropine 0.3mg or glycopyrronium bromide 200mcg IV. If the arrhythmia fails to respond, 0.6mg followed by 1.0mg atropine may be given. Failure to respond to drugs requires temporary pacing. This may be accomplished rapidly with an external system if there is haemodynamic compromise or by transvenous placement. Other indica-tions for temporary pacing are shown opposite. Higher degrees of heart block after an anterior myocardial infarction will usually require perma-nent pacing.

Indications for temporary pacing
- Persistent symptomatic bradycardia.
- Blackouts associated with:
  - 3° heart block.
  - 2° heart block.
  - RBBB and left posterior hemiblock.
- Cardiovascular collapse.
- Inferior myocardial infarction with symptomatic 3° heart block.
- Anterior myocardial infarction with:
  - 3° heart block.
  - RBBB and left posterior hemiblock.
  - Alternating RBBB and LBBB.

See also:

Temporary pacing (1), p96; Temporary pacing (2), p98; ECG monitoring, p162; Chronotropes, p274; Basic resuscitation, p338.

Acute coronary syndrome (1)

Anginal pain

Ischaemic or, rarely, spasmodic constriction of coronary arteries resulting in pain, usually precordial, pressing or crushing, and ± radiation to jaw, neck, or arms. The sedated, ventilated patient will not usually complain of pain, but signs of discomfort may be apparent, e.g. sweating, hypertension, tachycardia. Regularly scrutinise the ECG for ST segment and/or T wave changes.

A spectrum of severity is present, ranging from stable angina to myocardial infarction. Anginal attacks may have recently increased in frequency and/or severity, persist longer, respond less to nitrates, and occur at rest or after minimal exertion.

Pathophysiology

- Myocardial oxygen supply-demand imbalance usually due to coronary artery atheroma ± disruption of plaque or new non-occlusive thrombus formation. Spasm (Prinzmetal angina) is uncommon.
- Vasopressor drugs may compromise myocardial perfusion by further constricting an already stenosed vessel.
- Vasodilator drugs may also compromise myocardial perfusion by a 'coronary steal' phenomenon where blood flow is re-distributed away from stenosed vessels.

Diagnosis

- Symptoms, especially chest pain but also non-specific, e.g. sweating.
- ECG changes: ST segment elevation/depression, T wave inversion.
- No rise in cardiac enzymes or troponin above the myocardial infarction threshold.
- Dyskinetic areas of myocardium may be seen on echocardiography or angiography.

Treatment

- Ensure adequate oxygenation.
- Correct hypotension and tissue hypoperfusion.
- Consider drug causes, e.g. vasopressors.
- Glyceryl trinitrate (0.5mg SL) or nitrolingual spray (0.4–0.8mg), repeated as necessary.
- If symptoms are severe and/or persisting, maintain bed rest.
- Aspirin 75mg od PO (unless contraindicated).

For continuing angina

- IV nitrate infusion, e.g. glyceryl trinitrate, isosorbide trinitrate.
- Consider β-blocker (unless contraindicated), e.g. metoprolol.
- Consider calcium antagonist if β-blocker contraindicated though not on its own, e.g. diltiazem.
- LMW heparin and clopidogrel (unless contraindicated).
- Consider GP2b3a inhibitor (IV eptifibatide or tirofiban) in addition to aspirin + clopidogrel, if considered at high-risk of MI or death.
- If symptoms or ST segment changes persist despite optimal pharmacological intervention, inform cardiologist with a view to angiography and possible angioplasty or surgery.

Key papers

Yusuf S for the Clopidogrel in Unstable Angina to Prevent Recurrent Events Trial Investigators. (2001) Effects of clopidogrel in addition to aspirin in patients with acute coronary syndromes without ST-segment elevation. *N Engl J Med* **345**: 494–502.

Task Force for Diagnosis and Treatment of Non-ST-Segment Elevation Acute Coronary Syndromes of European Society of Cardiology. (2007) Guidelines for the diagnosis and treatment of non-ST-segment elevation acute coronary syndromes. *Eur Heart J* **28**: 1598–660.

See also:

Coronary revascularisation techniques, p104; ECG monitoring, p162; Echocardiography, p192; Cardiac function tests, p216; Vasodilators, p266; Anti-anginal agents, p276; Acute coronary syndrome (2), p390; Heart failure—assessment, p392.

Acute coronary syndrome (2)

Diagnosis of myocardial infarction
Rise and/or fall of cardiac biomarkers (preferably troponin) above upper reference limit plus evidence of myocardial ischaemia with ≥1 of:
- Symptoms of ischaemia.
- ECG changes of new ischaemia (new ST–T changes or new LBBB).
- Pathological Q waves on ECG.
- New loss of myocardium or new regional wall motion abnormality.

Management of uncomplicated infarction
- Oxygen—to maintain SaO_2 ≥98%.
- Good venous access and continuous ECG monitoring.
- Appropriate and prompt monitoring plus investigations as indicated, e.g. echocardiography, angiography, cardiac output monitoring.
- Adequate pain relief.
- Aspirin.
- Urgent referral for percutaneous coronary intervention (PCI) or, if not available, early thrombolysis.
- Early β-blockade.
- Gradual mobilisation.
- Do not delay arterial or central venous cannulation if clinically indicated. An experienced operator should perform these procedures to minimise the risk of bleeding. Avoid the subclavian route.

Complications of myocardial infarction
- Cardiopulmonary arrest.
- Continuing chest pain—may be ischaemic or pericarditic in origin.
- Pump failure.
- Hypotension—apart from cardiogenic shock, consider hypovolaemia (e.g. post-diuretics) or a reaction to a thrombolytic agent.
- Tachyarrhythmias/bradyarrhythmias.
- Valve dysfunction—predominantly mitral.
- Pericardial tamponade (rare).
- Ventricular septal defect (unusual, often presents 2–5 days later).
- Complications of thrombolytic therapy: arrhythmias, bleeding, hypotension, anaphylactoid reaction.

Management of complicated infarction
In addition to general measures for the uncomplicated infarction:
- Cardiopulmonary arrest—cardiopulmonary resuscitation.
- Continuing ischaemic chest pain—IV nitrate and heparin infusions, aspirin, clopidogrel, calcium antagonist, and β-blocker (unless contraindicated); consider urgent angiography ± stenting or surgery.
- Pericarditic chest pain—consider non-steroidal anti-inflammatory agent.
- Management of heart failure.
- Tachyarrhythmia—anti-arrhythmics, synchronised DC cardioversion.
- Bradycardias—chronotrope, consider temporary pacing.
- Valve dysfunction—heart failure management; consider surgery.
- Pericardial tamponade—pericardial aspiration.
- Ventricular septal defect—heart failure management, consider surgery.
- Management of thrombolysis complications.

Drug dosages

Diamorphine	2.5mg IV. Repeat PRN + anti-emetic
Streptokinase	1.5 million units in 100mL 0.9% saline IV over 1h
rtPA (alteplase)	15mg IV bolus, then 0.75mg/kg over 30min, then 0.5mg/kg over 1h to a maximal dose of 100mg. This is then followed by heparin for 24–48 h.
Tenecteplase	For acute MI: IV bolus of 0.5mg/kg over 10s, followed by heparin for 24–48h.
Reteplase	Two IV boluses of 10U given 30min apart, followed by heparin for 24–48h.
Aspirin	150mg PO od
Clopidogrel	300mg PO loading dose, then 75mg PO od
Atenolol	50mg PO od (increase to 100mg od if not hypotensive and HR exceeds 70bpm) or 5mg slow IV bolus
Propranolol	10–40mg PO qds (titrate to HR of 60bpm)
Isosorbide dinitrate	2–40mg/h IV
GTN	10–200mcg/min IV or 0.5–1mg SL
Diltiazem	60mg PO tds
Nifedipine	5–10mg SL or PO tds
Atropine	0.3mg IV. Repeat to maximum of 2mg
Lidocaine	1mg/kg slow IV bolus, then 2–4mg/min
Amiodarone	5mg/kg over 20min, then infused up to 15mg/kg/d in 5% glucose via central vein. (In emergency, give 150–300mg in 10–20mL 5% glucose over 3min.)

Key papers

Task Force on management of acute myocardial infarction of the European Society of Cardiology. (2003) Management of acute myocardial infarction in patients presenting with ST segment elevation. *Eur Heart J* **24**: 28–66.

Thygesen K for the Joint ESC/ACCF/AHA/WHF Task Force for the Redefinition of Myocardial Infarction. (2007) Universal definition of myocardial infarction. *Circulation* **116**: 2634–53.

See also:

Intra-aortic balloon counterpulsation, p102; Coronary revascularisation techniques, p104; ECG monitoring, p162; Echocardiography, p192; Cardiac function tests, p216; Vasodilators, p266; Anticoagulants, p316; Thrombolytics, p320; Basic resuscitation, p338; Cardiac arrest, p340; Hypotension, p380; Tachyarrhythmias, p384; Bradyarrhythmias, p386; Acute coronary syndrome (1), p388; Heart failure—assessment, p392.

Heart failure—assessment

Impaired ability of the heart to supply adequate oxygen and nutrients to meet the demands of the body's metabolising tissues.

Major causes
- Myocardial infarction/ischaemia.
- Drugs, e.g. β-blockers, cytotoxics.
- Tachyarrhythmias or bradyarrhythmias.
- Valve dysfunction.
- Sepsis.
- Septal defect.
- Cardiomyopathy/myocarditis.
- Pericardial tamponade.

Clinical features

Decreased forward flow leading to poor tissue perfusion
- Muscle fatigue leading ultimately to hypercapnia and collapse.
- Confusion, agitation, drowsiness, coma.
- Oliguria.
- Increasing metabolic acidosis, arterial hypoxaemia, and dyspnoea.

Increased venous congestion secondary to right heart failure
- Peripheral oedema.
- Hepatic congestion.
- Splanchnic ischaemia.
- Raised intracranial pressure.

Increased pulmonary hydrostatic pressure from left heart failure
- Pulmonary oedema, dyspnoea.
- Hypoxaemia.

Investigations

Test	Diagnosis
ECG	Myocardial ischaemia/infarction, arrhythmias
Chest X-ray	With left heart failure: pulmonary oedema (interstitial perihilar ('bat's wing') shadowing, upper lobe blood diversion, Kerley B lines, pleural effusion) ± cardiomegaly
Flow monitoring	Low cardiac output and stroke volume, low mixed venous oxygen saturation (<60%), raised PAWP (with left heart failure), raised RAP (with right heart failure). V waves with mitral or tricuspid regurgitation
Blood tests	Low SaO_2, variable $PaCO_2$, base deficit >2 mmol/L, hyperlactataemia, low venous O_2, (mixed or central venous), raised cardiac enzymes, troponin, BNP, thyroid function (if indicated)
Echocardiogram	Poor myocardial contractility, ventricular akinesia, hypokinesia or dyskinesia, pericardial effusion, valve stenosis or incompetence

Notes
Peripheral oedema implies total body salt and water retention, but not necessarily intravascular fluid overload.

See also:
IPPV—assessment of weaning, p60; Pulse oximetry, p144; Blood gas analysis, p154; Respiratory imaging, p158; ECG monitoring, p162; Blood pressure monitoring, p164; Central venous cateter—use, p170; Cardiac output—central thermodilution, p178; Cardiac output—peripheral thermodilution, p180; Cardiac output—indicator dilution, p182; Cardiac output—Doppler ultrasound, p184; Cardiac output—pulse contour analysis, p186; Cardiac output—other techniques, p188; Echocardiography, p192; Tissue perfusion monitoring, p194; Cardiac function tests, p216; Dyspnoea, p246; Respiratory failure, p350; Hypotension, p380; Tachyarrhythmias, p384; Bradyarrhythmias, p386; Acute coronary syndrome (1), p388; Acute coronary syndrome (2), p390; Heart failure—management, p392.

Heart failure—management

Basic measures

1. Determine likely cause and treat as appropriate, e.g. anti-arrhythmic.
2. Oxygen—to maintain SaO_2 ≥98%.
3. GTN spray SL, then commence IV nitrate infusion titrated rapidly until good clinical effect. Beware hypotension which, at low dosage, is suggestive of left ventricular underfilling, e.g. hypovolaemia, tamponade, mitral stenosis, pulmonary embolus.
4. If patient agitated or in pain, give diamorphine IV.
5. Consider early CPAP, BiPAP, and/or IPPV to reduce work of breathing and provide good oxygenation. Cardiac output will often improve. Do not delay until the patient is *in extremis*.
6. Furosemide is rarely needed as first-line therapy unless intravascular fluid overload is causative. Initial symptomatic relief is provided by its prompt vasodilating action; however, subsequent diuresis may result in marked hypovolaemia leading to compensatory vasoconstriction, increased cardiac work, and worsening myocardial function. Diuretics may be indicated for acute-on-chronic failure, especially if the patient is on long-term diuretic therapy, but should not be used if hypovolaemic. If furosemide is required, start at low doses, then reassess.

Directed management

1. Adequate monitoring (± cardiac output) and investigation (echocardiography).
2. Avoid hypovolaemia (e.g. diuretics given). Fluid challenge if necessary.
3. If vasoconstriction persists (high BP, low cardiac output), titrate nitrate infusion to optimise stroke volume. Allow BP to fall if well-perfused. If hypovolaemia is suspected (i.e. stroke volume falls), give fluid challenges to re-optimise stroke volume. Within 24 hours of nitrate infusion, commence ACE inhibition, initially at low dose but rapidly increased to appropriate long-term doses.
4. Inotropes are needed if tissue hypoperfusion, hypotension, or vasoconstriction persists despite optimal fluid loading and nitrate dosing. Consider epinephrine, dobutamine, or milrinone. Epinephrine may sometimes cause excessive constriction; dobutamine, and milrinone may excessively vasodilate. Levosimendan increases cardiac output through improving contractile efficiency.
5. Intra-aortic balloon counterpulsation augments cardiac output, reduces cardiac work, and improves coronary artery perfusion.
6. Angioplasty or surgical revascularisation is beneficial if performed early after myocardial infarct. Surgery may also be necessary for mechanical defects, e.g. acute mitral regurgitation.

Treatment endpoints

1. BP and cardiac output adequate to maintain organ perfusion (e.g. no oliguria, confusion, dyspnoea nor metabolic acidosis). Avoid treatment of blood pressure if organs are perfused.
2. Mixed (or central) venous oxygen saturation ≥60%. Excessive inotropes should be avoided as myocardial O_2 demand is increased.
3. Symptomatic relief.

Drug dosages

GTN	2–40mg/h IV or 0.4–0.8mg by SL spray
Isosorbide dinitrate	2–40mg/h IV
Nesiritide	2mcg/kg bolus followed by infusion of 0.01–0.03mcg/kg/min
Sodium nitroprusside	20–400mcg/min IV
Captopril	6.25mg PO test dose increasing to 25mg tds
Enalapril	2.5mg PO test dose increasing to 40mg od
Lisinopril	2.5mg PO test dose increasing to 40mg od
Epinephrine	Infusion starting from 0.05mcg/kg/min
Dobutamine	2.5–25mcg/kg/min IV
Dopamine	2.5–25mcg/kg/min IV
Milrinone	Loading dose of 50mcg/kg IV over 10min, followed by infusion from 0.375–0.75mcg/kg/min
Enoximone	Loading dose of 0.5–1mg/kg IV over 10min, followed by infusion from 5–20mcg/kg/min
Levosimendan	12–24 mcg/kg over 10min, followed by 0.1mcg/kg/min for 24h
Diamorphine	2.5mg IV. Repeat every 5min as necessary.
Furosemide	10–20mg IV bolus. Repeat or increase as necessary.

Key papers

Cotter G, Metzkor E, Kaluski E, et al. (1998) Randomised trial of high-dose isosorbide dinitrate plus low-dose furosemide versus high-dose furosemide plus low-dose isosorbide dinitrate in severe pulmonary oedema. Lancet **351**: 389–93.

Cuffe MS, Califf RM, Adams KF, et al. (2000) Rationale and design of the OPTIME CHF trial: outcomes of a prospective trial of intravenous milrinone for exacerbations of chronic heart failure. Am Heart J **139**: 15–22.

Follath F, Cleland JG, Just H, et al. (2002) Efficacy and safety of intravenous levosimendan compared with dobutamine in severe low-output heart failure (the LIDO study): a randomised double-blind trial. Lancet **360**: 196–202.

Nieminen MS, for the ESC Committe for Practice Guideline (CPG). (2005) Executive summary of the guidelines on the diagnosis and treatment of acute heart failure: the Task Force on Acute Heart Failure of the European Society of Cardiology. Eur Heart J **26**: 384–416.

Peter JV, Moran JL, Phillips-Hughes J, et al. (2006) Effect of non-invasive positive pressure ventilation (NIPPV) on mortality in patients with acute cardiogenic pulmonary oedema: a meta-analysis. Lancet **367**: 1155–63.

See also:

Oxygen therapy, p38; Endotracheal intubation, p42; Ventilatory support—indications, p44; Positive end expiratory pressure (1), p66; Positive end expiratory pressure (2), p68; Continuous positive

Renal disorders

Oliguria

Defined as a urine output <0.5mL/kg/h and caused by:
- Post-renal—urinary tract obstruction, e.g. blocked catheter, ureteric trauma, prostatism, raised intra-abdominal pressure, blood clot, bladder tumour.
- Renal—established acute renal failure, acute tubular necrosis (rare), glomerulonephritis.
- Pre-renal—hypovolaemia, low cardiac output, hypotension, inadequate renal blood flow.

Obstruction and pre-renal causes of oliguria must be excluded before resorting to diuretics.

Urinary tract obstruction

A full bladder should be excluded by palpation. Ensure a patent catheter is present. If obstruction is due to blood clot, the bladder should be irrigated. If obstruction is suspected higher in the renal tract, an ultrasound scan is required for diagnosis and possible intervention (e.g. nephrostomies). Raised intra-abdominal pressure may cause oliguria by impeding renal venous drainage (particularly if >20mmHg). Relief of the high pressure often promotes a diuresis.

Hypovolaemia

Once renal tract obstruction is excluded, it is mandatory to correct hypovolaemia by fluid challenge. Oliguria in hypovolaemic patients may be physiological or may be due to a reduced renal blood flow.

Inadequate renal blood flow and/or pressure

If cardiac output remains low despite correcting hypovolaemia, vasodilators and/or inotropes may be needed. If BP remains low after cardiac output is improved, vasopressors may be needed to achieve a mean BP of ≥60mmHg. In the elderly and those with pre-existing hypertension, a higher mean BP may be necessary to maintain urine output.

Persistent oliguria

Attempts to increase urine output with diuretics may follow the above measures if oliguria persists. Furosemide is given at a dose of 5–10mg IV with higher increments at 30min intervals to a maximum of 250mg. High doses or a low-dose infusion (1–5mg/h IV) may be needed if the patient has previously received diuretic.s. Mannitol (20g IV) may be considered though failure to promote diuresis may increase oedema formation. Failure to re-establish urine output may require renal support in the form of dialysis or haemofiltration. There is no point in continuing diuretic therapy if it is not effective; loop diuretics in particular may be nephrotoxic. Indications for renal support include fluid overload, hyperkalaemia, metabolic acidosis, creation of space for nutrition or drugs, persistent renal failure with rising urea and creatinine, and symptomatic uraemia.

Biochemical assessment
(not applicable if furosemide has been given previously)

	Pre-renal cause	Renal cause
Urine osmolality (mOsm/kg)	>500	<400
Urine Na (mmol/L)	<20	>40
Urine : plasma creatinine	>40	<20
Fractional Na excretion*	<1	>2

$$^*100 \times \frac{\text{urine : plasma Na}}{\text{urine : plasma creatinine}}$$

See also:
Urea and creatinine, p210; Electrolytes (Na$^+$, K$^+$, Cl$^-$, HCO$_3^-$), p212; Urinalysis, p232; Basic resuscitation, p338; Fluid challenge, p342; Acute renal failure—diagnosis, p400; Raised intra-abdominal pressure, p614; Post-operative critical care, p620.

Acute renal failure—diagnosis

Renal failure is defined as renal function inadequate to clear the waste products of metabolism despite absence or correction of haemodynamic or mechanical causes. Renal failure is suggested by:
- Uraemic symptoms (drowsiness, nausea, hiccough, twitching).
- Raised plasma creatinine (>200µmol/L).
- Hyperkalaemia.
- Hyponatraemia.
- Metabolic acidosis.

Persistent oliguria may be a feature of acute renal failure, but non-oliguric renal failure is common; 2–3L of poor quality urine per day may occur despite inadequate glomerular filtration. The prognosis is better if urine output is maintained. Clinical features may suggest the cause of renal failure and dictate further investigation. Acute tubular necrosis may occur following rapid loss of perfusion, e.g. major haemorrhage. However, it is a misnomer in renal failure due to sepsis, pancreatitis, etc., as minimal cell death is seen. Anaemia suggests chronic renal failure.

Post-operative renal failure

Risk factors include hypovolaemia, haemodynamic instability (particularly hypotension), major abdominal surgery in those >50 years, major surgery in jaundiced patients, biliary and other sepsis. Surgical procedures (particularly gynaecological) may be complicated by damage to the lower urinary tract with an obstructive nephropathy. Abdominal aortic aneurysm surgery may be associated with renal arterial disruption and should be investigated urgently with renography and possible arteriography or re-exploration.

Other causes

- Nephrotoxins—may cause renal failure via acute tubular necrosis, interstitial nephritis, or renal tubular obstruction. All potential nephrotoxins should be withdrawn.
- Rhabdomyolysis—suggested by myoglobinuria and raised CPK in patients who have suffered a crush injury, coma, or seizures.
- Glomerular disease—red cell casts, haematuria, proteinuria, and systemic features (e.g. hypertension, purpura, arthralgia, vasculitis) are all suggestive of glomerular disease. Renal biopsy or specific blood tests (e.g. Goodpasture's syndrome, vasculitis) are required to confirm diagnosis and appropriate treatment.
- Haemolytic uraemic syndrome—suggested by haemolysis, uraemia, thrombocytopaenia, and neurological abnormalities.
- Crystal nephropathy—suggested by the presence of crystals in the urinary sediment. Microscopic examination of the crystals confirms the diagnosis (e.g. urate, oxalate). Release of purines and urate are responsible for acute renal failure in the tumour lysis syndrome.
- Renovascular disorders—loss of vascular supply may be diagnosed by renography. Complete loss of arterial supply may occur in abdominal trauma or aortic disease (particularly dissection). More commonly, the arterial supply is partially compromised (e.g. renal artery stenosis) and blood flow is further reduced by haemodynamic instability or locally via drug therapy (e.g. NSAIDs, ACE inhibitors). Renal vein obstruction may be due to thrombosis or external compression (e.g. raised intra-abdominal pressure).

Nephrotoxins

The following are some common nephrotoxins:

Allopurinol	Aminoglycosides
Amphotericin	Cephalosporins
Dextran 40	Furosemide
Heavy metals	Herbal medicines
Narcotics	NSAIDs
Organic solvents	Paraquat
Penicillins	Pentamidine
Phenytoin	Radiographic contrast
Sulphonamides	Tetracyclines
Thiazides	Vancomycin

Key papers

Thurau K, Boylan JW. (1976) Acute renal success. The unexpected logic of oliguria in acute renal failure. *Am J Med* **61**: 308–15.

Wan L, Bagshaw SM, Langenberg C, et al. (2008) Pathophysiology of septic acute kidney injury: what do we really know? *Crit Care Med* **36**(4 Suppl): S198–203.

See also:

Blood pressure monitoring, p164; Urea and creatinine, p210; Electrolytes (Na$^+$, K$^+$, Cl$^-$, HCO$_3^-$), p212; Full blood count, p220; Urinalysis, p232; Hypotension, p380; Heart failure—assessment, p392; Oliguria, p398; Acute renal failure—management, p402; Intra-abdominal bowel perforation and obstruction, p418; Abdominal sepsis, p422; Pancreatitis, p424; Jaundice, p428; Acute liver failure, p430; Vasculitis, p574; Rhabdomyolysis, p612; Raised intra-abdominal pressure, p614; Post-operative critical care, p620.

Acute renal failure—management

- Identify and correct reversible causes.
- Attend to fluid management and nutritional support carefully.
- Early use of renal replacement techniques allow normal fluid and nutritional intake and may improve outcome.

Mortality in the setting of acute renal failure in the critically ill is high (50–60%). In surviving patients, permanent renal failure is rare with recovery usually seen within 1–6 weeks.

Urinary tract obstruction

- Decompress lower urinary tract obstruction with a urinary catheter (suprapubic if there is urethral disruption).
- Decompress ureteric obstruction by nephrostomy or stent.

Massive diuresis is common after urinary tract decompression so ensure an adequate circulating volume to prevent secondary pre-renal failure.

Haemodynamic management

- The circulating volume must be corrected first.
- Prompt restoration of circulating volume, and any necessary inotrope or vasopressor support may reverse pre-renal failure.
- Diuretics (furosemide, mannitol) may establish a diuresis if oliguria persists after pre-renal factors have been corrected.

Urgent treatment of hyperkalaemia

- 10–20mL 10% calcium chloride by slow IV injection.
- 100mL 8.4% sodium bicarbonate IV (centrally).
- Glucose (50g) and insulin (10–20IU) IV with careful blood glucose monitoring.
- Urgent renal replacement therapy.

Metabolic management

- Hypocalcaemia is best treated with renal replacement and calcium supplementation.
- Hyponatraemia is usually due to water excess although salt-losing nephropathies may require sodium chloride supplements.
- Hyperphosphataemia may be treated with renal replacement or aluminium hydroxide PO.
- Metabolic acidosis (not due to tissue hypoperfusion) may be corrected with dialysis, filtration, or a 1.26% sodium bicarbonate infusion.

Renal replacement therapy

Continuous haemofiltration forms the mainstay of replacement therapy in critically ill patients who may not tolerate haemodialysis.

Nephrotoxins and crystal nephropathies

Nephrotoxic agents should be withheld if possible. Drug dosage should be modified according to GFR. In some cases, urinary excretion of nephrotoxins and crystals may be encouraged by urinary alkalinisation.

Glomerular disease

Immunosuppressive therapy may be useful. Dialysis is often required for the more severe forms despite steroid responsiveness.

General indications for dialysis or haemo(dia)filtration

- Fluid excess (e.g. pulmonary oedema).
- Hyperkalaemia (>6.0mmol/L).
- Metabolic acidosis (pH<7.2) due to renal failure.
- Clearance of dialysable nephrotoxins and other drugs.
- Creatinine rising >100μmol/L/d.
- Creatinine >300–600μmol/L.
- Urea rising >16–20mmol/L/d.
- To create space for nutrition or drugs.

See also:

Haemo(dia)filtration (1), p108; Haemo(dia)filtration (2), p110; Peritoneal dialysis, p112; Plasma exchange, p114; Urea and creatinine, p210; Electrolytes (Na$^+$, K$^+$, Cl$^-$, HCO$_3^-$), p212; Crystalloids, p242; Colloids, p246; Diuretics, p280; Oliguria, p398; Acute renal failure—diagnosis, p400; Electrolyte management, p482; Hyperkalaemia, p488; Metabolic acidosis, p502.

Gastrointestinal disorders

Vomiting/gastric stasis

While vomiting per se is relatively rare in the ICU patient, large volume gastric aspirates are commonplace and probably represent the major reason for failure of enteral nutrition.

General principles

- Seek an underlying cause.
- Ensure volaemic and total body fluid status is adequate, especially as aspirates can exceed several litres/day.
- Monitor and correct electrolyte abnormalities, e.g. metabolic alkalosis, hypokalaemia.
- Oesophageal rupture (Boerhaave's syndrome) should be considered if vomiting forceful.

Ileus

Ileus affects the stomach more frequently than the rest of the GI tract. Abdominal surgery, drugs (particularly opiates), gut dysfunction as a component of multi-organ dysfunction, hypoperfusion, and prolonged starvation may all contribute to gastric ileus. Early and continued use of the bowel for feeding appears to maintain forward propulsive action. Management consists of treating the cause where possible. Consider the use of motility stimulants such as metoclopramide or erythromycin, and in resistant cases, bypassing the stomach with a nasoduodenal/nasojejunal tube or a jejunostomy. Caution should be exercised with efforts to establish enteral feeding if the patient has increasing abdominal distension and/or pain, or an explained and increasing metabolic acidosis. Bowel rest and/or parenteral feeding may be indicated if symptoms fail to settle.

Upper bowel obstruction

Relatively unusual; apart from primary surgical causes such as neoplasm or adhesions, the predominant cause in the ICU is gastric outlet obstruction. This may be related to longstanding peptic ulcer disease or occur in the short term from pyloric and/or duodenal swelling consequent to gastritis or duodenitis. This can be diagnosed endoscopically and treated by bowel rest plus an H_2 antagonist, proton pump inhibitor, or sucralfate.

Gastric irritation

Drugs or chemicals, either accidental or adverse reaction (e.g. corticosteroids, aspirin), intentional (e.g. alcohol, bleach) or therapeutic (e.g. ipecacuanha syrup) may induce vomiting. Treatment, where appropriate, may comprise: (i) removal of the cause, (ii) dilution with copious amounts of fluid, (iii) neutralisation with alkali and/or H_2 antagonist or proton pump inhibitor, and (iv) administration of an anti-emetic, e.g. metoclopramide.

Neurological

Stimulation of the emetic centre may follow any neurological event (e.g. trauma, CVA), drug therapy (e.g. chemotherapy), pain and metabolic disturbances. Management is by treating the cause where possible and by judicious use of anti-emetics, initially metoclopramide or prochlorperazine. Consider ondansetron if these are unsuccessful.

See also:
Upper gastrointestinal endoscopy, p120; Enteral feeding and drainage tubes, p122; Enteral nutrition, p128; Electrolytes (Na^+, K^+, Cl^-, HCO_3^-), p212; Anti-emetics, p292; Gut motility agents, p294; Upper gastrointestinal haemorrhage, p412; Bleeding varices, p414; Oesophageal perforation, p416; Intra-abdominal bowel perforation and obstruction, p418; Intracranial haemorrhage, p448; Subarachnoid haemorrhage, p450; Stroke, p452; Raised intracranial pressure, p454; Hypokalaemia, p490; Metabolic alkalosis, p504; Diabetic ketoacidosis, p510; Head injury (1), p586; Head injury (2), p588; Pain, p618; Effects of chemo- and radiotherapy, p626.

Diarrhoea

The definition of diarrhoea in the ICU patient is problematic as the amount of stool passed daily is difficult to measure. Frequency and consistency may also vary significantly. Loose/watery and frequent (≥4x per day) stool will often require investigation and/or treatment.

Common ICU causes

- Infection—*Clostridium (C.) difficile*, gastroenteritis (e.g. *Salmonella, Shigella*), rarer tropical causes (e.g. cholera, dysentry, giardiasis).
- Drugs, e.g. antibiotics, laxatives.
- Gastrointestinal—feed (e.g. lactose intolerance), coeliac disease, other malabsorption syndromes, inflammatory bowel disease, diverticulitis, pelvic abscess, bowel obstruction with overflow.

Enteral feed is often implicated but rarely causative.

For bloody diarrhoea consider infection, ischaemic or inflammatory bowel disease.

Diagnosis

- Rectal examination to exclude impaction with overflow. Consider sigmoidoscopy if colitis or *C. difficile* suspected (in the latter, a pseudomembrane is seen).
- Stool sent to laboratory for M, C & S, *C. difficile* toxin.
- Fat estimation (malabsorption) is rarely necessary in the ICU patient.
- If ischaemic or inflammatory bowel disease suspected, perform a CT or supine abdominal X-ray and inspect for dilated loops of bowel (NB. toxic megacolon), thickened walls (increased separation between loops), and 'thumbprinting' (suggestive of mucosal oedema). Fluid levels seen on erect or lateral abdominal X-ray may be seen in diarrhoea or paralytic ileus and do not necessarily indicate obstruction. Diarrhoea is often, but not always, bloody.
- If abscess suspected, perform ultrasonography or CT scan.

Management

- Treat cause where possible, e.g. for *C. difficile,* metronidazole plus colestyramine (binds the toxin). Anecdotal success has been reported with immunoglobulin therapy for *C. difficile* colitis.
- Consider temporary (12–24h) cessation of enteral feed if very severe. Consider changing feed if appropriate, e.g. coeliac disease, lactose intolerance.
- Consider stopping antibiotics.
- Give anti-diarrhoeal if infection excluded.
- Careful attention to fluid and electrolyte balance (in particular Na^+, K^+, Mg^{2+}).
- Request surgical opinion for possible colectomy if infarcted or inflamed bowel, toxic dilatation, or abscess suspected.

failure to open bowels

Common ICU causes

- Prolonged ileus occurs post-surgery or colonic pseudo-obstruction
- Lack of enteral nutrition
- Bowel obstruction: the 3 cardinal symptoms are constipation, vomiting, and abdominal pain. Post-operatively, these are very common and cause diagnostic difficulties.

Management

- Consider obstruction and exclude this (plain abdominal X-ray, CT scan)
- Avoid and reduce opioids
- Add a pro-kinetic
- If not contraindicated consider use of a laxative and/or enema
- Consider the use of a colonic decompression tube if obstruction is not present
- Mobilise and stop dropping if possible
- Adequate hydration but not fluid overload

See also:
Enteral nutrition, p128; Electrolytes (Na$^+$, K$^+$, Cl$^-$, HCO$_3^-$), p212; Bacteriology, p224; Virology, serology, and assays, p226; Antidiarrhoeals, p296; Lower intestinal bleeding and colitis, p420.

Failure to open bowels

Common ICU causes

- Prolonged ileus/decreased gut motility (e.g. opiates, post-surgery).
- Lack of enteral nutrition.
- Bowel obstruction—this is a relatively uncommon secondary event and is mainly seen post-operatively, either after a curative procedure or with development of adhesions.

Management

- Clinically exclude obstruction and confirm presence of stool per rectum.
- Ensure adequate hydration.
- Anti-constipation therapy may be given, usually starting with laxatives (e.g. lactulose or, for more urgent response, magnesium sulphate), then proceeding to glycerin suppositories, and finally, enemata if gentler measures prove unsuccessful.
- Consider reducing/stopping dose of opiate if possible.
- For colonic pseudo-obstruction, consider 2mg IV neostigmine.

Key paper

Robert J. Ponec RJ, Saunders MD, et al. (1999) Neostigmine for the treatment of acute colonic pseudo-obstruction. *N Engl J Med* **341**: 137–41.

See also:

Anti-constipation agents, p298; Intra-abdominal bowel perforation and obstruction, p418; Abdominal sepsis, p422; Pancreatitis, p424.

Upper gastrointestinal haemorrhage

Causes
- Peptic ulceration.
- Oesophagitis/gastritis/duodenitis.
- Varices.
- Mallory–Weiss lower oesophageal tear.
- Neoplasms.

Pathophysiology
Peptic ulceration is related to protective barrier loss leading to acid or biliary damage of the underlying mucosa and submucosa. Barrier loss occurs secondary to critical illness, alcohol, and drugs, e.g. non-steroidals, poisons, including corrosives. Direct damage, especially at the lower oesophagus, may occur from feeding tubes. Mucosal damage ('stress ulcers') may also occur as a consequence of tissue hypoperfusion. Gastric hypersecretion is uncommon in critically ill patients; indeed, gastric acid content and secretion are often reduced.

Prophylaxis
- Small-bore feeding tubes.
- Nasogastric enteral nutrition (even nasojejunal and parenteral feeding have also been shown to reduce the incidence of stress ulcer bleeding).
- Adequate tissue perfusion (flow and pressure).
- Prophylactic drug therapy (proton pump inhibitor, H_2 antagonist) decreases the incidence of stress ulceration though this is largely based on historic data when gut hypoperfusion was more prevalent. Patients at highest risk for stress ulcers are those requiring prolonged mechanical ventilation or with a concurrent coagulopathy.

Treatment of major haemorrhage
- Fluid resuscitation with colloid and blood, with blood products as appropriate to correct any coagulopathy. Maintain Hb >7–10g/dL and have adequate crossmatched blood available should further large haemorrhages occur.
- If possible, discontinue any ongoing anticoagulation, e.g. heparin.
- Urgent diagnostic fibreoptic endoscopy. Local injection of epinephrine or a sclerosant into (or thermal sealing of) a bleeding peptic ulcer base may halt further bleeding. Banding or sclerosant injection may arrest bleeding varices.
- If oesophageal varices are known or highly suspected, consider vasopressin or terlipressin ± a Sengstaken-type tube for severe haemorrhage, either as a bridge to endoscopy or if banding/injection is unsuccessful. Remember that sources of bleeding other than varices may be present, e.g. peptic ulcer.
- For peptic ulceration and generalised inflammation, commence H_2 antagonist or proton pump inhibitor. Give IV to ensure effect. Enteral antacid may also be beneficial.
- For continued bleeding, contact interventional radiologist with view to angiographic embolisation.
- Surgery is now rarely necessary, but should be considered if bleeding continues, e.g. >6–10 unit transfusion need and embolisation is not available or fails. Inform surgeon of any patient with major bleeding.

Bleeding varices

See also:
Sengstaken-type tube, p118; Full blood count, p220; Coagulation monitoring, p222; Colloids, p246; Blood transfusion, p248; Blood products, p250; H$_2$ blockers and proton pump inhibitors, p286; Sucralfate, p288; Antacids, p290; Basic resuscitation, p338; Bleeding varices, p414.

Bleeding varices

Varices develop following a prolonged period of portal hypertension, usually related to liver cirrhosis. Approximately one third will bleed. They are commonly found in the lower oesophagus, but occasionally in the stomach or duodenum. Torrential haemorrhage may occur. Approximately 50% of patients die within six weeks of presentation of their first bleed; each subsequent bleed carries a 30% mortality.

Management

1. If airway and/or breathing are compromised, perform endotracheal intubation and institute mechanical ventilation. This facilitates Sengstaken-type tube placement and endoscopy though may be associated with severe hypotension secondary to covert hypovolaemia. If possible, ensure adequate intravascular filling before intubation.

2. Fluid resuscitation with colloid and blood with blood products as appropriate to correct any coagulopathy. Ensure good venous access (at least two 14G cannulae). Group-specific or O-negative blood may be needed for emergency use. Maintain Hb >7–10g/dL and have at least four units of crossmatched blood available for urgent transfusion. There is a theoretical risk that over-transfusion may precipitate further bleeding by raising portal venous pressure. Cardiac output monitoring should be considered if the patient remains haemodynamically unstable or there is a history of heart disease.

3. If bleeding is torrential, insert a Sengstaken-type tube and commence administration of IV vasopressin/terlipressin (q.v.).

4. Gentle placement of a large-bore nasogastric tube is a reasonably safe procedure that facilitates drainage of blood, lessens the risk of aspiration, and can be used to assess continuing blood loss.

5. Perform urgent fibreoptic endoscopy to exclude other sources of bleeding. This also allows variceal banding or local injection of sclerosing agent. Bleeding is arrested in approximately 90% of cases. Endoscopy may be impossible if bleeding is too severe, and may have to be delayed for 6–24h until a period of tamponade by the Sengstaken-type tube ± vasopressin has enabled some control of the bleeding.

6. Either vasopressin, terlipressin, or octreotide can be administered for severe bleeding or prophylaxis against fresh bleeding. Vasopressin controls bleeding in approximately 60% of cases and its efficacy and safety appears to be enhanced by concurrent GTN. The side effect profile of terlipressin is lower as it does not appear to precipitate as much mesenteric, cardiac, or digital ischaemia. Octreotide is a somatostatin analogue, but longer-acting than its parent compound; like somatostatin, it is probably as effective as vasopressin but without the side effects.

7. If bleeding continues after prolonged balloon tamponade (2–3 days) and repeated endoscopy, consider transjugular intrahepatic portosystemic stented shunt (TIPSS). This can be performed quickly and carries a relatively low mortality compared to surgery although the risk of encephalopathy is increased.

8. The traditional alternative to TIPSS is oesophageal transection (now performed with a staple gun) with or without devascularisation. Mortality in the acute situation is of the order of 30%.

Drug dosages

Octreotide	50mcg bolus, then 50mcg/h infusion
Vasopressin	20 units over 20min, then 0.4 units/min infusion
	Also give glyceryl trinitrate 2–20mg/h to counteract myocardial and mesenteric ischaemia.
Terlipressin	2 mg IV, followed by 1–2mg IV 4–6 hourly until bleeding controlled for up to 72h

See also:

Oesophageal perforation

Causes
- Iatrogenic—typically as a complication of endoscopy, placement of a feeding tube, or surgery. This accounts for 85–90% of cases.
- Boerhaave's syndrome—oesophageal rupture related to forceful vomiting or, rarely, forceful coughing or obstruction by food.
- External trauma (usually penetrating injuries).
- Corrosive liquids.

Diagnosis
- Chest X-ray showing mediastinal emphysema and widening due to oedema.
- CT scan.
- Gastrografin® swallow.

Complications
- Pneumomediastinum.
- Mediastinitis.
- Sepsis.
- High mortality, especially with late diagnosis.

Management
- Immediate antibiotic therapy.
- Intravascular volume replacement.
- Surgical repair of the perforation (± oesophageal exclusion and cervical oesophagostomy). Surgery must be performed within 24h before tissues become too friable. Mediastinal drains are usually placed.
- Successful thoracoscopic closure is reported.
- In selected cases, the patient may be managed conservatively.
- Nil by mouth and parenteral nutrition for several weeks.
- Analgesia.

See alo:

Upper gastrointestinal endoscopy, p120; Enteral feeding and drainage tubes, p122; Parenteral nutrition, p130; Antimicrobials, p326; Basic resuscitation, p338; Fluid challenge, p342; Systemic inflammation/multi-organ failure —causes, p556; Sepsis and septic shock—treatment, p560; Multiple trauma (1), p582; Multiple trauma (2), p584.

Intra-abdominal bowel perforation and obstruction

Patients with bowel perforation or obstruction may be admitted to the ICU after surgery, for preoperative resuscitation, and cardiorespiratory optimisation, or for conservative management. Although rarely occurring *de novo* in the ICU patient, these conditions may be difficult to diagnose because of sedation ± muscle relaxation. Consider when there is:

- Abdominal pain, tenderness, peritonism.
- Abdominal distension.
- Agitation.
- Increased nasogastric aspirates, vomiting.
- Increasing metabolic acidosis.
- Signs of hypovolaemia or sepsis.

A firm diagnosis may not be made until laparotomy, although supine and either erect or lateral abdominal X-ray may reveal either free gas in the peritoneum (perforation) or dilated bowel loops with multiple fluid levels (obstruction). Ultrasound is usually unhelpful though faecal fluid may occasionally be aspirated from the peritoneum following perforation. CT may identify the site of perforation or obstruction.

It may be difficult to distinguish bowel obstruction from a paralytic ileus as: (i) bowel sounds may be present or absent in either, and (ii) X-ray and CT appearances may be similar.

Management

1. Correct fluid and electrolyte abnormalities. Resuscitation should be prompt and aggressive and usually consists of colloid replacement plus blood to maintain Hb >7–10g/dL. Inotropes or vasopressors may be required to restore an adequate circulation, particularly following perforation. Cardiac output monitoring should be considered if circulatory status remains unstable or vasoactive drugs are required.
2. The surgeon should be informed at an early stage. A conservative approach may be adopted, e.g. with upper small bowel perforation; however, surgery is usually required for large bowel perforation. Small or large bowel obstruction may sometimes be managed conservatively as spontaneous resolution may occur, e.g. adhesions. Prompt surgical exploration should be encouraged if the patient shows signs of systemic toxicity.
3. Both conservative and post-operative management of perforation and obstruction usually require continuous nasogastric drainage to decompress the stomach, nil by mouth, and parenteral nutrition.
4. Pain relief should not be withheld.
5. Broad-spectrum antibiotic therapy should be started for bowel perforation after appropriate specimens have been taken for laboratory analysis. Therapy usually comprises aerobic and anaerobic Gram-negative cover (e.g. 2nd/3rd generation cephalosporin, quinolone or carbapenem, plus metronidazole ± aminoglycoside).
6. Post-operative management of bowel perforation may involve repeated laparotomies to exclude collections of pus and bowel ischaemia/infarction; surgery should be expedited if the patient's condition deteriorates. Alternatively, regular ultrasonographic and/or CT examinations with percutaneous drainage may be adopted.

Lower intestinal bleeding and colitis

Causes of lower gastrointestinal bleeding
- Bowel ischaemia/infarction.
- Inflammatory bowel disease (ulcerative colitis, Crohn's disease).
- Infection, e.g. *Shigella*, *Campylobacter*, amoebic dysentery.
- Upper gastrointestinal source, e.g. peptic ulceration.
- Angiodysplasia.
- Neoplasm.

Although relatively rare, massive lower gastrointestinal haemorrhage can be life-threatening.

Ischaemic/infarcted bowel
Can occur following prolonged hypoperfusion or, occasionally, secondary to a mesenteric embolus. It usually presents with severe abdominal pain, bloody diarrhoea, and signs of systemic toxicity, including a rapidly increasing metabolic acidosis. Plasma phosphate levels may be elevated. CT or X-ray appearances of thickened, oedematous bowel loops ('thumb-printing') with an increased distance between bowel loops are suggestive. Treatment is by restoration of tissue perfusion, blood transfusion to maintain Hb >7–10g/dL and, if clinical features fail to settle promptly, laparotomy with a view to bowel excision.

Inflammatory bowel disease
Presents with weight loss, abdominal pain, and diarrhoea that usually contains blood. Complications of ulcerative colitis include perforation and toxic megacolon while complications of Crohn's disease include fistulae, abscesses, and perforations.
Management involves:
1. Fluid and electrolyte replacement.
2. Blood transfusion to maintain Hb >7–10g/dL.
3. High-dose corticosteroids IV and, if distal bowel involvement, by enema.
4. Nutrition (often parenteral).
5. Regular surgical review. Surgery may be indicated if symptoms fail to settle after 5–7 days, or for toxic megacolon, perforation, abscesses, or obstruction.
6. Antidiarrhoeal drugs should be avoided.

Angiodysplasia
Usually presents as fresh bleeding per rectum and this may be considerable. It is due to an arterio-venous malformation and is more common in the elderly. Localisation and embolisation by angiography may be curative during active bleeding. Surgery may be required if bleeding fails to settle on conservative management and, occasionally, 'blind' laparoscopic embolisation of a mesenteric vessel. However, localisation of the lesion may be difficult at laparotomy, necessitating extensive bowel resection.

See also:

Full blood count, p220; Coagulation monitoring, p222; Bacteriology, p224; Virology, serology and assays, p226; Colloids, p246; Blood transfusion, p248; Blood products, p250; Antimicrobials, p326; Basic resuscitation, p338; Diarrhoea, p408; Abdominal sepsis, p422.

Abdominal sepsis

This is a common but difficult to diagnose condition in the ICU patient. A proportion of such patients are admitted following laparotomy, but others may develop abdominal sepsis *de novo* or as a secondary complication following abdominal surgery, in particular after bowel resection. Sepsis may either be localised to an organ, e.g. cholecystitis, or the peritoneal cavity (abscess); alternatively, there may be a generalised peritonitis. Non-bowel infection or inflammation can present in a similar manner, e.g. pancreatitis, cholecystitis, gynaecological infection, pyelonephritis.

Clinical features

- Non-specific signs, including pyrexia (especially swinging), neutrophilia, falling platelets, increasing metabolic acidosis, circulatory instability.
- Abdominal distension ± localised discomfort, peritonism.
- Abdominal mass, e.g. gallbladder, pseudocyst, abscess.
- Failure to tolerate enteral feed/large nasogastric aspirates.
- Pleural effusion (if subdiaphragmatic sepsis).
- Diarrhoea (if pelvic sepsis).

Diagnosis

- Ultrasound.
- CT scan.
- Laparotomy.

Samples should be taken for microbiological analysis from blood, urine, stool, abdominal drain fluid, and vaginal discharge if present. A sample of pus is preferred to a swab. Hyperamylasaemia may suggest pancreatitis though levels can be elevated with other intra-abdominal pathologies.

Treatment

- Antibiotic therapy providing aerobic and anaerobic Gram-negative cover (e.g. 2nd or 3rd generation cephalosporin, quinolone or carbapenem, plus metronidazole ± aminoglycoside). Treatment can be modified depending on culture results and patient response.
- Ultrasonic or CT-guided drainage of pus.
- Laparotomy with removal of pus, peritoneal lavage, etc.

A negative laparotomy should be viewed as a useful means of excluding intra-abdominal sepsis rather than an unnecessary procedure. Laparotomy should be encouraged if the patient deteriorates and a high suspicion of abdominal pathology persists.

Cholecystitis, with or without (acalculous) the presence of gallstones, may present with signs of infection. There is a characteristic ultrasound and CT appearance of an enlarged organ with a thickened, oedematous wall surrounded by fluid. Treatment is often conservative with antibiotics (as above) and percutaneous, ultrasound-guided drainage via a pigtail catheter. Cholecystectomy is rarely necessary in the acute situation unless the gallbladder has perforated, though some authorities argue that this is the treatment of choice for acalculous cholecystitis.

See also:
Enteral feeding and drainage tubes, p122; Electrolytes (Na$^+$, K$^+$, Cl$^-$, HCO$_3^-$), p212; Full blood count, p220; Bacteriology, p224; Virology, serology, and assays, p226; Antimicrobials, p326; Basic resuscitation, p338; Fluid challenge, p342; Vomiting/gastric stasis, p406; Diarrhoea, p408; Failure to open bowels, p410; Intra-abdominal bowel perforation and obstruction, p418; Pancreatitis, p424; Systemic inflammation/multi-organ failure—causes, p556; Sepsis and septic shock—treatment, p560; Post-operative critical care, p620.

Pancreatitis

The inflamed pancreas and surrounding retroperitoneal tissues may range from mildly oedematous to haemorrhagic and necrotising. A pseudocyst may develop which can become infected, and the bile duct may be obstructed causing biliary obstruction and jaundice. Though overall mortality is quoted at 5–10%, this is much higher (approximately 40%) in those with severe pancreatitis requiring intensive care. Pancreatitis is severe if APACHE II score >8.

Causes

- Alcohol.
- Gallstones.
- Miscellaneous, e.g. ischaemia, trauma, viral, hyperlipidaemia.
- Part of the multiple organ failure syndrome.

Diagnosis

- Non-specific features include central, severe abdominal pain, pyrexia, haemodynamic instability, vomiting, ileus. Discoloration around the umbilicus (Cullen's sign) or flanks (Grey Turner's sign) is rarely seen.
- Plasma enzymes—elevated levels of amylase (usually >1000IU/mL), and pancreatic lipase are suggestive but non-specific. The levels may be normal, even in severe pancreatitis.
- Ultrasound.
- CT scan.
- Laparotomy.

Complications

- Multi-organ dysfunction syndrome.
- Infection/abscess formation.
- Occasional massive bleeding from erosion of local artery or vein.
- Hypocalcaemia.
- Diabetes mellitus.

Management

- General measures, including fluid resuscitation, blood transfusion to maintain Hb 7–10g/dL, respiratory support, analgesia, and anti-emetics. Routine antibiotic prophylaxis is no longer recommended.
- Adequate monitoring should be instituted, including pulmonary artery catheterisation if cardiorespiratory instability is present.
- The patient is traditionally kept nil by mouth with continuous nasogastric drainage, and nutrition and vitamins provided parenterally. However, recent studies show safety and efficacy of distal nasojejunal (or even nasogastric) enteral feeding.
- Relieve gallstone obstruction either endoscopically or surgically.
- Hypocalcaemia, if symptomatic, should be treated by intermittent slow IV injection (or occasionally, infusion) of 10% calcium chloride.
- Hyperglycaemia should be controlled by continuous IV insulin infusion.
- The role of surgery is controversial; advocates promote either a conservative approach with percutaneous drainage of infected and/or necrotic debris, or an aggressive, interventional strategy with regular (often daily) laparotomy for debridement and peritoneal lavage. Pseudocysts may resolve, or need drainage percutaneously or into the bowel.
- Probiotic therapy for pancreatitis is associated with worse outcomes.

Ranson's signs of severity in acute pancreatitis

On hospital admission	At 48h after admission
Age >55 years old	Haematocrit fall >10%
Blood glucose >11mmol/L	Blood urea rise >1mmol/L
Serum LDH >300U/L	Serum calcium <2mmol/L
Serum AST >250U/L	PaO_2 <8kPa
White blood count >16x10⁹/L	Arterial base deficit >4mmol/L
	Estimated fluid sequestration >6L

Pancreatitis severe if ≥2 criteria met within 48h of admission.

CT severity index

Element	Finding	Points
Grade of acute pancreatitis	Normal pancreas	0
	Pancreatic enlargement	1
	Inflammation of pancreas and peripancreatic fat	2
	Single fluid collection or phlegmon	3
	≥2 fluid collections or phlegmons	4
Degree of pancreatic necrosis	No necrosis	0
	Necrosis of one third of pancreas	2
	Necrosis of one half of the pancreas	4
	Necrosis of > one half of the pancreas	6

Add points for grade of acute pancreatitis + degree of pancreatic necrosis.

Severity index	Mortality	Complications
0–1	0%	0%
2–3	3%	8%
4–6	6%	35%
7–10	17%	92%

Pancreatitis Outcome Prediction (POP) score

Score	0	1	2	3	4	5	6	7	8	10
Age	16–29	30–39		40–49		50–59		60–69	≥70	
MAP	≥90	80–89		60–79	50–59		40–49		<40	
PaO_2/FIO_2	≥30			10–29.9	<10					
Arterial pH	>7.35	7.30–7.35	7.25–7.29		7.20–7.24	7.10–7.19	7.00–7.09			<7
Urea	<5	5–7.9		8–10.9	11–16.9		≥17			
Total serum calcium	2.0–2.29	1.8–1.99	1.6–1.79 or 2.3–2.49		<1.6 or 2.5					

Key paper

Harrison DA, D'Amico G, Singer M. (2007) The Pancreatitis Outcome Prediction (POP) Score: a new prognostic index for patients with severe acute pancreatitis. *Crit Care Med* **35**: 1703–8

See also:

APACHE score, p28; Enteral nutrition, p128; Parenteral nutrition, p130; Basic resuscitation, p338; Abdominal sepsis, p422; Hypocalcaemia, p496; Systemic inflammation/multi-organ failure—causes, p556; Sepsis and septic shock—treatment, p560.

Hepatic disorders

Jaundice

Jaundice is a clinical diagnosis of yellow pigmentation of sclera and skin resulting from a raised plasma bilirubin. It is usually visible when the plasma bilirubin exceeds 30–40µmol/L.

Common causes seen in the ICU
- Pre-hepatic—intravascular haemolysis (e.g. drugs, malaria, haemolytic uraemic syndrome), Gilbert's syndrome.
- Hepatocellular—critical illness, viral (hepatitis A, B, C, Epstein–Barr), alcohol, drugs (e.g. paracetamol, halothane), toxoplasmosis, leptospirosis.
- Cholestatic—critical illness, intrahepatic causes (e.g. drugs such as chlorpromazine, erythromycin and isoniazid, primary biliary cirrhosis), extrahepatic causes (e.g. biliary obstruction by gallstones, neoplasm, pancreatitis).

Diagnosis
- Urinalysis—unconjugated bilirubin does not appear in the urine.
- Measurement of conjugated and unconjugated bilirubin—conjugated bilirubin predominates in cholestatic jaundice; unconjugated bilirubin in pre-hepatic jaundice; a mixed picture is often seen in hepatocellular jaundice.
- Plasma alkaline phosphatase is usually markedly elevated in obstructive jaundice while prothrombin times, aspartate transaminase, and alanine aminotransferase are elevated in hepatocellular jaundice.
- Ultrasound or CT scan will diagnose extrahepatic biliary obstruction.

Management
1. Identify and treat cause. Where possible, discontinue any drug that could be implicated. If extrahepatic, consider percutaneous trans-hepatic drainage (under radiology guidance), ERCP ± bile duct stenting or, rarely, surgery.
2. Liver biopsy is rarely necessary in a jaundiced ICU patient unless the diagnosis is unknown and the possibility exists of liver involvement in the underlying pathology, e.g. malignancy.
3. Non-obstructive jaundice usually settles with conservative management as the patient recovers.
4. An antihistamine and topical calamine lotion may provide symptomatic relief for pruritus if troublesome. Colestyramine 4g tds PO may be helpful in obstructive jaundice.

See also:
Liver function tests, p218; Coagulation monitoring, p222; Acute liver failure, p430; Chronic liver failure, p434; Haemolysis, p476.

Acute liver failure

This results from massive damage to liver cells leading to severe liver dysfunction and encephalopathy. Survival rates for liver failure with grade 3 or 4 hepatic encephalopathy vary from 10–40% on medical therapy alone to 60–80% with orthotopic liver transplantation.

Major causes

- Alcohol.
- Drugs, particularly paracetamol overdose.
- Viral hepatitis, particularly hepatitis B, hepatitis C.
- Poisons, e.g. carbon tetrachloride.
- Decompensation of chronic disease, e.g. infection or variceal bleed.

Diagnosis

- Consider in any patient presenting with jaundice: generalised bleeding, encephalopathy, or marked hypoglycaemia.
- Prolonged PT or INR and hyperbilirubinaemia. In severe liver failure, plasma enzyme levels may not be elevated.

Management

- General measures include fluid resuscitation and blood transfusion to keep Hb 7–10g/dL. The circulation is usually hyperdynamic and dilated; vasopressors may be needed to maintain an adequate BP.
- Correct coagulopathy in patients who are bleeding or about to undergo an invasive procedure. Otherwise, withhold as this provides a good guide to recovery or the need for transplantation.
- Institute adequate monitoring for cardiorespiratory instability.
- Mechanical ventilation may be necessary for airway protection (e.g. encephalopathy, variceal bleed) or respiratory failure (e.g. lung shunts—hepatopulmonary syndrome in cirrhotics).
- Infection is common and may be Gram-positive, Gram-negative, or fungal. Clinical signs are often lacking. Samples of blood, sputum, urine, wound and catheter site swabs, drain fluid, and ascites should be sent for regular microbiological surveillance. Ascitic white blood count >250/hpf suggests spontaneous bacterial peritonitis. Systemic antimicrobial ± antifungal prophylaxis is often used to reduce infection rates, though confirmatory multicentre trial data are lacking.
- Monitor closely for hypoglycaemia. Treat with enteral (or parenteral) nutrition or 10–50% glucose infusion to maintain normoglycaemia.
- Renal failure occurs in 30–70% of cases. The incidence may be reduced by careful maintenance of intravascular volume. Vasopressin/terlipressin can be used to maintain urine output in hepatorenal syndrome.
- Upper gastrointestinal bleeding is common. Prophylactic H_2-blockers or proton pump inhibitors are routinely given.
- N-acetylcysteine increases transplant free survival in early stage acute liver failure.
- Extracorporeal systems that bind circulating toxins via albumin dialysis (e.g. MARS—Molecular Adsorbent Recirculation System) or adsorption columns (fractionated plasma separation and adsorption, charcoal haemoperfusion) have yet to show outcome benefit.
- Corticosteroid therapy is used in selected cases (e.g. alcoholic hepatitis) when bleeding and infection are absent.

Drug dosages

N-acetylcysteine	
Loading dose	150mg/kg IV infused over 1h diluted in 250mL 5% glucose
First maintenance dose	50mg/kg IV infused over 4h diluted in 500mL 5% glucose
Second maintenance dose	100mg/kg IV infused over 16h dilute in 1000mL 5% glucose
Continuing treatment	Consider 150mg/kg over 24h until liver failure improves or transplant.

Each infusion immediately follows the previous; total treatment time 21h).

See also:

Liver function tests, p218; Coagulation monitoring, p222; Lactate, p234; Acute renal failure—diagnosis, p400; Acute renal failure—management, p402; Hepatic encephalopathy, p432; Chronic liver failure, p434; Hypoglycaemia, p506; Paracetamol poisoning, p524; Infection—diagnosis, p552; Infection—treatment, p554.

Hepatic encephalopathy

Grading

1. Confused, altered mood.
2. Inappropriate, drowsy.
3. Stuporose but rousable, very confused, agitated.
4. Coma, unresponsive to painful stimuli.

The risk of cerebral oedema is far higher at grades 3 and 4 (50–85%). Suggestive signs include systemic hypertension, progressive bradycardia, and increasing muscle rigidity at ICP >30mmHg.

Management

- Correct/avoid potential aggravating factors, e.g. gut haemorrhage, over-sedation, hypoxia, hypoglycaemia, infection, electrolyte imbalance.
- Consider (ICP) monitoring. CT and clinical features correlate poorly with ICP though no controlled studies have yet been performed to show outcome benefit from ICP monitoring which carries its own complication rate (bleeding, infection).
- Maintain patient in slight head-up position (20–30°).
- Regular lactulose, e.g. 20–30mL qds PO, to achieve 2–3 bowel motions/day.
- Dietary restriction of protein is now not encouraged as this promotes endogenous protein utilisation.
- Hyperventilation to achieve a $PaCO_2$ of 3.5–4kPa is no longer recommended. It may also compromise cerebral blood flow.
- Give mannitol (0.5–1mg/kg over 20–30min) if serum osmolality <320mOsm/kg and either a raised ICP or clinical signs of cerebral oedema persist. If severe renal dysfunction is present, use renal replacement therapy in conjunction with mannitol. Consider maintaining Na^+ 145–155mmol/L.
- Sodium benzoate (2g tds PO) may be considered if the patient is severely hyperammonaemic.
- If still no response, consider possibility of liver transplantation.
- Exercise caution with concomitant drug usage.

Identification of patients unlikely to survive without transplantation

- Prothrombin time >100s.

Or any three of the following:

- Age <10 or >40y.
- Aetiology is seronegative hepatitis, Wilson's disease, halothane, or other drug reaction.
- Duration of jaundice pre-encephalopathy >7d.
- Prothrombin time >50s.
- Serum bilirubin >300μmol/L.

If paracetamol-induced:

- pH <7.3 or prothrombin time >100s and creatinine >200μmol/L plus grade 3 or 4 encephalopathy.

As only 50–85% of patients identified as requiring transplantation will survive long enough to receive one, the regional Liver Unit should be informed soon after diagnosis of all possible candidates.

See also:
Intracranial pressure monitoring, p200; Electrolytes (Na$^+$, K$^+$, Cl$^-$, HCO$_3^-$), p212; Liver function tests, p218; Coagulation monitoring, p222; Upper gastrointestinal haemorrhage, p412; Bleeding varices, p414; Acute liver failure, p430; Coma, p438; Raised intracranial pressure, p454.

Chronic liver failure

Patients admitted to intensive care with chronic liver failure may develop specific associated problems:

- Acute decompensation—may be secondary to infection, sedation, hypovolaemia, hypotension, diuretics, gastrointestinal haemorrhage, excess dietary protein, and electrolyte imbalance.
- Infection—the patient may transmit infection, e.g. hepatitis A, B, or C, and by being immunosuppressed, is also more prone to acquiring infections (including TB and fungi).
- Drug metabolism—many drugs are metabolised in whole or in part by the liver and/or excreted into the bile. Drug actions may be prolonged or slowed depending on whether the metabolites are active or not. In particular, sedatives may have a greatly prolonged duration of action.
- Portal hypertension—results in ascites, varices, and splenomegaly. Ascites may produce diaphragmatic splinting and may become infected. Drainage may incur a considerable protein loss. Varices may bleed while splenomegaly may result in thrombocytopaenia. Renal failure may occur from high intra-abdominal pressure (or hepatorenal syndrome).
- Bleeding—increased risk due to reduced production of clotting factors (II, VII, IX, X), varices, and splenomegaly-related thrombocytopaenia.
- Alcohol—the most frequent cause of cirrhosis in the western world, acute withdrawal may lead to delirium tremens with severe agitation, hallucinations, seizures, and cardiovascular disturbances.
- 2° hyperaldosteronism—results in oliguria, salt and water retention.
- Increased tendency to jaundice, especially during critical illness.

Management

1. Ascites.
- Take specimens for microbiological analysis (including TB), protein, and cytology. If WBC >250/hpf, give antibiotic cover (particularly covering Gram-negative bacteria).
- If present in large quantity: (i) decrease sodium and water intake, (ii) commence spironolactone PO (or potassium canrenoate IV) ± furosemide. Paracentesis ± colloid replacement or ascitic reinfusion (if uninfected/non-pancreatitic in origin) may be considered, particularly if diaphragmatic splinting occurs.
2. Coagulopathy.
- Vitamin K 10mg/day slow IV bolus for 2–3 days.
- Fresh frozen plasma, platelets as necessary.
3. Hypoglycaemia—should be prevented by adequate nutrition or 10% or 20% glucose infusion.
4. Adequate nutrition and vitamin supplementation. As patients are often malnourished and at risk of beriberi, thiamine should be given.
5. Acute decompensation—avoid any precipitating causes, e.g. infection, sedation, hypovolaemia, electrolyte imbalance.
6. Drug administration—review type and dose regularly.

See also:
Liver function tests, p218; Coagulation monitoring, p222; Virology, serology, and assays, p226; Acute liver failure, p430; Hypoglycaemia, p506.

Neurological disorders

Coma

Causes

- Brain injury—e.g. trauma, cerebrovascular accident, meningo-encephalitis, malaria, ictal (or post-ictal), space-occupying lesion.
- Metabolic—hypoglycaemia or hyperglycaemia, severe electrolyte disturbance (e.g. Na^+), renal failure, liver failure.
- Sepsis.
- Drug-related or poisoning—e.g. opiates, benzodiazepines, carbon monoxide poisoning, recreational drugs, alcohol.
- Haemodynamic—related to poor cerebral perfusion (cardiac arrest, severe heart failure, arrhythmia, hypotension).
- Respiratory—low PaO_2 and/or high $PaCO_2$.
- Endocrine—e.g. myxoedema, Addison's disease.
- Temperature disturbance (hyperpyrexia, hypothermia).

Investigation

- This is dictated by presenting history and examination findings.
- Urgent blood sugar testing (at the bedside).
- Urea and electrolytes, sugar (lab-measured), calcium, liver function.
- FBC and clotting screen to exclude coagulopathy.
- Urgent blood gas analysis (including COHb if indicated).
- Blood and urine poison/drug screen/alcohol level.
- Plasma creatine kinase and test urine for 'positivity' for blood if rhabdomyolysis possible (immobility, recreational drugs, hyperpyrexia).
- Metabolic screen (thyroid function, cortisol).
- Septic screen ± malaria screen.
- Lumbar puncture (± preceding CT scan if concerned about raised ICP).
- CT scan.
- Other neurological tests, e.g. EEG. MRI.

Management

- ABC—ensure adequate (protected) airway, breathing, circulation.
- Correct rapidly remediable causes promptly, e.g. hypoglycaemia, status epilepticus, specific antidote (e.g. naloxone for opiate toxicity).
- If meningitis suspected, give antibiotics immediately (e.g. ceftriaxone).
- Prioritise investigations based on likely diagnosis; treat accordingly.
- Institute measures to lower intracranial pressure if concerned about coning.
- Urgent referral to neurosurgeon if CT demonstrates space-occupying lesion (e.g. haematoma) or for brain decompression (craniectomy).
- Urgent consideration of thrombolysis if cerebral infarct or embolus.
- Consider duration of coma when treating metabolic abnormality. Correction of Na^+ and glucose may need to be more gradual.
- Unconscious patients involved in a traumatic event have an unstable spine until specifically excluded, and should be managed accordingly.
- Consider active warming (for hypothermia) or cooling (for prolonged cardiac arrest or, possibly, head injury).
- If rhabdomyolysis present, ensure adequate circulating volume, urinary alkalinisation, and relief of any compartment syndrome.
- DVT prophylaxis.
- Nursing measures to prevent contractures and pressure sores.

See also:

Acute weakness

Severe acute weakness may require urgent intubation and mechanical ventilation if the FVC <1L or gas exchange deteriorates acutely. Critical illness neuromyopathy presents with generalised weakness ± loss of sensation. It becomes apparent on reducing sedation in critically ill patients and is likely to be a neuromuscular manifestation of multiple organ failure.

Causes

- Critical illness neuromyopathy.
- New onset CVA—usually unilateral—increased risk in critical care patients with cerebral hypoperfusion and/or coagulopathy.
- Metabolic myopathies—treat low K^+, Mg^{2+}, Ca^{2+}, phosphate.
- Prolonged effects of muscle relaxants—consider low pseudocholinesterase levels or myasthenia if occurs after suxamethonium use. Prolonged effects of non-depolarising muscle relaxants are suggested by response to an anticholinesterase (neostigmine 2.5mg slow IV bolus with an anticholinergic). Patients with myasthenia gravis also respond.
- Cord compression.
- Guillain–Barré syndrome—lumbar puncture will confirm raised CSF protein with normal cells. If not found but suspicion remains strong, nerve conduction studies may demonstrate segmental demyelination with slow conduction velocities.
- Myasthenia gravis—fatigable weakness or ptosis suggests myasthenia gravis; response to IV edrophonium (Tensilon® test) and a strongly positive acetylcholine receptor antibody titre are confirmatory. Myasthenic syndrome associated with malignancy (Eaton–Lambert syndrome) often involves pelvic and thigh muscles, and tends to spare ocular muscles.
- Other diagnoses are made largely on the basis of clinical suspicion and specialised tests.

Management

- Correction of electrolyte and metabolic abnormalities and removal (if possible) of potentially contributory factors, e.g. corticosteroids.
- For Guillain–Barré, monitor FVC 2–4 hourly; intubate and mechanically ventilate if FVC <1L. Give IV Ig and consider plasmapheresis. Other indices of respiratory function are less sensitive. In particular, arterial blood gases may be maintained up to the point of respiratory arrest.
- Weak respiratory muscles lead to progressive basal atelectasis and sputum retention. Chest infection is a significant risk; regular chest physiotherapy with intermittent positive pressure breathing is required for prevention where mechanical ventilation is not necessary.
- Give DVT prophylaxis to immobile patients. They also require attention to posture to prevent pressure sores and contractures.
- Weak bulbar muscles may compromise swallowing with consequent malnutrition or pulmonary aspiration. Enteral nutritional support via a nasogastric tube is necessary.
- In cases with coexistent autonomic neuropathy, enteral nutrition may be impossible, necessitating parenteral nutritional support. They may also suffer arrhythmias and hypotension requiring appropriate support.

Causes of severe generalised weakness

Common in ICU	Uncommon in ICU
Metabolic myopathies	Endocrine myopathy
Prolonged effects of muscle relaxants	Lead poisoning
Critical illness neuromyopathy	Organophosphorus poisoning
Guillain–Barré syndrome	Botulism
Myasthenia gravis	Chronic relapsing polyneuritis
Pontine CVA	Sarcoid neuropathy
Substance abuse (especially benzene ring compounds)	Poliomyelitis
Multiple sclerosis	Diphtheria
	Familial periodic paralysis
	Porphyria

See also:

Airway maintenance, p40; Endotracheal intubation, p42; Ventilatory support—indications, p44; IPPV—assessment of weaning, p60; Pulmonary function tests, p148; Guillain–Barré syndrome, p456; Myasthenia gravis, p458; Critical care neuromuscular disorders, p460; Tetanus, p462; Botulism, p466.

Delirium

In the ICU, agitation and/or confusion are predominantly related to loss of day-night rhythm and inability to sleep, sepsis, cerebral hypoperfusion, or drugs (or their withdrawal). Delirium is related to increased mortality. 'ICU psychosis' is a common occurrence in the patient recovering from severe illness. 'Silent delirium', usually presenting as a withdrawn, non-communicative patient, is significantly under-recognised.

Common ICU causes

- Infection: including generalised sepsis, chest, cannula sites, urinary tract. Cerebral infection such as meningitis, encephalitis and malaria are relatively rare but should always be considered.
- Drug-related: (i) adverse reaction (particularly in the elderly), e.g. to sedatives, analgesics, diuretics, (ii) withdrawal, e.g. sedatives, analgesics, ethanol, (iii) abuse, e.g. opiates, amphetamines, alcohol, hallucinogens.
- Metabolic: e.g. hypoglycaemia or hyperglycaemia, hyponatraemia or hypernatraemia, hypercalcaemia, uraemia, hepatic encephalopathy, hypothermia or hyperthermia, dehydration.
- Respiratory: infection, hypoxaemia, hypercapnia.
- Neurological: infection (meningo-encephalitis, malaria), post-head injury/seizure/cardiac arrest, space-occupying lesion (e.g. haematoma).
- Haemodynamic: low output state, hypotension, endocarditis.
- Pain: full bladder (blocked Foley catheter), abdominal pain.
- Psychosis: 'ICU psychosis', other psychiatric states.

Principles of management

1. Examine and investigate for signs of: (i) infection, (ii) cardiovascular in-stability, (iii) covert pain, e.g. full bladder, (iv) focal neurology, e.g. men-ingism, unequal pupils, hemiparesis, respiratory failure (arterial blood gases), (v) metabolic derangement (biochemical screen).
2. If any of the above are found, treat as appropriate. Psychosis should not be assumed until treatable causes are excluded.
3. Reassure and calm the patient. Maintain quiet atmosphere and reduce noise levels. Attempt to restore day-night rhythm, e.g. by changing am-bient lighting and use of oral hypnotic agents, e.g. temazepam, a tot of alcohol, chloral.
4. Consider starting, changing, or increasing dose of sedative or major tranquilliser to control patient. If highly agitated and likely to endan-ger themselves, rapid short-term control can be achieved by a slow IV bolus of sedative. Consider propofol, a benzodiazepine, haloperidol, or chlorpromazine in the smallest possible dose to achieve the desired effect; observe for hypotension, respiratory depression, arrhythmias, and extrapyramidal effects. Opiates may be needed, especially if pain or withdrawal is a factor. An ethanol infusion can be considered for delirium tremens resulting from alcohol withdrawal, but this generally cannot be managed on a general ward on ICU discharge.
5. Sedation can be maintained by continuous infusion or intermittent in-jection, either regularly or as required. The less agitated patient may respond to IM injections of a major tranquilliser, though these should be avoided with concurrent coagulopathy.
6. There is no strong evidence for the use of antidepressants in ICU.

Drug dosages for severe agitation

Haloperidol	2.5mg by slow IV bolus. Repeat, doubling dose, every 10–15min until effect. For regular prescription, give qds.
Chlorpromazine	12.5mg by slow IV bolus. Repeat, doubling dose, every 10–15min until effect. May need up to 100mg. For regular prescription, give qds.
Midazolam/diazepam	2–5mg by slow IV bolus
Propofol	30–100mg by slow IV bolus
Morphine	2.5–5mg by slow IV bolus

NB. Beware excessive central and respiratory depression with opiates, benzodiazepines, and propofol.

Confusion assessment method for the ICU

CAM-ICU is a validated delirium monitoring instrument for use in ICU patients. For more details, see <www.icudelirium.org>.

Feature 1: Acute onset or fluctuating course
Different to baseline mental status or any fluctuation in mental status in the past 24h as evidenced by fluctuation on a sedation scale (e.g. RASS), GCS, or previous delirium assessment?

Feature 2: Inattention
Positive if cannot provide correct answers to number or picture test.

Feature 3: Disorganised thinking
Positive if fails to answer correctly logical statements (e.g. can you use a hammer to cut wood?) or to perform simple repetitive commands.

Feature 4: Altered level of consciousness
Positive if RASS or other sedation score is anything other than normal.

Overall CAM-ICU score:
Presence of features 1 and 2 and either feature 3 or 4 is positive for delirium.

Key papers

Ely EW, Inouye SK, Bernard GR et al. (2001) Delirium in mechanically ventilated patients: validity and reliability of the confusion assessment method for the intensive care unit (CAM-ICU). *JAMA* **286**: 2703–10.

Sessler CN, Gosnell M, Grap MJ et al. (2002) The Richmond Agitation-Sedation Scale: validity and reliability in adult intensive care patients. *Am J Respir Crit Care Med* **166**: 1338–44.

Girard TD, Kress JP, Fuchs BD, et al. (2008) Efficacy and safety of a paired sedation and ventilator weaning protocol for mechanically ventilated patients in intensive care (Awakening and Breathing Controlled trial): a randomised controlled trial. *Lancet* **371**: 126–34.

See also:

IPPV—failure to tolerate ventilation, p52; Toxicology, p228; Sedatives and tranquilisers, p308; Coma, p438; Generalised seizures, p444; Meningitis, p446; Infection—diagnosis, p552; Malaria, p568; Head injury (1), p586; Head injury (2), p588; Pain, p618; Pain and comfort, p624.

Generalised seizures

Control of seizures is necessary to prevent ischaemic brain damage, reduce cerebral oxygen requirements, and reduce intracranial pressure. Where possible, correct the cause and give specific treatment. A CT scan may be necessary to identify structural causes. Common causes include:

- Hypoxaemia.
- Hypoglycaemia.
- Abnormal plasma Ca^{2+}, Na^+, and Mg^{2+} levels.
- Space-occupying lesions.
- Metabolic and toxic disorders, e.g. liver failure, renal failure.
- Drug withdrawal, e.g. alcohol, benzodiazepines, anticonvulsants.
- Infection, especially meningo-encephalitis.
- Trauma.
- Idiopathic epilepsy.

Most seizures are self-limiting, simply needing protection from injury (coma position, protect head). Do not force anything into the mouth.

Specific treatment

- Correct hypoxaemia with oxygen (FIO_2 0.6–1.0).
- Intubate and ventilate if the airway is unprotected or the patient remains hypoxaemic despite breathing a high FIO_2.
- Urgently measure blood glucose and treat hypoglycaemia with 50% glucose 25–50mL IV.
- Correct anticonvulsant levels in known epileptics.
- Manage cerebral oedema with sedation, induced hypothermia, controlled hyperventilation, and osmotic diuretics.
- In patients with a known tumour, arteritis, or parasitic infection, high-dose dexamethasone may be given.
- Give thiamine 100mg IV to alcoholics and malnourished individuals.
- Consider surgery for space-occupying lesions, e.g. blood clot, tumour.

Anticonvulsants

Treatment should be commenced after 5 mins of continuous seizure activity.

- Benzodiazepines (e.g. lorazepam, diazepam) are first-line treatment.
- Phenytoin: give a loading dose IV if patient has not previously received phenytoin. Phenytoin may not provide immediate control of seizures within the first 24h.

If seizures continue, other appropriate anticonvulsants include:

- Magnesium sulphate.
- Clonazepam, which is particularly useful for myoclonic seizures.
- Propofol infusion.
- Thiopental infusion in severe intractable epilepsy.

With all anticonvulsants, care should be taken to avoid hypoventilation and respiratory failure. Mechanical ventilation will be required to maintain oxygenation in cases of continued seizures.

Other supportive treatment

Muscle relaxants prevent muscular contraction during seizures, but will not prevent continued seizures. They may be necessary to facilitate mechanical ventilation, but continuous (or repeated) EEG monitoring should be used to judge seizure control. Maintain optimal circulation and cerebral blood flow.

Drug dosages

Lorazepam	4mg IV
Diazepam	Initially 2.5–5mg IV or PR. Further increments as necessary to a maximum of 20mg.
Midazolam	Initially 2.5–5mg IV or PR. Further increments as necessary to a maximum of 20mg.
Phenytoin	Loading dose 18mg/kg IV at a rate <50mg/min with continuous ECG monitoring. Maintenance at 300–400mg/d IV, IM, or PO, adjusted according to levels.
Magnesium sulphate	Initially 20mmol over 3–5min, followed by 5–10mmol/h by infusion as necessary.
Clonazepam	1mg/h IV
Thiopental	1–3mg/kg IV, followed by lowest dose to maintain control
Propofol	0.5–2mg/kg IV, followed by 1–3mg/kg/h

Key paper

Treiman VA for the Veterans Affairs Status Epilepticus Cooperative Study Group. (1998) A comparison of four treatments for generalised convulsive status epilepticus. *N Engl J Med* **339**: 792–8.

See also:

Airway maintenance, p40; Endotracheal intubation, p42; Ventilatory support—indications, p44; EEG/CFM monitoring, p204; Electrolytes (Na$^+$, K$^+$, Cl$^-$, HCO$_3^-$), p212; Calcium, magnesium, and phosphate, p214; Anticonvulsants, p310; Respiratory failure, p350; Acute renal failure—diagnosis, p400; Acute liver failure, p430; Hepatic encephalopathy, p432; Chronic liver failure, p434; Meningitis, p446; Intracranial haemorrhage, p448; Stroke, p452; Raised intracranial pressure, p454; Hyponatraemia, p486; Hypomagnesaemia, p492; Hypocalcaemia, p496; Hypoglycaemia, p506; Head injury (1), p586; Head injury (2), p588.

Meningitis

A life-threatening condition demanding prompt treatment. As classical features of meningism may be absent, suspect in those presenting with obtundation, agitation, seizures, or focal neurology. Signs may be subtle or present insidiously in neutropaenics and the elderly. Meningococcaemia presents with a prominent rash in only 30% of cases, while *Listeria (L.) monocytogenes* may cause early seizures and focal neurology.

Diagnosis

- Bacterial meningitis is primarily diagnosed by CSF examination. Send lumbar puncture (LP) samples for urgent microscopy and culture, PCR, virology, protein and glucose estimation (+ concurrent plasma sample). Normal or lymphocytic CSF may be found in early pyogenic meningitis, especially *L. monocytogenes*.
- Raised ICP is common; LP (but not antibiotics) should be delayed until after the CT scan. A normal CT scan does not exclude raised ICP).
- Start empirical antibiotic therapy with concurrent corticosteroids immediately after taking blood cultures. CSF cultures are positive in 50% if antibiotics are given and 60–90% in untreated cases.
- CSF bacterial antigen testing is available for most infecting organisms; sensitivity varies from 50–100% while specificity is high.

Management

1. Antibiotic therapy, usually for ≥10 days though recent studies suggest equal efficacy with shorter courses.
2. Dexamethasone 10mg qds for four days should be started with or just before the first dose of antibiotic. Outcome benefit has been shown for pneumococcal meningitis though it is recommended for all.
3. General measures include attention to fluid and electrolyte replacement, adequate gas exchange, nutrition, and skin care.
4. Management of raised intracranial pressure if present.
5. Oral ciprofloxacin (adults only) or rifampicin should be given to family and close social contacts of meningococcal and haemophilus meningitis. The index case should also be treated before discharge.

Aseptic meningitis

No organisms are identified by routine CSF analysis despite a high neutrophil and/or lymphocyte count. Causes include viruses (e.g. mumps, measles), fungi, leptospirosis, listeriosis, brucellosis, atypical TB, SLE.

Encephalitis

Presenting features include drowsiness, coma, agitation, pyrexia, seizures, and focal signs; meningism need not necessarily be present.

Causes

- Bacterial (as for meningitis).
- Viruses (in particular, herpes simplex and up to 14 days exanthemata). Herpes simplex classically affects the temporal lobe and can be diagnosed by EEG. Aciclovir 10mg/kg tds IV is given for ten days.
- Rarer causes include leptospirosis and brucellosis; CSF reveals no organisms but a high lymphocyte count. If indicated, send CSF for acid fast stain (TB) and India Ink stain (*Cryptococcus*).

Typical CSF values in meningitis

	Pyogenic	Viral	Tuberculosis
Classical appearance	Turbid	Clear	Fibrin web
Predominant cell type	Polymorphs	Lymphocytes	Lymphocytes
Cell count/mm^3	>1000	<500	50–1500
Protein (g/L)	>1	0.5–1	1–5
CSF:blood glucose	<60%	>60%	<60%

Organisms and empirical starting antibiotic therapy

Organism	Patients often affected	Antibiotic and dosage regimen (alternatives in brackets)
Neisseria meningitidis (Meningococcus)	Young adults	Ceftriaxone 2–4g IV od (cefotaxime 50mg/kg IV 8-hourly) (benzylpenicillin 1.2g IV 2–4 hourly) (chloramphenicol 12.5mg/kg IV 6-hourly)
Streptococcus pneumoniae (Pneumococcus)	Older adults	Ceftriaxone 2–4g IV od (cefotaxime 50mg/kg IV 8-hourly) (chloramphenicol 12.5mg/kg IV 6 hourly)
Haemophilus influenzae	Children	Ceftriaxone 20–50mg/kg IV od (cefotaxime 50mg/kg IV 8-hourly) (chloramphenicol 12.5mg/kg IV 6-hourly)
Listeria monocytogenes	Elderly, immuno-compromised	Ampicillin 1g IV 4–6 hourly plus gentamicin 120mg IV stat, then 80mg 8–12 hourly (adjust by plasma levels)
Mycobacterium tuberculosis		Rifampicin/isoniazid/ethambutol/pyrazinamide
Cryptococcus neoformans	Immuno-compromised	Amphotericin B starting at 250mcg/kg IV od + flucytosine 50mg/kg IV 6-hourly
Staphylococcus aureus		Flucloxacillin 2g IV 6-hourly (vancomycin, teicoplanin, or linezolid (600mg IV 12hourly), often + rifampicin if MRSA)

Key papers

de Gans J, van de Beek D; European Dexamethasone in Adulthood Bacterial Meningitis Study Investigators. (2002) Dexamethasone in adults with bacterial meningitis. *N Engl J Med* **347**: 1549–56.

van de Beek D, de Gans J, McIntyre P, et al. (2007) Corticosteroids for acute bacterial meningitis. *Cochrane Database Syst Rev* **24**;(1): CD004405.

See also:

Bacteriology, p224; Virology, serology, and assays, p226; Antimicrobials, p326; Corticosteroids, p330; Basic resuscitation, p338; Coma, p438; Delirium, p442; Generalised seizures, p444; Raised intracranial pressure, p454; Infection control—general principles, p544; Infection control—dangerous pathogens, p548; Infection—diagnosis, p552; Infection—treatment, p554.

Intracranial haemorrhage

Extradural haemorrhage

Usually presents acutely after head injury. Characterised by falling Glasgow coma score progressing to coma, focal signs (lateralising weakness or anaesthesia, pupillary signs), visual disturbances, and seizures. Treatment by random burr holes has been supplanted by directed drainage following CT scan localisation.

A conservative approach may be adopted for small haematomata, but increasing size (assessed by regular CT scanning or clinical deterioration) are indications for surgical drainage.

Subdural haemorrhage

Classically presents days to weeks following head trauma with a fluctuating level of consciousness (35%), agitation, confusion, seizures, and signs of raised intracranial pressure, localising signs, or a slowly evolving stroke. Diagnosis is made by CT scan. Treatment is by surgical drainage.

Intracerebral haemorrhage

Causes include hypertension, neoplasm, vasculitis, coagulopathy, and mycotic aneurysms associated with bacterial endocarditis.

Clinical features include sudden onset coma, drowsiness and/or neurological deficit. Headache usually occurs only with cortical and intraventricular haemorrhage. The rate of evolution depends on the size and size of the bleed. The area affected is the putamen (55%), thalamus (10%), cerebral cortex (15%), pons (10%), and cerebellum (10%).

Diagnosis

CT scan is the definitive test. A coagulation and vasculitis blood screen may be indicated. Angiography is indicated if surgical repair is contemplated though not for drainage of blood clot.

Treatment

* Bed rest.
* Supportive (e.g. hydration, nutrition, analgesia, ventilatory support).
* Physiotherapy.
* Blood pressure control (maintain systolic BP <220–230mmHg).
* Correct any coagulopathy.
* Control raised intracranial pressure.
* Surgery—contact Regional Centre, e.g. for evacuation of haematoma, repair/clipping of aneurysm.
* Corticosteroid therapy is ineffective.

See also:

Subarachnoid haemorrhage

Pathology

- In 15%, no cause is found; of the remainder, 80% are due to a ruptured aneurysm, 5% to arteriovenous malformations, and 15% follow trauma.
- The anterior part of the Circle of Willis is affected in 90–95% of subarachnoid haemorrhage (SAH) while 10–15% affect the vertebrobasilar system.
- There is a 30% risk of rebleeding for which the mortality is 40%. Those surviving a month have a 90% chance of surviving a year.
- Cerebral vasospasm occurs in 30–40% of patients at 4–12 days after the bleed. This is the most important cause of morbidity and mortality.
- Hydrocephalus, seizures, hyponatraemia, and inappropriate ADH secretion are recognised complications.

Clinical features

- SAH may be preceded by a prodrome of headache, dizziness, and vague neurological symptoms.
- Often there is rapid onset (minutes to hours) presentation, including collapse, severe headache ± meningism.
- Cranial nerve palsies, drowsiness, and hemiplegia may also occur.

Diagnosis

Diagnosis is usually made by CT scan; if there is no evidence of raised intracranial pressure, a lumbar puncture may be performed revealing bloodstained CSF with xanthochromia.

Management

- Bed rest.
- Maintain adequate hydration, nutrition, analgesia, sedation.
- Cerebral vasospasm is prevented by nimodipine infusion and maintenance of a full intravascular volume.
- Systemic hypertension should only be treated if severe (e.g. systolic pressure >220–230mmHg) and prolonged.
- Surgery: the timing is controversial with either early or delayed (7–10 days) intervention being advocated. The Regional Neurosurgical Centre should be consulted for local policy.
- Antifibrinolytic therapy (e.g. tranexamic acid) reduces the incidence of rebleeding, but has no beneficial effect on outcome.

Key paper

Allen GS, Ahn HS, Preziosi T J, et al. (1983) Cerebral arterial spasm—a controlled trial of nimodipine in patients with subarachnoid haemorrhage. *N Engl J Med* **308**: 619–24.

Stroke

Pathology

- Haemorrhagic, embolic or thrombotic.
- 'Secondary' stroke may occur with meningitis, bacterial endocarditis, subarachnoid haemorrhage, and vasculitis.
- Dissection and cerebral venous thrombosis need to be considered, as anticoagulation is indicated for both (unless a large infarct is established as there is an increased risk of bleeding). Dissection should be suspected in younger patients, often presenting with severe headache or neck pain ± Horner's syndrome ± seizures after trauma or neck manipulation. Cerebral venous thrombosis may mimic stroke, tumour, subarachnoid haemorrhage, or meningo-encephalitis, and may present with headache, seizures, focal signs, or obtundation.

Urgent CT scan

Indicated when the diagnosis is in doubt, for continuing deterioration, suspicion of subarachnoid haemorrhage, hydrocephalus or trauma, or for patients who are anticoagulated or who have a bleeding tendency.

Aims of treatment

- To protect the penumbra with close attention to oxygenation, hydration, tight glycaemic control, and avoidance of pyrexia.
- Blood pressure control is needed for severe hypertension (e.g. >200/120mmHg) and for hypotension.
- Aspirin is given early for thrombotic stroke. The evidence for full anticoagulation is contentious as there is an increased risk of bleeding and no consistent subgroup benefit has been shown. Early anticoagulation probably benefits intracranial stenosis, stroke-in-evolution, complete vessel occlusion with minimal deficit, and in low-risk patients with a high probability of recurrence (secondary prevention).
- For thrombolysis, reperfusion extent depends on aetiology with basilar > middle cerebral artery > internal carotid, and embolic > thrombotic. Studies with rtPA (0.9mg/kg) given within 3h of stroke onset (and tight BP control) show favourable outcomes. However, there was a 6-fold increase in haemorrhage (to 5.9%), of whom 60% died. This was more common in the elderly and with more severe stroke.
- Some centres perform intra-arterial or ultrasound-enhanced thrombolysis.
- Neurosurgical intervention ± decompression may be considered for cerebellar haematoma, cerebellar infarction, and the 'malignant middle cerebral artery syndrome' (for massive infarction on the non-dominant side).
- Therapeutic hypothermia is theoretically beneficial but no large trial has yet been performed. Concerns include an increased risk of haemorrhage and rebound intracranial hypertension on rewarming.

Key paper

Hacke W , Donnan G, Fieschi C, et al. (2004) Association of outcome with early stroke treatment: pooled analysis of ATLANTIS, ECASS, and NINDS rt-PA stroke trials. *Lancet* **363**: 768–74.

See also:
Oxygen therapy, p38; Ventilatory support—indications, p44; Therapeutic hypothermia, p100;
Tight glycaemic control/intensive insulin therapy, p132; Blood pressure monitoring, p164;
Neuroprotective agents, p312; Thrombolytics, p316; Basic resuscitation, p338; Coma, p438;
Generalised seizures, p444; Intracranial haemorrhage, p448; Subarachnoid haemorrhage, p450;
Raised intracranial pressure, p454.

Raised intracranial pressure

Clinical features

- Headache, vomiting, dizziness, visual disturbance.
- Seizures, focal neurology, papilloedema.
- Increasing blood pressure, bradycardia (late responses).
- Agitation, increasing drowsiness, coma.
- Slow deep breaths, Cheyne–Stokes breathing, apnoea.
- Ipsilateral progressing to bilateral pupillary dilatation.
- Decorticate progressing to decerebrate posturing.

Diagnosis

- CT scan or MRI.
- Intracranial pressure (ICP) measurement >20mmHg.

Lumbar puncture should be avoided because of the risk of coning. Neither CT scan nor absence of papilloedema will exclude a raised ICP.

Management

1. Bed rest, 20–30° head-up tilt, sedation, quiet environment, minimal suction and noise. Sedation and β-blockade are often necessary to overcome a hyperadrenergic state, but sedative-induced hypotension should be avoided. The tape tethering the endotracheal tube in place should not occlude jugular venous drainage.
2. Ventilate if GCS ≤8, airway unprotected, or excessively agitated.
3. Maintain $PaCO_2$ at 4–4.5kPa and avoid rapid rises. CSF bicarbonate levels re-equilibrate within 4–6h, negating any benefit from hyperventilation.
4. If available and not contraindicated, monitor ICP. Aim to maintain ICP <20mmHg and cerebral perfusion pressure (= MAP – ICP) >70mmHg. Vasopressor therapy may be needed. Do not treat systemic hypertension unless very high (e.g. systolic >220–230mmHg).
5. Other monitoring techniques, e.g. jugular bulb venous saturation (SjO_2) and lactate, may be useful though they do not detect regional ischaemia.
6. Give mannitol 0.5mg/kg IV over 15min. Repeat at 4-hourly intervals depending on cerebral perfusion pressure (CPP) measurements and/or clinical signs of deterioration. Stop when plasma osmolality reaches 310–320mOsm/kg.
7. Avoid severe alkalosis as cerebral vascular resistance rises and cerebral ischaemia increases.
8. Consider specific treatment, e.g. for meningo-encephalitis, malaria, hepatic encephalopathy, surgery. Some neurosurgeons will decompress the cranium for generalised oedema by removing a skull flap. Seek local advice. Dexamethasone 4–16mg qds IV is beneficial for oedema surrounding a tumour or abscess and for herpes simplex encephalitis.

Acute deterioration/risk of imminent coning

1. Mechanically ventilate to $PaCO_2$ 3.0–3.5kPa for 10–20min.
2. Give mannitol 0.5g/kg IV over 15min. Repeat 4-hourly as necessary and stop when plasma osmolality >310–320mOsm/kg. Consider therapeutic hypothermia.
3. If no response in ICP, CPP and/or clinical features, give thiopental (successful in 50% of resistant cases).
4. Consider repeat CT scan and refer for urgent surgery if a surgically-amenable space-occupying lesion is diagnosed.

Causes of raised intracranial pressure
- Space-occupying lesion (e.g. neoplasm, blood clot, abscess).
- Increased capillary permeability (e.g. trauma, infection, hepatic encephalopathy).
- Cell death (e.g. hypoxia).
- Obstruction (e.g. hydrocephalus).

See also:
Oxygen therapy, p38; Ventilatory support—indications, p44; Therapeutic hypothermia, p100; Blood pressure monitoring, p164; Intracranial pressure monitoring, p200; Jugular venous bulb saturation, p202; Other neurological monitoring, p206; Neuroprotective agents, p312; Basic resuscitation, p338; Acute liver failure, p430; Hepatic encephalopathy, p432; Coma, p438; Generalised seizures, p444; Meningitis, p446; Intracranial haemorrhage, p448; Subarachnoid haemorrhage, p450; Stroke, p452; Head injury (1), p586; Head injury (2), p588; Brain stem death, p652.

Guillain–Barré syndrome

- An immunologically mediated acute demyelinating polyradiculopathy.
- Viral infections and immunisations are common antecedents.
- It includes a progressive, areflexic motor weakness (often symmetrical, ascending, and involving cranial nerves, including facial, bulbar, and extraocular weakness) with progression over a few days to weeks.
- There are often minor sensory disturbances (e.g. paraesthesiae).
- Autonomic dysfunction is not unusual.
- There is no increase in cell count on CSF examination, but protein levels usually rise progressively (>0.4g/L).
- Nerve conduction studies show slow conduction velocities with prolonged F waves.
- Other features include muscle tenderness and back pain.
- The major contributors to morbidity and mortality are respiratory muscle weakness and autonomic dysfunction (hypotension, hypertension, arrhythmias, ileus, and urinary retention).

Differential diagnosis

Other causes of acute weakness must be excluded before a diagnosis of Guillain–Barré syndrome can be made.

Specific treatment

- Intravenous immunoglobulin (0.4g/kg/d for five days) or plasma exchange (five 50mL/kg exchanges over 8–13 days) is effective if started within 14 days of onset of symptoms.
- Corticosteroids have not been shown to be beneficial.

Supportive treatment

Respiratory care

Regular chest physiotherapy and spirometry are required. Mechanical ventilation is needed if FVC <1L or $PaCO_2$ is raised. An early tracheostomy is useful since mechanical ventilation is likely to continue for several weeks. Patients with bulbar involvement or inadequate cough should have a tracheostomy even if spontaneous breathing continues.

Cardiovascular care

Continuous cardiovascular monitoring is required due to the effects of autonomic involvement. Arrhythmias are particularly likely with anaesthesia (especially with suxamethonium). Hypertensive and hypotensive responses are generally exaggerated with vasoactive drugs.

Nutritional support

Parenteral nutrition will be required in cases where there is ileus. Enteral nutrition is preferred if possible, but it should be noted that energy and fluid requirements are reduced in Guillain–Barré syndrome.

Analgesia

Analgesia is required for muscle, abdominal, and back pain. Although NSAIDs may be useful, opiates are often required.

Other support

Particular attention is required to pressure areas and deep vein thrombosis prophylaxis.

Key papers

Plasma Exchange/Sandoglobulin Guillain-Barré Syndrome Trial Group. (1997) Randomised trial of plasma exchange, intravenous immunoglobulin, and combined treatments in Guillain-Barré syndrome. *Lancet* **349**: 225–30.

van Koningsveld R, for the Dutch GBS study group. (2004) Effect of methylprednisolone when added to standard treatment with intravenous immunoglobulin for Guillain-Barré syndrome: randomised trial. *Lancet* **363**: 192–6.

Hughes RA, Swan AV, Raphaël JC, et al. (2007) Immunotherapy for Guillain-Barré syndrome: a systematic review. *Brain* **130**: 2245–57.

See also:

Airway maintenance, p40; Endotracheal intubation, p42; Ventilatory support—indications, p44; Plasma exchange, p114; Pulmonary function tests, p148; ECG monitoring, p162; Blood pressure monitoring, p164; Respiratory failure, p350; Hypotension, p380; Hypertension, p382; Tachyarrhythmias, p384; Bradyarrhythmias, p386; Acute weakness, p440.

Myasthenia gravis

- Myasthenia gravis is an autoimmune disease associated with acetylcholine receptor and, rarely, anti-striated muscle antibodies.
- It is associated with autoimmune thyroid disease, SLE, and rheumatoid arthritis.
- Painless weakness with normal tendon reflexes, deteriorating after exertion, and recovering after rest. Weakness deteriorates during stress, infection, or trauma.
- Younger (<45y), predominantly female patients may have a thymoma which, if resected, may provide remission.

Diagnosis of myasthenia

- Edrophonium is a short-acting anticholinesterase used in the diagnosis.
- In myasthenic patients with an acute deterioration, the test may distinguish a myasthenic from a cholinergic crisis.
- In cholinergic crisis, edrophonium may cause further deterioration so atropine and facilities for urgent intubation and ventilation should be available. To minimise the risk, a test dose of 1mg is administered. After one minute, give an additional 4mg and, if no change is apparent in one minute, give another 5mg.
- A positive test is judged by improvement of weakness within 3min compared to no improvement with saline injection.
- The test may be combined with objective assessment of respiratory function by measuring the FVC response or by assessing the response to repetitive stimulation with an EMG.

Maintenance treatment

Anticholinesterase drugs provide the mainstay of symptomatic treatment, but corticosteroids, immunosuppressives, and plasma exchange may provide pharmacological remission. Anticholinesterases may produce improvement in some muscle groups and cholinergic deterioration in others due to differential sensitivity.

Myasthenic crisis

- Mechanical ventilatory support if FVC <1L or $PaCO_2$ is raised.
- New myasthenics should be started on corticosteroids ± azathioprine and pyridostigmine. Plasmapheresis may reduce antibody load.
- Known myasthenics require corticosteroids and increased pyridostigmine or neostigmine ± IV immunoglobulin.
- If the condition deteriorates drug therapy should be stopped; plasma exchange may be life-saving.

Cholinergic crisis

- Mechanical ventilatory support if FVC <1L or $PaCO_2$ is raised.
- Cholinergic symptoms (e.g. sweating, salivation, lacrimation, colic, fasciculation, confusion, ataxia, small pupils, bradycardia, hypertension, seizures) are usually most severe 2h after the last anticholinesterase.
- Atropine given prophylactically in the treatment of myasthenia may mask some of the cholinergic symptoms.
- If a deterioration fails to respond to edrophonium, all drugs should be stopped and atropine given.
- Repeat edrophonium test every 2h and reintroduce anticholinesterases when positive.

Drug dosages

Prednisolone	80mg/d orally
Azathioprine	2.5mg/kg/d orally
Pyridostigmine	60–180mg 6-hourly orally
Neostigmine	1–2.5mg 2–4 hourly IV
Atropine	1mg 6-hourly IV, repeated every 30min to maximum of 8mg

Drugs causing deterioration in myasthenia gravis

- Aminoglycosides.
- Streptomycin.
- Tetracyclines.
- Local anaesthetics.
- Muscle relaxants.
- Opiates.

See also:
Airway maintenance, p40; Endotracheal intubation, p42; Ventilatory support—indications, p44; Plasma exchange, p114; Pulmonary function tests, p148; ECG monitoring, p162; Blood pressure monitoring, p164; Corticosteroids, p328; Respiratory failure, p350; Hypertension, p382; Bradyarrhythmias, p386; Acute weakness, p440; Generalised seizures, p444; Vasculitides, p574.

Critical care neuromuscular disorders

Neuromuscular disorders in the critically ill have long been recognised, particularly in those mechanically ventilated. First suspicions are often raised when patients fail to wean from mechanical ventilation or limb weakness is noted on stopping sedation. This may be profound and can persist for weeks to months. Occasionally, it may be permanent. Variable degrees of neuropathy and myopathy are found on EMG, nerve conduction studies, and biopsy. Corticosteroids and prolonged use of paralysing agents are implicated, but this remains unproven. Disuse atrophy, catabolic states, and drug therapy (e.g. high-dose corticosteroids, muscle relaxants) are probably responsible for some cases, but do not explain all. A neuromyopathic component of multi-organ dysfunction syndrome may be relevant.

Critical illness neuropathy

- Neurophysiological studies have demonstrated an acute, idiopathic, axonal degeneration in patients with flaccid weakness following a prolonged period of intensive care.
- Sensation may be affected, alone or in combination with motor fibres.
- Nerve conduction velocities are normal indicating no demyelination. CSF is normal unlike Guillain–Barré syndrome.
- The neuropathy is self-limiting, but prolongs the recovery phase of critical illness. Recovery may take weeks to years.
- Recovery requires multidisciplinary teamwork for rehabilitation and management of neuropathic pain.
- Pyridoxine (100–150mg daily PO) has been used in the treatment, but supporting evidence is not strong.

Critical illness myopathy

- Disuse atrophy and drug induced myopathy are common in critically ill patients.
- Corticosteroid-induced myopathy is less common as the indications for high-dose corticosteroids have been reduced.
- Muscle relaxants may have a prolonged effect and may be potentiated by β_2 agonists. They may be associated with structural myopathic changes when used in asthma.
- Muscle histological studies have demonstrated abnormalities (fibre atrophy, mitochondrial defects, myopathy, and necrosis) which could not be associated with corticosteroid or muscle relaxant therapy. Myopathy may cause renal damage via myoglobinuria.
- Critical illness myopathy is associated with various forms of muscle degeneration, but is usually self-limiting. Recovery may take weeks to years. Occasionally, residual deficit remains.
- Recovery requires multidisciplinary teamwork for rehabilitation.

See also:

IPPV—assessment of weaning, p60; Sedatives and tranquilisers, p308; Muscle relaxants, p310; Acute weakness, p440; Systemic inflammation/multi-organ failure —causes, p556.

Tetanus

The clinical syndrome caused by the exotoxin tetanospasmin from the anaerobe, *Clostridium tetani*, in contaminated or devitalised wounds. Tetanospasmin ascends intra-axonally in motor and autonomic nerves, blocking the release of inhibitory neurotransmitters. The disease may be modified by previous immunisation such that milder or localised symptoms may occur with heavier toxin loads.

Clinical features

- Gradual onset of stiffness, dysphagia, muscle pain, hypertonia and rigidity, and muscle spasm.
- Laryngospasm often follows dysphagia.
- Muscle spasm is often provoked by minor disturbance, e.g. laryngospasm may be provoked by swallowing.
- Onset of symptoms within five days of injury implies a heavy toxin load and severe disease.
- The disease is self-limiting so treatment is supportive, but may need to continue for several weeks.

Management of the wound

If a contaminated wound is present, it should be debrided surgically after 250IU human tetanus immunoglobulin has been given (in a different site to any tetanus toxoid immunisation). Benzylpenicillin 1.2g 6-hourly and metronidazole 500mg 8-hourly IV are appropriate antibiotics. Tetanus-prone wounds include:

- Any wound or burn sustained more than 6h before surgical treatment.
- Any wound or burn with a significant degree of devitalised tissue, puncture-type wounds, contact with soil or manure, or clinical evidence of sepsis.

Mild tetanus

Patients with mild symptoms, no respiratory distress, and a delayed onset of symptoms should be nursed in a quite environment with mild sedation to prevent tetanic spasms.

Severe tetanus

- Intubate and ventilate since asphyxia may occur due to prolonged respiratory muscle spasm.
- Sedate with diazepam (PO or IV as necessary).
- Muscle rigidity is best treated with magnesium sulphate 20mmol/h IV or benzodiazepines, with the addition of muscle relaxants if necessary.
- Autonomic hyper-reactivity (arrhythmias, hypotension, hypertension, and myocardial ischaemia) is often seen. It is minimised by sedation, anaesthesia, and treated by atropine 1–20mg/h IV, propranolol 10mg 8-hourly IV or NG, and magnesium sulphate 20mmol/h IV.
- Human tetanus immunoglobulin 1000–1500 units IM may shorten the course of the disease by removing circulating toxin. Rapid fixation of the toxin to tissues limits the usefulness of this approach.

Tetanus toxoid prophylaxis

The disease confers no immunity so patients must be immunised prior to hospital discharge.

- Last dose of tetanus toxoid <5 years   No further dose
- Last dose of tetanus toxoid <10 years   One dose
- No previous immunisation   3 doses

See also:

Airway maintenance, p40; Endotracheal intubation, p42; Ventilatory support—indications, p44; Sedatives and tranquilisers, p308; Antimicrobials, p326; Respiratory failure, p350; Hypotension, p380; Hypertension, p382; Tachyarrhythmias, p384; Bradyarrhythmias, p386.

Botulism

An uncommon, lethal disease caused by exotoxins of the anaerobe *Clostridium (C.) botulinum*. Botulism is most commonly a foodborne disease, especially associated with canned foods. It may be contracted by wound contamination with aquatic soils or from skin popping (*C. novyi* or *C histolyticum* introduced from drug abusers injecting into skin or muscle). Deliberate release of the toxin or contamination of foodstuff with *C. botulinum* is considered a potential biological weapon with the adult lethal dose of toxin being <1mcg. The toxin is carried in the blood to cholinergic neuromuscular junctions where it binds irreversibly. Symptoms begin between six hours and eight days after contamination and are more severe with earlier onset. Botulism is diagnosed by isolating *C.* from the stool, gastric aspirate or wound, or by mouse bioassay (survival of immunised mice and death of non-immunised mice when infected serum is injected).

Clinical features

- Symptoms include gastrointestinal disturbance, sore throat, fatigue, dizziness, paraesthesiae, cranial involvement, and a progressive, descending flaccid weakness.
- Parasympathetic symptoms are common.
- The disease is usually self-limiting within several weeks.

Management

Antibiotics are not indicated for the management of botulism unless there is a contaminated wound.

Respiratory care

Regular spirometry and mechanical ventilation if FVC <1L. Patients with bulbar palsy need intubation for airway protection.

Toxin removal

If there is no ileus, the use of non-magnesium containing cathartics (e.g. sorbitol) may remove the toxin load. Magnesium may enhance the effect of the toxin.

Antitoxin

Prevents further paralysis but does not reverse existing paralysis. May shorten the course of the disease if given early. There is a risk of anaphylactoid reactions, but usually treatment is limited to two doses minimising the risk.

Wound botulism

Surgical debridement (after antitoxin treatment to neutralise any toxin released during sugery), benzylpenicillin 1.2g IV 6-hourly and metronidazole 500mg IV 8-hourly, and antitoxin are the mainstays of treatment for contaminated wounds.

Key paper

Brett MM, Hallas G, Mpamugo O. (2004) Wound botulism in the UK and Ireland. *J Med Microbiol* **53**: 555–61.

See also:

Airway maintenance, p40; Endotracheal intubation, p42; Ventilatory support—indications, p44; Antimicrobials, p326; Respiratory failure, p350; Bradyarrhythmias, p386.

Haematological disorders

Bleeding disorders

A common problem in the critically ill, this may be due to: (i) large vessel bleeding—usually 'surgical' or following a procedure (e.g. chest drain, tracheostomy, accidental arterial puncture, removal of intravenous or intra-arterial catheter); peptic ulcer bleeding is now relatively uncommon due to improved attention to perfusion and nutrition; (ii) around vascular catheter sites or from intubated/instrumented lumens and orifices—usually related to severe multisystem illness or excess anticoagulant therapy, including thrombolytics; (iii) small vessel bleeding, e.g. skin petechiae, gastric erosions—usually related to anticoagulation or severe generalised illness, including disseminated intravascular coagulation.

Common ICU causes

- Decreased platelet production, e.g. sepsis- or drug-induced.
- Decreased production of coagulation factors, e.g. liver failure.
- Increased consumption, e.g. DIC, trauma, bleeding, heparin-induced thrombocytopaenia, antiplatelet antibodies, extracorporeal circuits.
- Impaired or deranged platelet function.
- Drugs, e.g. heparin, aspirin, antibiotics.

Principles of management

1. Transfuse platelets according to indications in the table.
2. Antiplatelet medication taken in the past 1–2 weeks may affect platelet function, resulting in bleeding despite a normal platelet count. One pool of platelets may be occasionally indicated. Abciximab, acting on glycoprotein 2b/3a, has an antiplatelet effect so patients may be at increased risk of surgical bleeding. Platelets should be made available, but used only for excessive oozing/bleeding.
3. Abnormalities of the prothrombin time (PT) may be due to liver impairment or poor nutritional status. Vitamin K, orally or IV, is indicated. FFP is not needed unless significant bleeding occurs.
4. In patients on warfarin, urgent reversal of INR may be indicated. 1mg vitamin K will reverse warfarin within 4–6h while 10mg will saturate liver stores, preventing warfarin activity for >1 week. Prothrombin complex (e.g. Octaplex®, Beriplex®) will correct INR within 20–30min. Vitamin K (2mg) must be given with the infusion. In a life-threatening bleed due to warfarin, 5mg vitamin K and 50U/kg of prothrombin complex is required. FFP should not be used to reverse warfarin or to correct a slightly increased PT, unless associated with active bleeding, e.g. DIC.
5. For bleeding related to thrombolysis: (i) stop the drug infusion; (ii) give tranexamic acid 10mg/kg, repeated 6–8 hourly; (iii) give 4 units FFP.
6. Cryoprecipitate is rarely needed. Consider when thrombin time is elevated and fibrinogen is reduced, e.g. with DIC. Standard FFP contains fibrinogen and may be satisfactory. However, with fibrinogen levels <1.0 and especially <0.5, consider cryoprecipitate. The aim is to increase fibrinogen levels >1.5. Cryoprecipitate is never indicated in patients with von Willebrand's disease or haemophilia.
7. Factor VIIa may be useful for severe, intractable bleeding once a standard clotting screen and platelet levels have been fully corrected. Further studies are needed to confirm its efficacy.

Management of major bleeding

1. If external, direct occlusion/deep suture.
2. Urgent expert opinion, e.g. for surgery, endoscopy + injection, etc.
3. Correct coagulopathy. Consider use of factor VIIa if very severe and not surgically remediable.

Management of vascular catheter or percutaneous drain site bleeding

1. Direct pressure/occlusive dressing.
2. Correct coagulopathy; consider use of tranexamic acid.
3. Surgical intervention is rarely necessary although perforation/laceration of local artery/vein should be considered if bleeding fails to stop or becomes significant.

Indications for platelet transfusion

Platelet count	Situation
<10 x 10⁹/L	Always
<20 x 10⁹/L	Acute bleeding, sepsis, concurrent use of antibiotics, or other abnormalities of haemostasis. A single pool is normally enough.
<50 x 10⁹/L	DIC or invasive procedures, e.g. insertion of indwelling catheters, transbronchial biopsy, laparotomy
<80 x 10⁹/L	Epidurals and lumbar punctures
<100 x 10⁹/L	Procedures involving closed sites such as surgery to the eyes or brain

See also:

Full blood count, p220; Coagulation monitoring, p222; Blood transfusion, p248; Blood products, p250; Coagulants and antifibrinolytics, p322.

Clotting disorders

Although critically ill patients often tend to be auto-anticoagulated, the risk of major venous thrombosis increases with long-term immobility and paralysis and in specific pro-thrombotic conditions such as pregnancy, thrombotic thrombocytopaenic purpura, SLE (lupus anticoagulant), sickle cell crisis, hyperosmolar diabetic coma, heparin-induced thrombocytopaenia syndrome (HITS), and congenital or acquired protein C or protein S deficiency.

Disseminated intravascular coagulation is associated with microvascular clotting, a consumption coagulopathy, and increased fibrinolysis.

Clotting of extracorporeal circuits, e.g. for renal replacement therapy, may be due to: (i) mechanical obstruction to flow, e.g. kinked catheter; (ii) inadequate anticoagulation; or (iii) in severe illness, a decrease in endogenous anticoagulants (e.g. antithrombin III); this may result in circuit blockage despite a coexisting thrombocytopaenia and/or coagulopathy.

Axillary vein or subclavian vein thrombosis may result from indwelling intravenous catheters.

Management

1. All patients should be given TED (thromboembolic disease) stockings (grade II), preferably above the knee. Exceptions are patients with arterial vascular disease or those in whom the stockings do not fit.
2. If the patient is not auto-anticoagulated, give prophylactic LMW heparin (5000IU od SC) for long-term immobility/paralysis, and to high-risk patients (e.g. previous DVT, femoral fractures).
3. For pulmonary embolism or deep vein thrombosis, give 200IU/kg SC daily (or 100 IU/kg bd if at risk of bleeding).
4. Partial thromboplastin times (PTT) should be checked regularly if giving unfractionated heparin and maintained at approximately 2–3x normal. Monitoring is not necessary for LMW heparin though anti-factor Xa levels can be used.
5. Intra-arterial clot can be treated with local infusion of thrombolytics, usually followed by heparinisation. Seek vascular surgical advice.
6. Axillary vein or subclavian vein thrombosis should be managed by elevation of the affected arm, e.g. in a Bradford sling, and heparinisation.
7. Specific conditions may require specific therapies e.g. plasma exchange for SLE and TTP, whole blood exchange for sickle cell crisis.
8. If HITS is suspected, stop all heparin infusions (including arterial catheter flush) and treat with either danapranoid or hirudin. Confirm with an antibody test.
9. Warfarinisation should be avoided until the platelet count is within the normal range as it may exacerbate the prothrombotic risk.

See also:
Full blood count, p220; Coagulation monitoring, p222; Anticoagulants, p318.

Anaemia

Defined as a low haemoglobin due to a decreased red cell mass, it may also be 'physiological' due to dilution from an increased plasma volume, e.g. pregnancy, vasodilated states.

Major causes in the ICU patient

- Blood loss, e.g. haemorrhage, regular blood sampling.
- Severe illness—analogous to the 'anaemia of chronic disease', there is decreased marrow production and, possibly, a decreased lifespan.

Rarer causes include:

- Microcytic anaemia—predominantly iron deficiency.
- Normocytic—chronic disease.
- Bone marrow failure (idiopathic, drugs, neoplasm, radiation).
- Haemolysis.
- Renal failure.
- Macrocytic—vitamin B_{12} and folate deficiency, alcoholism, cirrhosis, sideroblastic anaemia, hypothyroidism.
- Congenital diseases—sickle cell, thalassaemia.

Management

1. Treatment of the cause where possible.
2. Blood transfusion:
- The ideal haemoglobin level for optimal oxygen carriage and viscosity remains contentious. A multicentre trial showed improved outcomes if a trigger of 7g/dL was used though this was with non-leukodepleted blood which is now rarely used. A higher transfusion threshold, e.g. 9–10g/dL or higher, may potentially benefit those with cardiorespiratory disease although prospective trial data are lacking.
- Transfusion is usually given as packed cells. This may need to be given rapidly during active blood loss or slowly (over 4h) for correction of a gradually falling haemoglobin level.
- In patients needing massive blood transfusion, ensure adequate correction of plasma and platelets to prevent dilutional coagulopathy. For each 6–8 units of packed red cells, give FFP 10–15mL/kg (approx. three bags for a 70kg person), a pool of platelets, and 1 unit of cryoprecipitate.
- Rarely, patients admitted with a chronically low haemoglobin, e.g. <4–5g/dL, which often follows long-term malnutrition or vitamin deficiency, will need a much slower elevation in haemoglobin level to avoid precipitating acute heart failure. Thiamine should be co-administered. An initial target of 7–8g/dL is often acceptable. Obviously, this may need to be altered in the light of any concurrent acute illness, where elevation of oxygen delivery is deemed necessary, or with a concurrent acute haemorrhage. In patients with B_{12} deficiency, blood transfusion should not be given without discussion. Treat with B_{12} injections.
- Erythropoietin reduces the need for blood transfusion in long-term ICU patients, and may be useful in those with multiple antibodies or declining transfusion for religious reasons. Prospective studies found no mortality benefit except in the subgroup admitted following trauma. However, there was a significant increase in thrombotic events.

Key papers

Hébert PC, Wells G, Blajchman MA, et al. for the Transfusion Requirements in Critical Care Investigators, Canadian Critical Care Trials Group. (1999) A multicentre, randomised, controlled clinical trial of transfusion requirements in critical care. *N Engl J Med* **340**: 409–17.

Corwin HL, Gettinger A, Fabian TC, et al. for the EPO Critical Care Trials Group. (2007) Efficacy and safety of Epoetin Alfa in critically ill patients. *N Engl J Med* **357**: 965–76.

See also:

Full blood count, p220; Blood transfusion, p248.

Sickle cell disease

A chronic, hereditary disease almost entirely confined to the black population where the gene for Hb S is inherited from each parent. The red blood cells lack Hb A; when deprived of oxygen, these cells assume sickle shapes, resulting in erythrostasis, occlusion of blood vessels, thrombosis, and tissue infarction. After stasis, cells are more fragile and prone to haemolysis. Occasionally, there may be bone marrow failure.

Chronic features

Patients with sickle cell disease are chronically anaemic (7–8g/dL) with a hyperdynamic circulation. Splenomegaly is common in youth, but with progressive episodes of infarction, splenic atrophy occurs leading to an increased risk of infection, particularly pneumococcal.

Chronic features include skin ulcers, renal failure, avascular bone necrosis (± supervening osteomyelitis, especially *Salmonella*), hepatomegaly, jaundice, and cardiomyopathy. Sudden cardiac death is not uncommon, usually before the age of 30.

Sickle cell crises

Crises are precipitated by various triggers, e.g. hypoxaemia (air travel, anaesthesia, etc.), infection, cold, dehydration, and emotional stress.

Thrombotic crisis

This occurs most frequently in the bones or joints, but also affect chest and abdomen, giving rise to severe pain. Occasionally, neurological symptoms (e.g. seizures, focal signs), haematuria, or priapism may be present. Pulmonary crisis is common; secondary chest infection or ARDS may supervene, worsening hypoxaemia, and further exacerbating the crisis.

Aplastic crisis

Related to parvovirus infection, it is suggested by worsening anaemia and a reduction in the normally elevated reticulocyte count (10–20%).

Haemolytic crisis

Intravascular haemolysis with haemoglobinuria, jaundice, and renal failure sometimes occurs.

Sequestration crisis

Rapid hepatic and splenic enlargement due to red cell trapping with severe anaemia. This condition is particularly serious.

Management

Prophylaxis against crisis includes avoidance of hypoxaemia, other known precipitating factors, prophylactic penicillin, and pneumococcal vaccine.

1. Painful crises usually require prompt opiate infusions. Although psychological dependence is a risk in a small number of patients, analgesia should not be withheld.
2. Give oxygen to maintain SaO_2 at 97–99%. Avoid hyperoxia.
3. Rehydrate with intravenous fluids and keep warm.
4. If infection is suspected, antibiotics should be given as indicated.
5. Transfuse blood if haemoglobin falls. In central nervous respiratory crisis, perform red cell exchange (manual or via apheresis).
6. Lower proportion of sickle cells to <30% by exchange transfusion.
7. Mechanical ventilation may be necessary for chest crises.

Haemolysis

Shortening of erythrocyte lifespan below the expected 120 days. Marked intravascular haemolysis may lead to jaundice and haemoglobinuria.

Causes

- Blood transfusion reactions.
- Malaria.
- Sickle cell haemolytic crisis.
- Drugs, e.g. high-dose penicillin, methyl dopa.
- Autoimmune (cold or warm antibody-mediated)—may be idiopathic or secondary, e.g. lymphoma, SLE, mycoplasma.
- Haemolytic uraemic syndrome/thrombotic thrombocytopaenic purpura (microangiopathic haemolytic anaemia).
- Trauma (cardiac valve prosthesis).
- Glucose-6-phosphate dehydrogenase deficiency—oxidative crises occur following ingestion of fava beans or administration of drugs (e.g. primaquine, sulphonamides) leading to rapid onset anaemia and jaundice.

Diagnosis

- Unconjugated hyperbilirubinaemia, increased urinary urobilinogen (increased RBC breakdown).
- Reticulocytosis (increased RBC production).
- Splenic hypertrophy (extravascular haemolysis).
- Methaemoglobinaemia, haemoglobinuria, free plasma haemoglobin (intravascular haemolysis), reduced serum haptoglobins.
- RBC fragmentation (microangiopathic haemolytic anaemia).
- Coombs' test (immune-mediated haemolysis).
- Other (including haemoglobin electrophoresis, bone marrow biopsy).

Management

1. Identification and specific treatment of the cause where possible.
2. Blood transfusion to maintain haemoglobin >7g/dL.
3. Massive intravascular haemolysis may lead to acute renal failure. Maintain a good diuresis and haemo(dia)filter if necessary.

See also:
Full blood count, p220; Blood transfusion, p248; Anaemia, p472; Sickle cell disease, p474; Malaria, p568; SARS, VHF, and H5N1, p570.

Platelet disorders

Thrombocytopaenia

Rarely symptomatic until the platelet count <50 x 10^9/L; spontaneous bleeding is more likely when the count <20 x 10^9/L. Although bleeding is often minor, e.g. skin petechiae, oozing at intravascular catheter sites, it may be massive or life-threatening, e.g. haemoptysis, intracranial haemorrhage.

Causes
- Sepsis—a common cause of a low platelet count in the critically ill; it is often a barometer of either recovery or deterioration.
- Disseminated intravascular coagulation.
- Drugs.
- Related to antiplatelet antibody production, e.g. heparin (heparin-induced thrombocytopaenia syndrome, HITS), sulphonamides, quinine.
- Resulting in bone marrow suppression, e.g. chemotherapy agents.
- Others, e.g. aspirin, chlorpromazine, prochlorperazine, digoxin.
- Following massive bleeding and multiple blood transfusions.
- Bone marrow failure, e.g. tumour infiltration, drugs.
- Splenomegaly.
- Thrombotic thrombocytopaenic purpura (TTP), haemolytic uraemic syndrome (HUS).
- Idiopathic thrombocytopaenic purpura (ITP).
- Specific infections, e.g. measles, infectious mononucleosis, typhus.
- Collagen vascular diseases, e.g. SLE.

Management
1. Treat the cause, e.g. antibiotics for sepsis, stopping offending drugs, plasma exchange for TTP, splenectomy and corticosteroids for ITP.
2. Platelet support:
- Platelet transfusions in an otherwise well person with no significant bleeding can be withheld until the count falls <10 x 10^9/L.
- Give 1–2 pools if count <50 x 10^9/L and either bleeding, septic or due to undergo surgery/invasive procedure. For CNS or eye surgery, aim for counts >100 x 10^9/L.
- Platelet transfusion is contraindicated in TTP, HUS, and HITS.

Deranged platelet function

Function may be deranged albeit with normal counts, e.g. following aspirin within past 1–2 weeks, epoprostenol, uraemia. Fresh platelets may be required if the patient is symptomatic. In uraemia, one dose of vasopressin (20mcg IV over 30min) may be useful before surgery.

Thrombocythaemia

Rare in ICU patients; platelet counts often exceed 800 x 109/L.

Causes
Prolonged low level bleeding, post-splenectomy, myeloproliferative disorders. Essential (idiopathic) thrombocythaemia is unusual.

Management
As the major risk is thrombosis, management is based upon mobilising the patient and administration of either prophylactic aspirin (150mg bd PO) or LMW heparin (5000IU od SC). Dipyridamole (300–600mg tds PO) is occasionally used.

See also:
Plasma exchange, p114; Full blood count, p220; Blood products, p250; Anticoagulants, p318;
Corticosteroids, p328.

Metabolic disorders

Electrolyte management

A balance must be achieved between electrolyte intake and output. In electrolyte disturbance consider:
- Altered intake.
- Impaired renal excretion.
- Increased body losses.
- Body compartment redistribution (e.g. increased capillary leak, secondary hyperaldosteronism).

As well as Na^+ and K^+, consider Mg^{2+}, Ca^{2+}, Cl^- and PO_4^{3-} balance.

Plasma electrolyte values are poorly reflective of whole body stores; however, excessively high or low plasma levels may induce symptoms, and deleterious physiological and metabolic sequelae.

Water balance must also be taken into account; depletion or excess repletion may, respectively, concentrate or dilute electrolyte levels.

Gravitational peripheral oedema implies increased total body Na^+ and water though intravascular salt and water depletion may coexist.

The usual daily requirements of Na^+ and K^+ are 60–80mmol.

Electrolyte losses
- Large nasogastric aspirate, vomiting Na^+, Cl^-
- Sweating Na^+, Cl^-
- Polyuria Na^+, Cl^-, K^+, Mg^{2+}
- Diarrhoea Na^+, Cl^-, K^+, Mg^{2+}
- Ascitic drainage Na^+, Cl^-, K^+

Principles of management
1. Establish sources and degree of fluid and electrolyte losses.
2. Assess patient for signs of: (i) intravascular fluid depletion—hypotension (e.g. following changes in posture, PEEP, vasodilating drugs), oliguria, increasing metabolic acidosis, thirst; (ii) total body NaCl and water overload—i.e. gravitational oedema.
3. Measure urea, creatinine, osmolality, and electrolyte content of plasma and urine.
4. As appropriate, either replace estimated fluid and electrolyte deficit or increase excretion (with diuretics, haemofiltration). For rate of fluid and specific electrolyte replacement, see individual sections.

Hypernatraemia

Clinical features

Thirst, lethargy, coma, seizures, muscular tremor and rigidity, and an increased risk of intracranial haemorrhage. Thirst usually occurs when the plasma sodium rises 3–4mmol/L above normal. Lack of thirst is associated with central nervous system disease.

Management

Depends upon the cause and whether total body sodium stores are normal, low or elevated, and body water is normal or low.

Rate of correction

- If hyperacute (<12h), correction can be rapid.
- Otherwise, aim for gradual correction of plasma sodium levels (over 1–3 days), particularly in chronic cases (>2 days' duration), to avoid cerebral oedema through sudden lowering of osmolality. A rate of plasma sodium lowering <0.7mmol/h has been suggested.

Hypovolaemia

- If hypovolaemia is accompanied by haemodynamic alterations, restore the circulation with colloid or (less efficiently) with a crystalloid such as isotonic saline or (perhaps, preferably to avoid hyperchloraemia), Ringer's lactate.
- Artificial colloid solutions consist of hydroxyethyl starches or gelatins usually dissolved in saline solution.

Normal total body Na⁺ (water loss)

- Water replacement either added to enteral feed or as 5% glucose IV. Up to 5L/d may be necessary.
- If cranial diabetes insipidus is present, restrict salt and give thiazide diuretics. Cranial diabetes insipidus (CDI) may be complete or partial. Complete CDI will require desmopressin (10mcg bd intranasal or 1–2mcg IV bd), whereas partial CDI may require desmopressin but often responds to drugs that increase the rate of ADH secretion or end-organ responsiveness to ADH, e.g. chlorpropamide, hydrochlorthiazide.
- Nephrogenic diabetes insipidus is managed by a low salt diet and thiazides. High-dose desmopressin may be effective. Consider removal of causative agents, e.g. lithium, demeclocycline.

Low total body Na⁺ (Na⁺ and water losses)

- Treat hyperosmolar non-ketotic diabetic crisis or uraemia as appropriate.
- Otherwise consider 0.9% saline or hypotonic (0.45%) saline. Up to 6L/d may be needed.

Increased total body Na⁺ (Na⁺ gain)

- Water replacement either added to enteral feed or as 5% glucose IV. Up to 5L/d may be necessary.
- In addition, furosemide 10–20mg IV prn may be necessary.

Causes of hypernatraemia

Type	Aetiology	Urine
Low total body Na$^+$	Renal losses: Diuretic excess, osmotic diuresis (glucose, urea, mannitol) Extra-renal losses: Excess sweating	[Na$^+$] >20mmol/L Iso- or hypotonic [Na$^+$] <10mmol/L Hypertonic
Normal total body Na$^+$	Renal losses: diabetes insipidus Extra-renal losses: Respiratory and renal insensible losses	[Na$^+$] variable Hypo-, iso-, or hypertonic [Na$^+$] variable Hypertonic
Increased total body Na$^+$	Conn's syndrome, Cushing's syndrome, excess NaCl, hypertonic NaHCO$_3$	[Na$^+$] >20mmol/L Iso- or hypertonic

See also:

Electrolytes (Na$^+$, K$^+$, Cl$^-$, HCO$_3^-$), p212; Urinalysis, p232; Diuretics, p280; Hyperosmolar diabetic emergencies, p512.

Hyponatraemia

Clinical features

Nausea, vomiting, headache, fatigue, weakness, muscular twitching, obtundation, psychosis, seizures, and coma. Symptoms depend on the rate as well as the magnitude of fall in the plasma $[Na^+]$.

Management

Rate and degree of correction

- In chronic (>48h) asymptomatic hyponatraemia, correction should not exceed 4mmol/L per 24h at a rate <0.3mmol/L/h.
- In chronic symptomatic hyponatraemia, increase plasma Na^+ at 1–1.5mmol/L/h until symptoms resolve, then as per asymptomatic cases.
- In acute (<48h) hyponatraemia, the ideal rate of correction is controversial but should be < 20 mmol/L/24h.
- A plasma Na^+ of 125–130mmol/L is a reasonable target for initial correction of both acute and chronic states.
- Neurological complications, e.g. central pontine myelinolysis, may be related to the degree of correction and (in chronic hyponatraemia) the rate. Premenopausal women are more prone to complications.

Extracellular fluid (ECF) volume excess

- If symptomatic (e.g. seizures, agitation) and not oedematous, give 100mL aliquots hypertonic (1.8%) saline.
- If symptomatic and oedematous, consider furosemide (10–20mg IV bolus prn), mannitol (0.5g/kg IV over 15–20min), and replacement of urinary sodium losses with aliquots of hypertonic saline.
- If not symptomatic, restrict water to 1–1.5L/d. If hyponatraemia persists, consider inappropriate ADH (SIADH) secretion.
- If SIADH likely, give isotonic saline and consider demeclocycline.
- If SIADH unlikely, consider furosemide (10–20mg IV bolus prn), mannitol (0.5g/kg IV over 15–20min), and replacement of urinary sodium losses with aliquots of hypertonic saline.
- Check plasma levels every 2–3 h. Haemofiltration or dialysis may be necessary if renal failure is established.

Extracellular fluid volume (ECF) depletion

- If symptomatic (e.g. seizures, agitation), give isotonic (0.9%) saline; consider hypertonic (1.8%) saline.
- If not symptomatic, give isotonic (0.9%) saline.

General points

- Equations that calculate excess water are unreliable. It is safer to perform frequent estimations of plasma sodium levels.
- Hypertonic saline may be dangerous in the elderly and those with impaired cardiac function. An alternative is to use furosemide with replacement of urinary sodium (and potassium) losses each 2–3h. Thereafter, simple water restriction is usually sufficient.
- Many patients achieve normonatraemia by spontaneous diuresis.
- Use isotonic solutions for reconstituting drugs, etc.
- Hyponatraemia may intensify the cardiac effects of hyperkalaemia.
- True hyponatraemia may occur with a normal osmolality in the presence of abnormal solutes e.g. ethanol, ethylene glycol, glucose.

Causes of hyponatraemia

Type	Aetiology	Urine [Na⁺]
ECF volume depletion	Renal losses:	>20mmol/L
	Diuretic excess, osmotic diuresis (glucose, urea, mannitol), renal tubular acidosis, salt-losing nephritis, mineralocorticoid deficiency	
	Extra-renal losses:	
	Vomiting, diarrhoea, burns, pancreatitis	<10mmol/L
Modest ECF volume excess (no oedema)	Water intoxication:	>20mmol/L
	(NB. Post-operative, TURP syndrome), inappropriate ADH secretion, hypothyroidism, drugs (e.g. carbamazepine, chlorpropamide), glucocorticoid deficiency, pain, emotion	
	Acute and chronic renal failure	
		>20mmol/L
ECF volume excess (oedema)	Nephrotic syndrome, cirrhosis, heart failure	<10mmol/L

Causes of inappropriate ADH secretion

- Neoplasm, e.g. lung, pancreas, lymphoma.
- Most pulmonary lesions.
- Most central nervous system lesions.
- Surgical and emotional stress.
- Glucocorticoid and thyroid deficiency.
- Idiopathic.
- Drugs, e.g. chlorpropamide, carbamazepine, narcotics.

See also:

Electrolytes (Na⁺, K⁺, Cl⁻, HCO₃⁻), p212; Urinalysis, p232; Diuretics, p280; Vomiting/gastric stasis, p406; Diarrhoea, p408; Pancreatitis, p424; Chronic liver failure, p434; Hyperosmolar diabetic emergencies, p512; Burns—fluid management, p592.

Hyperkalaemia

Plasma potassium depends on the balance between intake, excretion, and the distribution of potassium across cell membranes. Excretion is normally controlled by the kidneys.

Causes

- Reduced renal excretion (e.g. chronic renal failure, adrenal insufficiency, diabetes, potassium sparing diuretics).
- Intracellular potassium release (e.g. acidosis, rapid transfusion of old blood, cell lysis—including rhabdomyolysis, haemolysis, tumour lysis, K$^+$ channel openers (nicorandil, isoflurane, ciclosporin).
- Potassium poisoning and iatrogenic overload. A rapid rate of rise of potassium is more dangerous than a chronically elevated level. Cardiac arrest has been seen following 40mmol KCl infused over 1 hour.

Clinical features

Hyperkalaemia may cause dangerous arrhythmias, including cardiac arrest. Arrhythmias are more closely related to the rate of rise of K$^+$ than the absolute level. Clinical features such as paraesthesiae and areflexic weakness are not clearly related to the degree of hyperkalaemia, but usually occur after ECG changes (tall 'T' waves, flat 'P' waves, prolonged PR interval, and wide QRS).

Hypotension, often resistant to high doses of catecholamines, frequently occurs with hyperkalaemia related to excess K$^+$ channel activation.

Management

After confirmation of hyperkalaemia, potassium restriction is needed for all cases and haemodiafiltration or haemodialysis may be needed for resistant cases. An ECG should be performed looking for features of hyperkalaemia. Potassium-containing drugs should be stopped.

Cardiac arrest associated with hyperkalaemia

Sodium bicarbonate (8.4%) 50–100mL should be given in addition to standard CPR and other treatment detailed below.

Potassium >7mmol/L

Calcium chloride (10%) 10mL should be given urgently under ECG guidance in addition to treatment detailed below. Although calcium chloride does not reduce plasma potassium levels, it stabilises the myocardium against arrhythmias.

Clinical features of hyperkalaemia or potassium >6mmol/L with ECG changes

Glucose (50mL 50%) and soluble insulin (10IU) should be given IV over 20min. Blood glucose should be monitored every 15min and more glucose given if necessary. In addition, calcium resonium 15g qds PO or 30g bd PR can be considered.

If resistant to medical treatment, haemodialyse or haemodiafilter (more effective than haemofiltration).

Hyperkalaemia related to K$^+$ channel opening drug

Give glibenclamide (glyburide) 5–10mg via the nasogastric tube. An effect is often seen within 30 minutes.

Key paper

Singer M, Coluzzi F, O'Brien A, et al. (2005) Reversal of life-threatening, drug-related potassium-channel syndrome by glibenclamide. *Lancet* **365**: 1873–5.

Hypokalaemia

Plasma potassium depends on the balance between intake, excretion, and the distribution of potassium across cell membranes. Excretion is normally controlled by the kidneys.

Causes
- Inadequate intake or replacement.
- Gastrointestinal losses (e.g. vomiting, diarrhoea, fistula losses).
- Renal losses (e.g. diabetic ketoacidosis, Conn's syndrome, secondary hyperaldosteronism, Cushing's syndrome, renal tubular acidosis, metabolic alkalosis, hypomagnesaemia, drugs—including diuretics, corticosteroids, theophyllines).
- Haemofiltration losses.
- Potassium transfer into cells (e.g. acute alkalosis, glucose infusion, insulin treatment, familial periodic paralysis).

Clinical features
- Arrhythmias (SVT, VT, and Torsades de Pointes).
- ECG changes (ST depression, 'T' wave flattening, 'U' waves).
- Metabolic alkalosis.
- Constipation.
- Ileus.
- Weakness.

Management
1. Wherever possible, the cause of potassium loss should be treated.
2. Potassium replacement should be intravenous with ECG monitoring when there is a clinically significant and compromising arrhythmia (give 20mmol over 30min, repeated according to levels).
3. Slower IV replacement (20mmol over 1–2h) can be used otherwise.
4. Oral supplementation (to a total intake of 80–120mmol/d, including nutritional input) can be given where there are no clinical features and enteral absorption is satisfactory.

See also:
Electrolytes (Na$^+$, K$^+$, Cl$^-$, HCO$_3^-$), p212; Urinalysis, p232; Diuretics, p280; Corticosteroids, p328; Metabolic alkalosis, p504; Diabetic ketoacidosis, p510.

Hypomagnesaemia

Causes

- Excess loss, e.g. diuretics, other causes of polyuria (including poorly controlled diabetes mellitus), severe diarrhoea, prolonged vomiting, large nasogastric aspirates,
- Inadequate intake, e.g. starvation, parenteral nutrition, alcoholism, malabsorption syndromes

Clinical features

Magnesium is primarily an intracellular ion involved in the production and utilisation of energy stores and in the mediation of nerve transmission. Normal plasma levels range from 0.7–1.0mmol/L; severe symptoms do not usually occur until levels drop below 0.5mmol/L. Low plasma levels, which do not necessarily reflect either intracellular or whole body stores, may thus be associated with features related to these functions:

- Confusion, irritability.
- Seizures.
- Muscle weakness, lethargy.
- Arrhythmias.
- Symptoms related to hypocalcaemia and hypokalaemia which are resistant to calcium and potassium supplementation, respectively.

Management

- Where possible, identify and treat the cause.
- For severe, symptomatic hypomagnesaemia, 10mmol of magnesium sulphate can be given IV over 3–5min. This can be repeated as needed.
- In less acute situations or for asymptomatic hypomagnesaemia, 10–20mmol $MgSO_4$ solution can be given over 1–2h and repeated as necessary, or according to repeat plasma levels.
- Continuous IV infusion (e.g. 3–5mmol $MgSO_4$ solution/h) can be given; however, this is usually reserved for therapeutic indications where supranormal plasma levels (1.5–2mmol/L) of magnesium are sought, e.g. treatment of supraventricular and ventricular arrhythmias, pre-eclampsia and eclampsia, bronchospasm.
- Oral magnesium sulphate has a laxative effect and may cause severe diarrhoea.
- High plasma levels of magnesium may develop in renal failure; caution should be applied when administering IV magnesium.

See also:
Calcium, magnesium, and phosphate, p214; Bronchodilators, p254; Diuretics, p280; Asthma—general management, p364; Tachyarrhythmias, p384; Generalised seizures, p444.

Hypercalcaemia

Causes

- Malignancy (e.g. myeloma, bony metastatic disease, hypernephroma).
- Hyperparathyroidism.
- Sarcoidosis.
- TB.
- Excess intake of calcium, vitamin A or D.
- Drugs, e.g. thiazides, lithium.
- Immobilisation.
- Rarely, thyrotoxicosis, Addison's disease.

Clinical features

Usually become apparent when total (ionised and unionised) plasma levels >3.5mmol/L (normal range 2.2–2.6mmol/L) or the ionised fraction >1.7mmol/L (normal range 1.05–1.25). Symptoms depend on the patient's age, the duration and rate of increase of plasma calcium, and the presence of concurrent medical conditions.

- Nausea, vomiting, weight loss, pruritus.
- Muscle weakness, fatigue, lethargy.
- Depression, mania, psychosis.
- Drowsiness, coma.
- Abdominal pain, constipation.
- Acute pancreatitis.
- Peptic ulceration.
- Polyuria, renal calculi, renal failure.
- Arrhythmias.

Management

1. Identify and treat cause where possible.
2. Monitor haemodynamics, urine output, and ECG morphology with frequent estimations of plasma Ca^{2+}, PO_4^{3-}, Mg^{2+}, Na^+, and K^+.
3. Intravascular volume repletion—inhibits proximal tubular reabsorption of calcium and often lowers plasma calcium by 0.4–0.6mmol/L. It should precede diuretics or other therapy. Either colloid or 0.9% saline should be used, depending on the presence of hypovolaemia-related features.
4. Calciuresis—after adequate intravascular volume repletion, a forced diuresis with furosemide plus 0.9% saline (6–8L/d) may be attempted. An effect is usually seen within 12h. Loop diuretics inhibit calcium reabsorption in the ascending limb of loop of Henlé. More aggressive furosemide regimens can be attempted but can potentially result in complications. Thiazides should not be used as tubular reabsorption may be reduced and hypercalcaemia worsened.
5. Dialysis/haemofiltration—may be indicated at an early stage if the patient is in established oligo-anuric renal failure ± fluid overloaded.
6. Corticosteroids reduce hypercalcaemia in haematological cancers (lymphoma, myeloma), vitamin D overdose, and sarcoidosis.
7. Calcitonin has the most rapid onset of action within 12–24h. Its action is usually short-lived and rebound hypercalcaemia may occur. It generally does not drop the plasma level more than 0.5mmol/L.
8. Bisphosphonates (e.g. pamidronate) and IV phosphate should only be given after specialist advice is taken in view of their toxicity and potential complications.

Drug dosages

Diuretics	Furosemide 10–40mg IV 2–4h (may be increased to 80–100mg IV every 1–2h)
Corticosteroids	Hydrocortisone 100mg qds IV or prednisolone 40–60mg PO for 3–5d
Pamidronate	15–60mg slow IV bolus
Calcitonin	3–4U/kg IV followed by 4U/kg SC bd

See also:

Calcium, magnesium, and phosphate, p214; Diuretics, p280; Corticosteroids, p328; Acute renal failure—diagnosis, p400; Acute renal failure—management, p402; Pancreatitis, p424; Diabetic ketoacidosis, p510; Thyroid emergencies, p524; Hypoadrenal crisis, p526.

Hypocalcaemia

Causes

- Associated with hyperphosphataemia.
- Renal failure.
- Rhabdomyolysis.
- Hypoparathyroidism (including surgery), pseudohypoparathyroidism.
- Associated with low/normal phosphate.
- Critical illness, including sepsis, burns.
- Hypomagnesaemia.
- Pancreatitis.
- Osteomalacia.
- Over-hydration.
- Massive blood transfusion (citrate-binding).
- Hyperventilation and resulting respiratory alkalosis may reduce ionised plasma Ca^{2+} levels and induce clinical features of low calcium.

Clinical features

These usually appear when total plasma calcium levels <2mmol/L and the ionised fraction is <0.8mmol/L.
- Tetany (including carpopedal spasm).
- Muscular weakness.
- Hypotension.
- Perioral and peripheral parasthesiae.
- Chvostek and Trousseau's signs.
- Prolonged QT interval.
- Seizures.

Management

1. If respiratory alkalosis is present, adjust ventilator settings or, if spontaneously hyperventilating and agitated, calm ± sedate. Rebreathing into a bag may be beneficial.
2. If symptomatic, give 5–10mL 10% calcium chloride solution over 2–5min. Repeat as necessary.
3. Correct hypomagnesaemia or hypokalaemia if present.
4. If asymptomatic and in renal failure or hypoparathyroid, consider enteral/parenteral calcium supplementation and vitamin D analogues.
5. If hypotensive or cardiac output is decreased following administration of a calcium antagonist, give 5–10mL 10% calcium chloride solution over 2–5min.

See also:

Calcium, magnesium, and phosphate, p214; Diuretics, p280; Hypotension, p380; Acute renal failure—diagnosis, p400; Acute renal failure—management, p402; Pancreatitis, p424; Hypomagnesaemia, p492; Hypophosphataemia, p498; Rhabdomyolysis, p612.

Hypophosphataemia

Causes
- Critical illness.
- Inadequate intake.
- Loop diuretic therapy (including low-dose dopamine).
- Parenteral nutrition—levels may fall rapidly during high-dose IV glucose therapy, especially with insulin.
- Alcoholism.
- Hyperparathyroidism.
- Refeeding syndrome—occurs when malnourished patients are given high carbohydrate loads, with rapidly falling phosphate, magnesium and potassium, and fluid retention. This can precipitate acute heart failure due to an increase in cardiac work and a sudden rise in CO_2 production due to the diet-induced increase in RQ.

Clinical effects
Hypophosphataemia is associated with muscle weakness, rhabdomyolysis, paresthesiae, haemolysis, platelet dysfunction, and cardiac failure. However, this is rarely clinically apparent, even in patients with severe hypophosphataemia where plasma levels may drop <0.1mmol/L.

Management
Phosphate supplements (5–10mmol) should be given by intravenous infusion over 6h and repeated according to the plasma phosphate level.
To prevent refeeding syndrome, recognise the possibility and start feed slowly with aggressive supplementation of K^+, Mg^{2+}, and phosphate.

See also:

Enteral nutrition, p128; Parenteral nutrition, p130; Tight glycaemic control/intensive insulin therapy, p132; Calcium, magnesium and phosphate, p214; Diuretics, p280.

General acid-base principles

In the Stewart theory, blood pH is determined by PCO_2, the strong ion difference, and the concentration of non-volatile weak acids. Weak acids dissociate to produce weak anions (predominantly albumin, phosphate). Bicarbonate, though produced according to PCO_2, is also a weak anion and is not a dependent determinant of pH. Strong ions are completely ionised with pKa <4. Normally, there is a surfeit of strong cations—the strong ion difference that balances weak anions to maintain electrical equilibrium.

$$\text{Strong ion difference} = (Na^+ + K^+ + Mg^{2+} + Ca^{2+})$$
$$- (Cl^- + Lactate + SO_4^{2-})$$

A change in charge equilibrium by altering strong ion difference or weak anion concentration is compensated by a change in concentration of H^+ ions with resulting acid base disturbance. With time, respiratory and renal adjustments. correct pH towards normal by altering plasma PCO_2 and strong ion difference.

Factors changing pH

In addition to changes in $PaCO_2$, the following will affect pH:

Increased strong ion difference (alkalosis)
- Chloride loss, e.g. vomiting, large gastric aspirates, diuretics, hyper-aldosteronism, corticosteroids.
- Potassium retention, e.g. renal failure, distal renal tubular acidosis.
- Sodium load.

Decreased strong ion difference (acidosis)
- Chloride increase, e.g. saline, acetazolamide.
- Hyperlactataemia.
- Na^+ or K^+ loss, e.g. diarrhoea, small bowel fistula, urethro-enterostomy, proximal renal tubular acidosis.
- Unmeasured anions, e.g. ketosis, salicylate poisoning.

Decreased weak acids (alkalosis)
- Hypoalbuminaemia.

Principles of management

1. Correct (where possible) the underlying cause, e.g. hypoperfusion.
2. Avoid large volume saline-based fluids. Consider balanced electrolyte solutions such as Hartmann's or Ringer's lactate.
3. NaCl infusion for vomiting-induced alkalosis; insulin, Na^+, and K^+ in diabetic ketoacidosis.
4. Correct pH in specific circumstances only, e.g. $NaHCO_3$ in renal failure.

See also:

Blood gas analysis, p154; Electrolytes (Na$^+$, K$^+$, Cl$^-$, HCO$_3^-$), p212; Lactate, p236; Crystalloids, p242; Sodium bicarbonate, p244; Metabolic acidosis, p502; Metabolic alkalosis, p504.

Metabolic acidosis

A subnormal arterial blood pH with a base deficit >2mmol/L, reduced strong ion difference and/or an increase in weak acids. Outcome in critically ill patients has been linked to severity, duration, and hyperlactataemia.

Causes

- Hyperlactataemia—may be due to tissue hypoperfusion (e.g. circulatory shock) or necrosis, cellular abnormalities (any cause of mitochondrial inhibition, e.g. sepsis, drug-related inhibition of aerobic respiration), and accelerated anaerobic respiration. The latter may be due to tissue hypoxia or to excess adrenergic tone/catecholamine infusion (notably epinephrine), increasing activity of muscle Na^+ pumps. High lactate may be seen with increased muscle activity (e.g. post-seizure). Lung lactate release is seen in acute lung injury.
- Hyperchloraemia, e.g. excessive saline infusion.
- Ketoacidosis—high levels of β-hydroxybutyrate and acetoacetate related to uncontrolled diabetes mellitus, starvation, and alcoholism.
- Renal failure—accumulation of organic acids.
- Drugs—in particular, aspirin (salicylic acid) overdose, acetazolamide (carbonic anhydrase inhibition), ammonium chloride, drugs inhibiting mitochondrial function (e.g. highly active antiretroviral therapy). Vasopressor agents may be implicated, possibly by inducing regional ischemia or, in the case of epinephrine, accelerated glycolysis.
- Ingestion of poisons, e.g. paraldehyde, ethylene glycol, methanol.
- Cation loss, e.g. severe diarrhoea, small bowel fistulae, ileostomy.
- Glucose-6-phosphatase deficiency.
- Thiamine deficiency (affects glycolysis and the Krebs' cycle).
- Prolonged seizures.
- Excessive muscular activity.

Clinical features

- Dyspnoea.
- Haemodynamic instability.
- A rapidly increasing metabolic acidosis (over minutes to hours) is not due to renal failure. Other causes, particularly severe tissue hypoperfusion, sepsis, or tissue necrosis, should be suspected when there is associated systemic deterioration.

Management

1. The underlying cause should be identified and treated where possible rather than administering alkali or manipulating minute volume to normalise the arterial pH.
2. Urgent haemo(dia)filtration may be necessary if oligoanuria persists.
3. Reversal of the metabolic acidosis (other than simple buffering with bicarbonate) is generally an indication of successful therapy. An increasing base deficit suggests that the therapeutic manoeuvres in operation are either inadequate or wrong.
4. Bicarbonate therapy may be appropriate when tissue hypoperfusion has been corrected/excluded. This is particularly the case for ongoing loss of alkali (e.g. biliary fistula, diarrhoea) or inability to acidify urine.
5. The benefits of buffers such as Carbicarb and THAM (tris-hydroxy-methyl-aminomethane) remain unproven.

Key paper

Levy B, Gibot D, Franck P, et al. (2005) Relation between muscle Na$^+$K$^+$ATPase activity and raised lactate concentrations in septic shock: a prospective study. *Lancet* **365**: 871–5.

See also:

Metabolic alkalosis

A supranormal arterial blood pH with a base excess >2mmol/L and an increased strong ion difference caused either by loss of (non-carbonic) acid or gain of base. As the kidney is usually efficient at excreting large quantities of bicarbonate, persistence of a metabolic alkalosis usually depends on either chronic renal failure or a diminished extracellular fluid volume with severe depletion of K^+, resulting in an inability to reabsorb Cl^- in excess of Na^+.

- The patient is usually asymptomatic although, if spontaneously breathing, will hypoventilate.
- A metabolic alkalosis will cause a left shift of the oxyhaemoglobin curve, reducing oxygen availability to the tissues.
- If severe (pH >7.6), metabolic alkalosis may result in encephalopathy, seizures, decreased coronary blood flow, and cardiac contractility.

Causes

- Diuretics.
- Large nasogastric aspirates, vomiting.
- Secondary hyperaldosteronism with potassium depletion.
- Use of haemofiltration replacement fluid containing excess buffer (e.g. lactate).
- Renal compensation for chronic hypercapnia (increasing strong ion difference). This can develop within 1–2 weeks. Though more apparent when the patient hyperventilates or is hyperventilated to normocapnia, an overcompensated metabolic alkalosis can occasionally be seen in the chronic state (i.e. a raised pH in an otherwise stable long-term hypercapnic patient).
- Excess administration of bicarbonate.
- Excess administration of citrate (large blood transfusion).
- Drugs, including laxative abuse, corticosteroids.
- Rarely, Cushing's, Conn's, Bartter's syndrome.

Management

1. Replacement of fluid, sodium chloride (i.e. give 0.9% saline), and potassium losses are often sufficient to restore acid-base balance.
2. With distal renal causes related to hyperaldosteronism, addition of spironolactone (or potassium canrenoate) can be considered.
3. Active treatment is rarely necessary. If so, give ammonium chloride 5g tds PO. Hydrochloric acid has been used on occasion for severe metabolic alkalosis (pH >7.7). It should be given via a central vein in a concentration of 1mmol HCl per mL water at a rate <1mmol/kg/h.
4. Compensation for a longstanding respiratory acidosis, followed by correction of that acidosis, e.g. with mechanical ventilation, will lead to an uncompensated metabolic alkalosis. This usually corrects with time though acetazolamide (or rarely, mechanical 'hypoventilation', i.e. maintaining hypercapnia) can be considered.

See also:

Haemo(dia)filtration (1), p108; Haemo(dia)filtration (2), p110; Blood gas analysis, p154; Electrolytes (Na⁺, K⁺, Cl⁻, HCO₃⁻), p212; Diuretics, p280; Sodium bicarbonate, p244; Blood transfusion, p248; Acute renal failure—diagnosis, p400; Vomiting/gastric stasis, p406; General acid-base principles, p500; Diabetic ketoacidosis, p510; Systemic inflammation/multi-organ failure—causes, p556; Sepsis and septic shock—treatment, p560.

Hypoglycaemia

Causes

- Inadequate intake of carbohydrate.
- Excess insulin or sulphonylurea.
- Liver failure with depletion of glycogen stores.
- Alcohol.
- Hypoadrenalism (including Addison's disease), hypopituitarism.
- Quinine, aspirin.

Clincal features

- Nausea, vomiting.
- Increased sympathetic activity, e.g. sweating, tachycardia.
- Altered behaviour and conscious level.
- Seizures, focal neurological signs.

Management

1. Monitor carefully with regular bedside estimations. The frequency should be increased in conditions known to precipitate hypoglycaemia, e.g. insulin infusion, liver failure, quinine treatment of malaria.
2. Administer 25mL 50% glucose solution if the blood glucose is:
   - ≤3mmol/L or
   - ≤4mmol/L and the patient is symptomatic or
   - Within the normal range, but the patient is symptomatic (usually longstanding, poorly controlled diabetics).

   Repeat as necessary every few minutes until symptoms abate and the blood glucose level has normalised.
3. If the blood glucose is 3–4mmol/L and the patient is non-symptomatic, either reduce the rate of insulin infusion (if present) or increase calorie intake (enterally or parenterally). In insulin-dependent diabetes mellitus, the insulin should continue with adequate glucose intake.
4. A continuous parenteral infusion of 10%, 20%, or 50% glucose solution, varying from 10–100mL/h, may be required, depending on the degree of continuing hypoglycaemia and the patient's fluid balance/urine output. 5% glucose solution only contains 20Cal/100mL and should not be used to prevent or treat hypoglycaemia.
5. In the rare instance of no venous access, hypoglycaemia may be temporarily reversed by glucagon 1mg given either IM or SC.
6. Continuing hypoglycaemia in the face of adequate treatment and lack of symptoms should be confirmed with formal laboratory blood sugar estimation to exclude malfunctioning of the bedside testing equipment.

See also:
Enteral nutrition, p128; Parenteral nutrition, p130; Tight glycaemic control/intensive insulin therapy, p132; Acute liver failure, p430; Generalised seizures, p444; Hypoadrenal crisis, p516.

Hyperglycaemia

Causes

- A common occurrence in critically ill patients due to a combination of impaired glucose tolerance, insulin resistance, high circulating levels of endogenous catecholamines and corticosteroids, and regular administration of such drugs which antagonise the effect of insulin.
- Pancreatitis resulting in islet cell damage.

Clinical features

None in the short term, other than polyuria from the osmotic diuresis. The patient may complain of thirst or show signs of hypovolaemia if fluid balance is allowed to become too negative.

Metabolic effects

Relative lack of insulin prevents cellular glucose uptake and utilisation resulting in:
- Increased lipolysis.
- Altered cellular metabolism.
- Increased oxidative damage.
- Increased risk of infection (decreased neutrophil action).

Prognostic significance

Strict maintenance of glycaemic control (approximately 4–6.5mmol/L) with a regimen of insulin and glucose resulted in significant outcome improvements in surgical and medical ICU population staying four days. Whether this is related to prevention of hyperglycaemia and/or an effect related to additional administration of insulin still remains uncertain. However, subsequent multicentre studies have failed to reproduce these findings. The increased risk of hypoglycaemia (and potential outcome detriment) has led some authorities to suggest an upper blood glucose level of 8mmol/L should be tolerated.

Management

1. Treatment should be given if blood glucose persists >7–8mmol/L.
2. Short-acting insulin infusion (e.g. Actrapid®) should be used and titrated to maintain normoglycaemia (4–7mmol/L). Usually 1–4U/h are required though may need to be much higher in diabetics who become critically ill. Regular bedside monitoring of blood sugar should be performed; this should be undertaken hourly if unstable.
3. Oral hypoglycaemic agents should be generally avoided in the ICU patient because of their prolonged duration of action and unpredictable absorption.

Key papers

Van den Berghe G, Wouters P, Weekers F, et al. (2001) Intensive insulin therapy in critically ill patients. *N Engl J Med* **345**: 1359–67.

Van den Berghe G, Wilmer A, Hermans G, et al. (2006) Intensive insulin therapy in the medical ICU. *N Engl J Med* **354**: 449–61.

Brunkhorst FM, Engel C, Bloos F, et al. (2008) Intensive insulin therapy and pentastarch resuscitation in severe sepsis. *N Engl J Med* **358**:125–39.

See also:

Enteral nutrition, p128; Parenteral nutrition, p130; Tight glycaemic control/intensive insulin therapy, p132; Diabetic ketoacidosis, p510; Hyperosmolar diabetic emergencies, p512.

Diabetic ketoacidosis

May occur *de novo* in a previously undiagnosed diabetic, or follow an acute insult (e.g. infection), or inadequate insulin in a known diabetic.

Clinical features

- Excess fat metabolism to fatty acids with ketone production.
- An osmotic diuresis with large losses of fluid (up to 6–10L), sodium (400–800mmol), potassium (250–800mmol), and magnesium.

Symptoms arise from hypovolaemia, metabolic acidosis, and electrolyte imbalance with polyuria. Hyperventilation is a prominent feature. Coma needs not necessarily be present to be life-threatening. Plasma amylase commonly exceeds 1000U/L, but does not indicate pancreatitis.

Monitoring

Adequate invasive monitoring is essential, particularly if the patient has circulatory instability or cardiac dysfunction. Urine output, blood gases, and plasma electrolytes should also be monitored frequently.

Fluid and electrolyte management

1. Fluid and electrolyte repletion should be tailored to individual needs. Traditional regimens (e.g. 3–4L within the first 3–4h) increase the risk of cerebral oedema, cardiac and/or renal failure.
2. Colloid fluid challenges should initally be given in states of hypotension and tissue hypoperfusion to restore the circulating blood volume.
3. Thereafter, replace fluid with 0.9% saline at a rate of 100–200mL/h until the salt and water debt has been replenished.
4. Hypotonic (0.45%) saline resuscitation may be appropriate in the non-shocked patient if the plasma sodium is rising rapidly (shift of water and potassium into cells and sodium out).
5. Use 5% glucose solution (100–200mL/h) after replacing the sodium debt.
6. Monitor K^+ replacement. Both acidosis and excessive K^+ administration cause hyperkalaemia while fluid and insulin will produce hypokalaemia. Check levels frequently to maintain normokalemia. Infusion of 10–40mmol/h KCl will be needed.
7. Monitor magnesium replacement. 3–5mmol/h is usually sufficient.

Hyperglycaemia

Correct at a rate of 2–4mmol/h by adjusting the insulin infusion (usually 1–5U/h). Monitor blood glucose hourly. Continue IV insulin until heavy ketonuria has disappeared and the base deficit normalised.

Other aspects of managing ketoacidosis

1. Seek and treat a precipitating cause, e.g. sepsis, myocardial infarction, stroke, gastroenteritis.
2. Only give antibiotics for proved or highly suspected infection.
3. Abdominal pain should not be dismissed as part of the syndrome.
4. If obtunded, a nasogastric tube should be inserted as gastric emptying is often delayed and acute gastric dilatation is common.
5. Avoid bicarbonate, even for severe acidosis (pH <7.0). It causes an increased intracellular acidosis, depressed respiration due to a relative CSF alkalosis and sodium overload.
6. LMW heparin 5000U od SC is indicated in immobile patients.

Hyperosmolar diabetic emergencies

This is more common in elderly, non-insulin dependent diabetics though can present *de novo* in young adults. Precipitating factors are similar to ketoacidosis, e.g. sepsis, myocardial infarction.

Clinical features

- Fluid depletion is greater, blood glucose levels often higher, coma more common, and mortality much higher than diabetic ketoacidosis.
- Confusion, agitation, and drowsiness that may persist for 1–2 weeks.
- A metabolic acidosis may be present but is not usually profound; ketoacidosis is not a major feature.
- Hyperosmolality may predispose to thrombotic events; this is the major cause of mortality. Hyperosmolality may not be severe.
- Focal neurological signs and disseminated intravascular coagulation are occasionally recognised.

Management

As for diabetic ketoacidosis, however:

1. Unless the patient shows signs of hypovolaemia and tissue hypoperfusion, in which case colloid challenges should be given for prompt resuscitation, fluid replacement should be more gradual as the risk of cerebral oedema is higher. This can be with either 0.9% saline or, if the plasma sodium is high, 0.45% saline at a rate of 100–200mL/h.
2. The plasma sodium rises with treatment, even with 0.45% saline, and can often increase in the first few days to 160–170mmol/L before gradually declining thereafter. Aim to correct slowly.
3. Serum phosphate and Mg^{2+} levels fall rapidly with this condition; replacement may be needed as guided by frequently taken plasma levels.
4. Patients may be hypersensitive to insulin and require lower doses.
5. Unless otherwise contraindicated and in view of the high risk of thromboembolism, these patients should be fully heparinised until full recovery (which may take ≥5 days).

Thyroid emergencies

Thyrotoxic crisis

Presents as an exacerbation of the clinical features of hyperthyroidism (e.g. pyrexia, hyperdynamic circulation, heart failure, confusion). There is usually a precipitating factor such as infection, surgery, ketoacidosis, myocardial infarction, or childbirth. It may present with exhaustion in the elderly with few features of hyperthyroidism. The diagnosis is confirmed by standard thyroid function tests.

Management

- Pyrexia should be controlled by surface cooling (avoid aspirin which displaces thyroxine from plasma proteins).
- Catecholamine effects should be reduced by β-blockade (e.g. propranolol 1–5mg IV, then 20–80mg PO qds). These should be used with caution if there is acute heart failure.
- Blockade of thyroxine synthesis is achieved by potassium iodide 200–600mg IV over 2h, then 2g/d PO and carbimazole 60–120mg/d PO.
- Blockade of peripheral T4 to T3 conversion is achieved by dexamethasone 2mg IV qds.
- Careful fluid and electrolyte management is essential.

Myxoedema coma

Presents as an exacerbation of the features of hypothyroidism (e.g. hypothermia, coma, bradycardia, metabolic and respiratory acidosis, anaemia). There may be a precipitating factor (e.g. cold, infection, surgery, myocardial infarction, CVA, central nervous system depressant drugs). Diagnosis is confirmed by thyroid function tests.

Management

- Treatment of complications of severe hypothyroidism (e.g. hypotension, heart failure, hypothermia, bradycardia, seizures) is more important than thyroid hormone replacement.
- Thyroxine replacement should be with low doses (0.1–0.2mg PO or PR and reduced in ischaemic heart disease).
- There are no definite advantages to using T3 replacement, high dose replacement regimens, or IV treatment.
- Corticosteroids (hydrocortisone 100mg qds IV) should be given since coexisting hypoadrenalism is masked by myxoedema.

Sick euthyroid /low T3 syndrome

This is a frequent complication of critical illness with low T3 and T4 and high reverse T3 (rT3) levels. These correlate with the severity of disease and a poor outcome. There is both reduced TSH secretion and altered peripheral thyroid metabolism. A trial of thyroxine administration in critically ill patients produced a negative outcome although those suffering from the sick euthyroid syndrome were not identified. Optimal treatment of this syndrome thus remains unknown.

See also:
Hypotension, p380; Tachyarrhythmias, p384; Bradyarrhythmias, p386; Acute coronary syndrome (1), p388; Heart failure—assessment, p392; Heart failure—management, p394; Hypothermia, p600; Pyrexia—causes, p602; Pyrexia—management, p604.

Hypoadrenal crisis

Clinical features

Primary hypoadrenalism

- Glucocorticoid deficiency (e.g. weakness, vomiting, diarrhoea, abdominal pain, hypoglycaemia).
- Mineralocorticoid deficiency (e.g. dehydration, hyponatraemia, weight loss, postural hypotension, hyperkalaemia).
- Skin pigmentation due to ACTH excess.

Secondary hypoadrenalism

- May be due to critical illness, corticosteroid withdrawal after 2 weeks' treatment, hypopituitarism, or etomidate use.
- No skin pigmentation.
- Features of mineralocorticoid deficiency may be absent.

Diagnosis

Diagnosis is confirmed by plasma cortisol, ACTH levels, and a negative Synacthen® (ACTH analogue) test, although treatment should begin on clinical suspicion. Synacthen® 250mcg IV should produce a >200nmol/L rise in plasma cortisol. In primary hypoadrenalism, levels remain below 600nmol/L. However, baseline levels may be normal or elevated in the relative adrenal deficiency seen in sepsis and other critical illnesses. Dexamethasone may be used for corticosteroid replacement for 48h before a Synacthen test is performed since other corticosteroid treatments may be detected in the plasma cortisol assay.

Management

- Salt and water deficiency should be corrected urgently. Initial fluid replacement should be with colloid if there is hypotension or evidence of poor tissue perfusion. Otherwise, 4–5L/d 0.9% saline will be needed for several days.
- Fluid management should be carefully monitored to ensure adequate replacement without fluid overload.
- Glucocorticoid replacement should be with hydrocortisone 50–100mg tds IV on day 1, then 20–50mg tds on days 2–3). Hydrocortisone may be changed to equivalent doses of dexamethasone when a Synacthen® test is performed.
- The relative hypoadrenalism related to sepsis can be treated with hydrocortisone 50mg qds for seven days, and then a reducing dose over the next 5–7 days. Studies have shown more rapid resolution of shock and an improved outcome in those showing a suboptimal response to synthetic ACTH.

See also:
Electrolytes (Na⁺, K⁺, Cl⁻, HCO₃⁻), p212; Corticosteroids, p328; Hyponatraemia, p486; Hyperkalaemia, p488; Hypoglycaemia, p506.

Poisoning

Poisoning—general principles

Consider poisoning in patients presenting with altered consciousness, respiratory or cardiovascular depression, vomiting, hypothermia, or seizures. Diagnosis is often obvious though the obtunded or truly suicidal patient may prevent an accurate history being taken. Clinical signs may be confused due to ingestion of multiple poisons or absent if effects are delayed. Poisons may also enter the body via routes other than ingestion, e.g. inhalation or transdermally. Salicylate and paracetamol are extremely common agents in self-poisoning and patients often present without alteration in conscious level.

Investigation

All patients require urea and electrolyte, baseline liver function, coagulation studies, blood glucose, and blood gas estimations. Urine samples and gastric aspirate should be saved for possible later toxicology analysis. Obtain salicylate and paracetamol levels urgently due to the common lack of early signs and to direct specific early treatment. Other drug levels may help in diagnosis but treatment is often supportive. Early support from the local Poisons Information Service should be solicited.

Supportive treatment

Treat cardiovascular and respiratory compromise and neurological disturbance as by standard intensive care methods. In the unconscious patient, opiates and benzodiazepines may be reversed temporarily to allow assessment of underlying neurological status though caution should be applied in epileptics.

Gastric emptying

Despite previous widespread use, there is little supporting evidence and it carries significant complication risks. Consider gastric emptying if the poison is not a corrosive or hydrocarbon, has been ingested <60min previously, and cannot be eliminated by other means (e.g. iron). Forced emesis (ipecacuanaha 30mL in 200mL water) is no longer recommended as vomiting may be delayed for 30min and may be intractable. Aspiration is a serious risk with either form of gastric emptying therapy; intubate the patient for airway protection if consciousness is at all impaired.

Prevention of absorption

Activated charcoal is probably more effective than gastric emptying to prevent drug absorption. A charcoal:poison weight ratio of 10:1 is recommended. Give activated charcoal (50–100g as a single dose) NG to adsorb poison remaining in the gut ± a cathartic agent.

Enhanced elimination

Forced diuresis is no longer recommended. Fluid repletion with mild urinary alkalinisation is useful for salicylates. Small molecules may be removed by haemodialysis (e.g. ethylene glycol, methanol, oxalic acid, formic acid, salicylates, lithium). Activated charcoal given to prevent absorption may also adsorb poison returned to the small bowel via the enterohepatic circulation. This may be useful in carbamazepine, phenobarbital, theophylline, quinine, and dapsone poisoning. Multiple doses of activated charcoal are probably ineffective.

Salicylate poisoning

Serious, life-threatening toxicity is likely after ingestion of >7.5g salicylate. Aspirin (acetyl salicylic acid) is the most common form ingested.

Loss of consciousness is rare but metabolic derangements are complex (e.g. respiratory alkalosis due to respiratory centre stimulation, dehydration due to salt and water loss, renal bicarbonate excretion and hyperthermia, hypokalaemia, metabolic acidosis due to interference with carbohydrate, lipid and amino acid metabolism, hyperthermia due to uncoupling of oxidative phosphorylation and increased metabolic rate).

There may also be pulmonary oedema due to capillary leak and bleeding due to reduced prothrombin levels. Although gastric erosions are common with aspirin treatment, bleeding from this source is rare in acute poisoning.

Management

Prevention of absorption

Give activated charcoal (50–100g) NG to adsorb salicylate remaining in the gut.

Salicylate levels

Repeat blood levels as they may continue to rise as absorption continues. Levels taken after 12h may underestimate the degree of toxicity due to tissue binding. If salicylate levels are <3.1mmol/L after 1h of ingestion and there is no metabolic derangement, then observation, fluids, and repeat levels are all that is required. Urine alkalinisation is required if levels >3.6mmol/L or there is metabolic derangement but no renal failure. Levels >5.1mmol/L (or >3.6mmol/L with renal failure) require haemodialysis.

Urine alkalinisation

Alkalinisation rather than forced diuresis is more important for salicylate excretion. Urinary pH must be >7.0 without arterial alkalosis (pH <7.5). Potassium loss occurs with a bicarbonate infusion due to the diuresis and as a toxic effect of the salicylate. Monitor and correct potassium levels in a high dependency environment. Fluid repletion is essential. Alkalinisation, if successful, should continue until salicylate levels fall <3.6mmol/L. Calcium levels may drop with prolonged alkalinisation.

Haemodialysis

Indications include salicylate levels >5.1mmol/L, renal failure, or marked metabolic acidosis.

See also:
Blood gas analysis, p154; Electrolytes (Na$^+$, K$^+$, Cl$^-$, HCO$_3^-$), p212; Calcium, magnesium and phosphate, p214; Toxicology, p228; Poisoning—general principles, p520.

Paracetamol poisoning

Serious, life-threatening toxicity is likely after ingestion of >10–15g paracetamol, particularly with co-ingestion of enzyme-inducing drugs (e.g. anticonvulsants, anti-TB therapy) and/or alcohol.

Paracetamol is rapidly absorbed and metabolised by conjugation in the liver. Hepatic necrosis occurs due to toxicity of an alkylating metabolite normally removed by conjugation with glutathione; glutathione is rapidly depleted with overdose and may already be low in starvation, alcoholics, and HIV disease, thus predisposing these groups to an increased risk of toxicity.

Toxicity is usually asymptomatic for 1–2 days although laboratory assessment of liver function may become abnormal after 18h.

Hepatic failure develops after 2–7 days.

Management

If ingestion of >12g has occurred <1h previously, activated charcoal (50–100g) should be given NG to adsorb paracetamol remaining in the bowel. Take blood levels to confirm ingestion, but should not be interpreted for toxicity unless taken four or more hours from ingestion. The mainstay of treatment is with N-acetylcysteine (NAC) to restore hepatic glutathione levels by increasing intracellular cysteine levels.

N-acetylcysteine

Treatment is most effective if started within 8h of ingestion, but is currently advised for up to 36h of ingestion. Start NAC if paracetamol levels are in the toxic range (see figure 30.1) or >12g paracetamol has likely been ingested. Continue NAC until paracetamol is not detected in the blood. It is given by continuous IV infusion (150mg/kg over 15min, 50mg/kg in 500mL 5% glucose over 4h, then 50mg/kg in 500mL 5% glucose 8-hourly).

Methionine

Methionine is an alternative to NAC, but absorption is unreliable if there is vomiting or activated charcoal administration. Give 2.5g methionine PO 4-hourly for four doses within 12h of ingestion.

Complications

The major complication is hepatic (± renal) failure. A rise in prothrombin time, INR, and bilirubin are early warning signs of significant hepatic damage and this should prompt early referral to a specialist centre.

Guidelines for referral to a Specialist Liver centre

- Arterial pH <7.3.
- INR >3 on day 2 or >4 thereafter.
- Oliguria and/or rising creatinine.
- Altered conscious level.
- Hypoglycaemia.

Guidelines for liver transplantation

- Arterial pH <7.3.

Or all the following:

- PT >100, INR >6.5.
- Creatinine >200µmol/L.
- Grade 3–4 encephalopathy.

High lactate levels (>3.5mmol/L at 4 and 12h) and low factor V levels are also associated with a poor outcome if not transplanted.

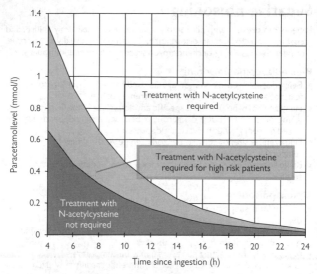

Fig. 30.1. Graph for predicting treatment requirement.

Treatment is required at lower levels if the patient is a known alcoholic, protein-depleted, HIV-positive, or is taking enzyme-inducing drugs, e.g. phenytoin.

See also:

Liver function tests, p218; Coagulation monitoring, p222; Toxicology, p228; Acute liver failure, p430; Poisoning—general principles, p520.

Sedative poisoning

Patients can present with alterated consciousness, respiratory failure, and sometimes, cardiovascular disturbance. Treatment is usually supportive. Consider the possibility of rhabdomyolysis after prolonged immobility.

Benzodiazepine poisoning

- Benzodiazepines are common agents used for self-poisoning, but severe features are uncommon, except at extremes of age.
- Flumazenil may be used as a specific antidote (0.2–1.0mg IV given in 0.1mg increments), but is dangerous in benzodiazepine dependence and mixed poisoning with tricyclic antidepressants.
- Flumazenil is short-acting so benzodiazepine reversal may be temporary.
- Rapid reversal of benzodiazepines may lead to anxiety attacks or seizures.

Opioid poisoning

- Treatment is supportive with attention particularly to respiratory depression and cardiovascular disturbance.
- Naloxone may be used as an antidote (0.2–0.4mg IV) although rapid reversal is not desired in opioid abusers.
- Naloxone is short-acting so reversal may be temporary.
- Consider HIV or other viral infection, and endocarditis in IV drug abusers.
- In iatrogenic poisoning, naloxone will reverse the pain relief that opioids were given for. In these cases, respiratory depression is better reversed by the non-specific respiratory stimulant, doxapram (1.0–1.5mg/kg over 30s IV followed by 1.5–4.0mg/min).

Barbiturates

Treatment is supportive with particular attention to respiratory and cardiovascular depression. Vasodilatation may be extreme requiring fluid support and, in some cases, inotropic support. Phenobarbital may be eliminated by forced alkaline diuresis.

See also:
Airway maintenance, p40; Respiratory stimulants, p256; Coma, p438; Poisoning—general
principles, p520.

Tricyclic antidepressant poisoning

Tricyclic antidepressants are prescribed to patients who are at greatest risk of a suicide attempt. They are rapidly absorbed from the gastrointestinal tract although gastric emptying is delayed.

Clinical features

- Anticholinergic effects (dilated pupils, dry mouth, ileus, urine retention).
- Arrhythmias (often associated with prolonged QT interval and broad QRS complex).
- Hypotension related to arrhythmias and/or cardiac depression through Na^+ channel blockade.
- Hyper-reflexia with extensor plantars, visual hallucinations, coma, and seizures. Drug levels do not correlate with severity.
- Metabolic acidosis in severe poisoning.
- Metabolism is usually rapid and improvement is usually within 24h.

Management

1. There is no specific treatment for tricyclic antidepressant poisoning.
2. Patients require ECG monitoring during the first 24h and until ECG changes have disappeared for 12h.
3. Activated charcoal (50g) via a nasogastric tube will adsorb tricyclics remaining in the bowel.
4. Cardiac arrhythmias are more common if there is an acidosis. Give bicarbonate to achieve an arterial pH of 7.5. If arrhythmias occur with no acidosis and fail to respond to treatment with amiodarone or phenytoin, bicarbonate (25–50mL 8.4% IV) may still be useful.
5. Seizures are best managed with benzodiazepines and phenytoin.

See also:
Airway maintenance, p40; Sodium bicarbonate, p244; Tachyarrhythmias, p384; Coma, p438;
Generalised seizures, p444; Poisoning—general principles, p520.

Amphetamines and Ecstasy

Amphetamines, e.g. 3,4-methylenedioxymethamphetamine (MDMA, 'Ecstasy') and 3,4-methylenedioxyethamphetamine ('Eve'), are stimulants taken predominantly for recreational use or as appetite suppressants. They are hallucinogenic at higher doses. MDMA cause rapid decreases in central nervous system 5-hydroxytryptamine and 5-hydroxyindole-3-acetic acid levels and increases in dopamine release.

Clinical features of overdose

- Agitation, hyperactivity, hypertension, hallucinations, paranoia followed by exhaustion, coma, convulsions, and hyperthermia.
- Idiosyncratic responses to Ecstasy and Eve are more common with numerous reports of mortality and major morbidity following ingestion of just 1–2 tablets.
- Ingestion in hot environments, e.g. nightclubs, and concurrent dehydration is more likely to be associated with idiosyncratic responses.
- Features include profound hyperthermia (>40°C), agitation, seizures, muscle rigidity, hypertension, tachycardia, sweating, coma, disseminated intravascular coagulation, and rhabdomyolysis.
- These complications lead to hypovolaemia, electrolyte imbalance (particularly hyperkalaemia), and a metabolic acidosis.
- Some patients taking Ecstasy or Eve have been admitted with water intoxication and acute hyponatraemia following ingestion of large amounts of water.

Management

1. Supportive care, including airway protection, fluid resuscitation, electrolyte correction, and if needed, mechanical ventilation.
2. Early stages of amphetamine poisoning can be often controlled with tepid sponging, chlorpromazine, β-blockade. Forced acid diuresis to increase urinary excretion is rarely needed.
3. Manage severe complications as they arise, e.g. rapid cooling for hyperpyrexia, anticonvulsants for seizures, urine alkalinisation ± fasciotomies for rhabdomyolysis, platelet, and fresh frozen plasma infusions for coagulopathy.
4. Dantrolene is sometimes given to treat hyperpyrexia at a dose of 1mg/kg IV, repeated to a cumulative maximum dose of 10mg/kg, particularly if the temperature is >40°C. However, no outcome benefit has been reported through its use and it can cause side effects.

See also:

Airway maintenance, p40; Hypertension, p382; Coma, p438; Delirium, p442; Generalised seizures, p444; Hyperkalaemia, p488; Metabolic acidosis, p502; Poisoning—general principles, p520; Hyperthermia, p600; Rhabdomyolysis, p612.

Cocaine poisoning

Modes of action

- Blocks reuptake of dopamine (causing euphoria, hyperactivity) and norepinephrine (causing vasoconstriction and hypertension). Arrhythmias may also result.
- Blocks Na^+ channels, resulting in a local anaesthetic action and myocardial depression.
- Platelet activation.
- Mitochondrial dysfunction leading to myocardial depression.

Complications

- Chest pain related to myocardial ischaemia or infarction, or to coronary artery spasm.
- Heart failure.
- Seizures.
- Cerebrovascular accidents.
- Pneumothorax.
- Rhabdomyolysis.
- Premature labour—abruption.
- Agitated delirium, hyperthermia.

Management

1. Local chest pain guidelines should be followed. ECG abnormalities often resolve within 12h. Arrhythmias should be treated conventionally, but avoiding β-blockers (leaving an unopposed α-action).
2. Verapamil or phentolamine may be useful for treating hypertension.
3. Oxygen.
4. Give benzodiazepine for agitation, delirium, chest pain.
5. Aspirin for chest pain, CVA.
6. Nitrates for chest pain.
7. Low molecular weight heparin or clopidogrel may also be given unless the blood pressure is very high.
8. Urinary alkalinisation for rhabdomyolysis.

See also:
Pneumothorax, p368; Hypertension, p382; Acute coronary syndrome (1), p388; Acute coronary syndrome (2), p390; Heart failure—assessment, p392; Heart failure—management, p394; Delirium, p442; Generalised seizures, p444; Stroke, p452; Poisoning—general principles, p520; Hyperthermia, p600; Rhabdomyolysis, p612.

Inhaled poisons

Carbon monoxide (CO)

CO poisoning should be considered in anyone found in a smoke-filled, enclosed space. CO displaces oxygen from haemoglobin to which it has 200 times greater affinity and thus prevents oxygen carriage. There is also a direct toxic effect on mitochondrial oxidative phosphorylation as it competes with oxygen for the same binding site on cytochrome oxidase.

Clinical features

- Fatigue, headache, vomiting, dizziness, confusion, dyspnoea, cerebral oedema in severe poisoning.
- A cherry red appearance of the skin and mucosae are classical.
- PaO_2 will be normal unless there is respiratory depression and pulse oximetry is misleading.
- The half-life of carboxyhaemoglobin is 4h when breathing room air and 50min when breathing 100% oxygen.

Management

- Carboxyhaemoglobin levels should be measured by a co-oximeter and treatment started immediately with oxygen at the maximum concentration that can be delivered (ideally FIO_2 1.0).
- If carboxyhaemoglobin levels >25% or there is associated mental disturbance, the optimal treatment is hyperbaric oxygen at 3 atmospheres for 30min, repeated 6-hourly if levels remain >25%. Death is likely with carboxyhaemoglobin levels >60%.
- High concentration oxygen treatment should continue until carboxyhaemoglobin levels <10%.

Cyanide

- Severe cyanide poisoning has an extremely rapid onset and occurs in some cases of smoke inhalation. Survival may be associated with anoxic brain damage.
- Diagnosis must be made clinically; cyanide levels take >3h to perform.

Clinical features

Clinical features include anxiety, agitation, hyperventilation, headache, loss of consciousness, dyspnoea, weakness, dizziness, and vomiting. The skin remains pink and hypotension may be severe. An unexplained metabolic acidosis is suggestive.

Management

- High concentration oxygen should be given, but is only truly effective when given at hyperbaric pressures.
- In mild cases, rapid, natural detoxification reduces cyanide levels by 50% within 1h, allowing supportive therapy only.
- Sodium thiosulphate (150mg/kg IV followed by 30–60mg/kg/h) converts cyanide to thiocyanate and should be used if there is unconsciousness. However, it is slow-acting.
- Nitrites produce methaemoglobinaemia (metHb) and may potentially worsen cyanide toxicity.
- Dicobalt edetate (300mg IV), the specific antidote is toxic (vomiting, urticaria, tachycardia, hypotension, dyspnoea, chest pain) in the absence of cyanide. It is best avoided unless cyanide toxicity is likely.

Key paper

Weaver LK, Hopkins RO, Chan KJ, et al. (2002) Hyperbaric oxygen for acute carbon monoxide poisoning. *N Engl J Med* **347**: 1057–67.

See also:
Oxygen therapy, p38; Blood gas analysis, p154; Poisoning—general principles, p520.

Household chemicals

Corrosives

Strong acids and alkalis are increasingly available in the household and ingestion may lead to shock and bowel perforation. Avoid gastric elimination techniques since aspiration of corrosives may cause severe lung damage. Early surgical repair of perforation may be necessary.

Petroleum

Access to petroleum in the home is easy.

Clinical features

Gut ingestion and absorption gives clinical features similar to those of alcohol intoxication with more severe neurological depression.

Management

- Avoid gastric elimination techniques since a few drops of petroleum spilling into the lungs can lead to a severe pneumonitis. This is due to the low surface tension and vapour pressure of petroleum allowing rapid spread through the lungs.
- Treatment involves supportive therapy and 250mL liquid paraffin orally.

Paraquat

Paraquat is widely available as a selective weedkiller which is inactivated on contact with the soil. A dose of 2–3g is usually fatal (equivalent to 80–120g of granules or 10–15mL of industrial liquid concentrate). It inhibits mitochondria and generates superoxide which damages lipid membranes.

Clinical features

- Very little of the ingested paraquat is absorbed from the gut, but a large dose will lead rapidly to shock with widespread tissue necrosis.
- A burning sensation in the mouth and abdomen, development of painful mouth ulcers and, after several days, a relentless, proliferative alveolitis leading to ARDS and death from pulmonary fibrosis. Liver, heart, and kidney may also be affected. Death may be slow and take up to 30 days following ingestion.

Management

- Treatment should begin on clinical grounds in view of the severity of toxicity and the time taken for laboratory confirmation.
- Remove patient from ongoing contact, decontaminate skin with large volumes of water, and remove their clothing. Staff should take care not to contaminate themselves.
- Urgently instill 1000mL water containing 150g Fuller's earth via a nasogastric tube. Alternatively, 1g activated charcoal may be given.
- A cathartic such as 25g magnesium sulphate should be given.
- Severe diarrhoea may ensue, requiring careful fluid management.
- If paraquat poisoning is confirmed, 200–500mL of 30% Fuller's earth is given 2-hourly for 24h via a nasogastric tube.
- Fluid repletion to encourage renal excretion.
- Pulmonary fibrosis is more severe when breathing high FIO_2. Oxygen should be avoided but, in severe hypoxaemia, give the lowest concentration possible accepting low PaO_2. Liposomal superoxide dismutase and glutathione peroxidase are used experimentally.

See also:
Poisoning—general principles, p520.

Methanol and ethylene glycol

Methanol

Toxicity mainly due to oxidation of methanol to formic acid and formaldehyde. The oxidative pathway is an enzymatic process involving alcohol dehydrogenase, but proceeds at 20% of the rate of ethanol oxidation.

Clinical features

Clinical features of poisoning include blindness (due to concentration of methanol in the vitreous humour), severe metabolic acidosis, headache, nausea, vomiting, and abdominal pain.

Management

- Metabolism of methanol is slow so treatment will need to be prolonged (several days).
- Treatment includes ethanol or, preferably, fomepizole, to inhibit alcohol dehydrogenase.
- On presentation 1mL/kg ethanol (50%) can given orally followed by 0.5mL/kg 2-hourly for 5 days. Alternatively, an infusion can be given (7.5mL/kg ethanol (10%) over 30min followed by 0.5–1.0mL/kg/h aiming for blood ethanol levels of 100–150mg/dL). Levels need to be repeated frequently to avoid under- or overdosing.
- Block metabolism with 4-methyl pyrazole (fomepizole) infused or injected 12-hourly IV. Though more expensive than alcohol, it is effective, well-tolerated, and there is no need for therapeutic monitoring.
- If methanol levels are >1000mg/L, haemodialysis is used until levels are <250mg/L.

Ethylene glycol

Ethylene glycol is partially metabolised by alcohol dehydrogenase to oxalic acid which is responsible for a severe metabolic acidosis, renal failure, and seizures.

Clinical features

Clinical suspicion is aroused by odourless drunkenness, oxalate crystals in the urine or blood, and the severe acidosis. As little as 50mL can be fatal.

Management

Treatment is as for methanol.

See also:
Blood gas analysis, p154; Metabolic acidosis, p502; Poisoning—general principles, p520.

Organophosphate poisoning

Organophosphates in pesticides are the major cause of suicidal poisoning in developing countries and are used as nerve agents in terrorist attacks (e.g. Sarin, Tabun, VX, GF). They can be absorbed through intact skin, gut, or inhaled. Their mode of toxicity is via inhibiting cholinesterase.

Cholinergic (anticholinesterase) syndrome
- Salivation, lacrimation, bronchorrhoea, sweating.
- Anxiety and restlessness.
- Vomiting, diarrhoea.
- Bradycardia.
- Bronchospasm.
- Pulmonary oedema.
- Miosis.
- Hyperglycaemia.
- Muscle weakness and fasciculation with paralysis.

Management
- Skin decontamination should never be neglected or hurried but must occur prior to critical care admission. The patient's clothes should be removed. The patient's body should then be thoroughly washed with soap and water to prevent further absorption from the skin. Staff should be protected from the organophosphate by wearing gloves, gowns, and eye protectors.
- The airway should be protected and oxygen given to avoid hypoxaemia (ventricular fibrillation more common with atropine in hypoxaemia).
- Atropine—antagonises acetylcholine at muscarinic receptors. A dose of 2mg should be given every 5–10 minutes until the mouth is dry. Severe poisoning may require >100mg atropine.
- Pralidoxime—reactivates inhibited enzymes if given before the agent permanently binds to the enzyme. A dose of 30mg/kg, repeated every 4–6 hours or an infusion of 8mg/kg/h to a maximum dose of 12g in 24 hours should be given.
- Diazepam—neuroprotection.

See also:
Bronchodilators, p254; Chronotropes, p274; Bradyarrhythmias, p386; Poisoning—general
principles, p520.

Infection and inflammation

Infection control—general principles

Nosocomial infection is a major cause of mortality, morbidity, and increased length of stay. Marked variations in infection control policies for isolation, microbiological surveillance, handwashing, glove and gown use, impregnated vascular catheter use, duration of indwelling catheters, and frequency of change of disposables reflect a weak evidence base. It is generally accepted that handwashing before and after patient contact and strict aseptic technique when performing procedures are mandatory.

Staff measures (universal precautions)

The authors currently use the following precautions:
- Remove watches and jewellery, remove long-sleeved white coats and jackets, roll shirt sleeves up to elbow.
- Hand and forearm washing before and after touching patient. Use alcohol-based gel after skin contact, but soap and water for body fluid contact or if patient has *C. difficile* (alcohol does not eradicate spores).
- Wear disposable aprons and gloves if in contact with patient.
- Wear gloves and aprons when handling any body fluid and eye protection when there is any danger of fluid or droplet splash.
- Use strict aseptic technique for invasive procedures (e.g. central venous catheter insertion) and clean technique for basic procedures, e.g. endotracheal suction, changing ventilator circuits, or drug infusions.
- Bedside equipment (including computer keyboards, infusion and syringe pumps, ventilators, and bed rails) should be cleaned regularly.
- Previous immunisation against hepatitis B, tuberculosis.
- Stethoscopes should be cleaned between patients.
- Clear signposting of precautions to be taken on access doors.

Visitors

- Non-ICU medical and paramedical staff, relatives, and friends should adhere to the policies in force, e.g. handwashing, aprons, and gloves.
- Traffic through the ICU should be minimised.

Cross-infection

- Inform the Infection Control team should cross-infection arise. It may be worthwhile typing the microorganism to confirm an outbreak.
- Source isolate the patient for multi-resistant or virulent organisms.
- If cross-infection persists/spreads, other sources should be sought, e.g. taps, sinks, reusable equipment (rebreathing bags, ventilators).

Isolation

- Source isolation—for patients carrying potentially contagious, virulent or multiresistant organisms, e.g. tuberculosis.
- Protective isolation—for immunosuppressed patients at risk of acquiring infection, e.g. when neutropaenic following chemotherapy

Microbiological surveillance

Policies vary; some routinely screen sputum, bronchoalveolar lavage, blood, urine, and drain fluid every 2–4 days while others screen only on clinical indication, e.g. deteriorating gas exchange, pyrexia, neutrophilia. Some perform routine MRSA surveillance of hairline ± nose ± groin with rapid PCR-based technologies where results are available within 6h.

See also:

Critical Care Unit layout, p2; Patient safety, p14; Bacteriology, p224; Virology, serology, and assays, p226; Infection control—dangerous pathogens, p548; Routine changes of disposables, p550; Infection—diagnosis, p552; Neutropaenia and infection, p628.

Infection control—HIV

Protection of staff from transmission of HIV follows standard universal precautions:
- Do not handle body fluids without gloves.
- Protect face and eyes where there is a risk of splash contamination.
- Dispose of needles in appropriate burn bins without re-sheathing.
- Clean up any fluid spillages immediately.

Robust procedures are usually adhered to when a patient is known to be HIV-positive; the real risk is in the patient of unknown HIV status. Patients presenting to critical care with non-HIV-related illness may also be unknown positives. It follows that precautions should be taken for all patients.

Staff exposure

Needlestick injury, eye or skin cut contact with the patient's bodily fluids should be prevented by strict infection control procedures. However, should exposure happen, wash the area thoroughly and contact the designated person within the hospital promptly (e.g. HIV specialist, microbiologist) who can advise on risk and the desirability of taking post-exposure anti-retroviral prophylaxis (typically two nucleoside reverse transcriptase inhibitors for four weeks). The chance of getting infected from a needlestick injury is <1 in 300.

Different countries have different policies with regard to testing HIV status on incapacitated patients whose blood or other bodily fluid has been in contact with a health care worker. Current UK General Medical Council policy has recently changed to not allow testing in such cases.

See also:
Critical Care Unit layout, p2; Patient safety, p14; Infection control—general principles, p544;
Multi-resistant infections, p562; SARS, VHF, and H5N1, p570.

Infection control—dangerous pathogens

Risk assessment

Before exposing staff to patients with dangerous pathogens, there must be a full assessment of the risks. Advice should be sought from communicable disease experts. This must include access to intelligence relating to likely pathogens in endemic areas visited or, if locally acquired, local infection surveillance data. Ideally, a risk assessment will have been performed in advance of the referral and should include:

- Which pathogen may be present (hazard identification).
- The likelihood of infection.
- The severity of infection if it occurs.
- Where the pathogen is likely to be present (e.g. in blood samples or spillages, on contaminated instruments and equipment, in waste, and on contaminated clothing).
- Ways in which staff may be exposed (e.g. through direct personal exposure to blood in invasive procedures, accidental exposure, handling contaminated items for cleaning or disposal).
- Estimate of exposure, i.e. number and range of sources and frequency of contact, taking account of systems of work and protective measures

Control measures

- Universal precautions.
- Airborne precautions (negative pressure isolation room and use of filter respirators conforming to European Standard EN 149:2001 or equivalent for people entering the room).
- Contact precautions (long-sleeved, fluid-repellent gown, and protective gloves with tight-fitting cuffs. In addition, there should be eye protection for organisms that can infect via eye splash).
- Clinical waste precautions (in addition to universal precautions for handling waste, leak-proof biohazard bags must be used for safe disposal).

See also:
Patient safety, p14; Infection control—general principles, p544; Infection control—dangerous pathogens, p548; HIV-related disease, p566.

Routine changes of disposables

Care of intravascular catheters

- Sites should be covered with transparent semi-permeable dressings to allow observation and prevent secretions from accumulating.
- Routine changes of intravascular catheters are no longer recommended. As the risk of infection increases considerably after a week *in situ*, catheters should be removed as soon as clinically feasible.
- Catheters should be changed to a fresh site if:
  - The old site appears infected.
  - The patient shows signs of severe infection.
  - A positive growth is obtained from a blood culture drawn through the catheter or from the tip of the previous catheter.
- Catheter changes over a guidewire are no longer recommended as sterility cannot be assured. This can be considered if new central venous access if difficult or the risk of insertion is high (e.g. coagulopathy).

Routine changes of disposables

	Frequency
Ventilator circuit with bacterial filters	Between patients unless soiled
Ventilator circuit with water bath humidifier	Daily
Endotracheal tube catheter mount and bacterial filter	Between patients unless soiled
Oxygen masks	Between patients unless soiled
CPAP circuits	Between patients unless soiled
Rebreathing bags and masks	Between patients unless soiled
Intravenous infusion giving sets	48h
Parenteral nutrition giving sets	Daily
Enteral feeding giving sets	Daily
Arterial/venous pressure transducer sets	48h
Urinary catheter bags	Weekly

See also:
Arterial cannulation, p166; Central venous catheter—insertion, p168; Infection control—general principles, p544.

Infection—diagnosis

Infection is a common cause of critical care admission and the major secondary complication. Critically ill patients are predisposed to further infection as many of their natural barriers and defence mechanisms are lost, altered, or penetrated. They are often heavily instrumented, sedated, and immobile. They often develop immune hyporesponsiveness as part of their critical disease process, notwithstanding any therapeutic immune suppression they may have received. The high antibiotic load encourages colonisation by pathogenic organisms and subsequent development of infections by multidrug resistant and/or atypical (e.g. fungi) organisms.

Sepsis is defined as the systemic inflammatory response to an infectious insult (either confirmed or highly likely). Whereas infection is a localised phenomenon, the septic process often affects distant organs.

Diagnosis

- Often problematic in the critically ill patient as focal signs may be lacking and/or camouflaged by concurrent disease (e.g. ventilator-associated pneumonia on top of ARDS). Symptoms are often not forthcoming due to the patient's state of mental incompetence.
- In addition, all of the traditional clinical and biochemical markers of infection are non-specific. These include pyrexia, neutrophilia, and altered sputum. Furthermore, the frequent presence of colonising organisms e.g. MRSA on skin, *Pseudomonas aeruginosa* in the respiratory tract, does not imply concomitant infection. As a consequence, many patients are overtreated with antibiotics, enhancing the risk of overgrowth of resistant/atypical organisms.
- Markers of inflammation (C-reactive protein, procalcitonin) may be useful, though studies have produced conflicting results as to their specificity/sensitivity in diagnosing underlying infection/sepsis.
- The value of routine screening (microbiological surveillance) is not proven though this may help to identify infecting organisms earlier.
- For cases of suspected infection, appropriate samples should be taken for analysis, including blood, sputum, wound swabs, drainage fluid, aspirated pus, catheter tips, cerebrospinal fluid, etc. These should generally be taken before new antibiotics are commenced.
- Consider less common causes of infection such as endocarditis or osteomyelitis, particularly if the patient fails to settle after a standard course of therapy.

Differential diagnosis of pyrexia

- Infection.
- Non-infective causes of inflammation, e.g. trauma, surgery, burns, myocardial infarction, vasculitis, hepatitis, cholecystitis, pancreatitis.
- Adverse drug reactions.
- Excessive ambient heating.
- Miscellaneous causes, e.g. neoplasm.

Definitions

Infection

Microbial phenomenon characterised by an inflammatory response to the presence of microorganisms or the invasion of normally sterile host tissue by those organisms.

Bacteraemia

The presence of viable bacteria in the blood.

Sepsis

The systemic response to infection. Definition as for systemic inflammatory response syndrome (SIRS) but as a result of infection.

SIRS

Two or more of:
- Temperature >38°C or <36°C.
- Heart rate >90bpm.
- Respiratory rate >20 breaths/min or $PaCO_2$ <32mmHg (4.3kPa).
- WBC >12,000cells/mm^3, <4000/mm^3, or >10% immature forms.

Sites of infection pre- and post-admission to critical care

Organ	Primary site of infection needing admission to Critical Care	Secondary site of infection acquired while in Critical Care
Brain	+	+
Sinuses	–	+
Cannula/wound sites	++	+++++
Other skin and soft tissue	++	+
Chest	++++	++++
Urogenital tract	++	+
Abdomen	++++	++
Bone	+	+
Heart valves	+	+

Key paper

American College of Chest Physicians/Society of Critical Care Medicine Consensus Conference. (1992) Definitions for sepsis and organ failure and guidelines for the use of innovative therapies in sepsis. *Crit Care Med* **20**: 864–74.

See also:

Bacteriology, p224; Virology, serology, and assays, p226; Acute chest infection (1), p356; Acute chest infection (2), p358; Systemic inflammation/multi-organ failure—causes, p556; Pyrexia—causes, p602; Pyrexia—management, p604.

Infection—treatment

Principles

- Drain pus.
- Change cannula sites, if necessary.
- Appropriate antibiotic therapy after laboratory specimens taken—may not be necessary for mild infections where cause has been removed, e.g. an infected catheter.
- Radiological and/or surgical intervention, if indicated.

Antimicrobials

Regular input from microbiology ± infectious disease specialists is recommended to advise on best options for empirical therapy and for possible modification based on early communication of laboratory results (including antibiotic sensitivity patterns).

Empirical antimicrobial therapy is guided on illness severity, the likely site of infection and infecting organism(s), whether the infection is community-acquired or nosocomial (including Critical Care acquired), immunosuppression status, and known antibiotic resistance patterns of hospital and local community organisms.

In general, critically ill patients should receive parenteral antibiotics at appropriate dosage, taking into account any impaired hepatic or renal clearance or concurrent renal replacement therapy. Broad-spectrum therapy may be initially needed, with refinement, cessation, or change after 2–3 days, depending on clinical response and sensitivity patterns of organisms subsequently isolated. The duration of treatment remains highly contentious. Apart from specific conditions such as endocarditis, tuberculosis, and meningitis where prolonged therapy is probably advisable, it may be sufficient to stop within 3–5 days provided the patient has shown adequate signs of recovery.

Patients not responding or deteriorating should be considered as either treatment failures or inappropriately treated (i.e. no infection was present in the first place). Commonly accepted markers of infection are not specific in the critically ill patient. Indeed, pyrexia may settle on stopping antibiotic treatment. Cessation or change of antibiotic therapy must be considered according to the patient's condition and any subsequent laboratory results. An advantage of ceasing therapy is the ability to take further specimens for culture in an antibiotic-free environment.

Other measures

It may be necessary to remove indwelling pacemakers, tunnelled vascular catheters, prosthetic joints, plates, implants, grafts, and stents if these are the suspected cause of infection. This should be done in consultation with microbiologists and the appropriate specialist as individual risk and benefit need to be carefully weighed up.

Specimen antibiotic regimens (organism unknown)

Sepsis of unknown origin	2nd/3rd generation cephalosporin OR quinolone OR carbapenem OR piptazobactam ± Aminoglycoside (if Gram-negative suspected) ± Metronidazole (anaerobic cover) ± Glycopeptide or linezolid (if MRSA suspected)
Pneumonia—community-acquired	2nd/3rd generation cephalosporin + macrolide
Pneumonia—nosocomial	3rd generation cephalosporin OR quinolone OR carbapenem OR piptazobactam ± aminoglycoside (if Gram-negative suspected) + Teicoplanin, vancomycin + rifampicin or linezolid (if MRSA likely)
Skin and soft tissue	Flucloxacillin (if MSSA likely) Glycopeptide or linezolid (if MRSA likely) Benzylpenicillin or clindamycin (if *Streptococcus* suspected)
Abdominal	2nd/3rd generation cephalosporin OR quinolone OR carbapenem OR piptazobactam ± Aminoglycoside ± metronidazole
Gynaecological	2nd/3rd generation cephalosporin OR quinolone OR carbapenem OR piptazobactam ± Aminoglycoside + Metronidazole
Nephro-urological	2nd/3rd generation cephalosporin OR quinolone OR carbapenem OR piptazobactam ± Aminoglycoside

NB. Local resistance patterns should be borne in mind when prescribing.

See also:

Antimicrobials, p326; Acute chest infection (1), p356; Abdominal sepsis, p422; Meningitis, p446; Tetanus, p462; Botulism, p464; Sepsis and septic shock—treatment, p560; Multi-resistant infections, p562; HIV-related disease, p566; Malaria, p568; SARS, VHF, and H5N1, p570.

Systemic inflammation/multi-organ failure—causes

Exposure to an exogenous insult can result in an exaggerated, generalised, and often inappropriate systemic inflammatory response syndrome ('SIRS'). Stimulation of inflammatory pathways leads to activation of macrophages, endothelium, neutrophils, platelets, coagulation, fibrinolytic and contact systems with release of inflammatory mediators and effectors (e.g. cytokines, prostanoids, proteases, free oxygen radicals, nitric oxide, endothelin). This results in microvascular abnormalities, blood flow redistribution, endothelial swelling, loss of tight junctions between cells, interstitial oedema and fibrosis, and mitochondrial dysfunction. The consequences of this may be organ dysfunction, varying from 'mild' to severe, and affecting single or multiple organs. This may result in combinations of cardiovascular collapse, gastrointestinal failure, renal failure, hepatic failure, encephalopathy, neuropathy, myopathy, and/or disseminated intravascular coagulation. Acute respiratory distress syndrome (ARDS) and its milder variant acute lung injury (ALI) are the respiratory components of this pathophysiological response.

Causes include:

- Infection.
- Trauma, burns.
- Pancreatitis.
- Inhalation injuries.
- Massive blood loss/transfusion.
- Miscellaneous including drug-related (including overdose), myocardial infarction, drowning, hyperthermia, pulmonary embolus.

Definitions

Systemic inflammatory response syndrome (SIRS)

Two or more of:
- Temperature >38°C or <36°C.
- Heart rate >90bpm.
- Respiratory rate >20 breaths/min or $PaCO_2$ <32mmHg (4.3kPa).
- WBC >12,000cells/mm^3, <4000/mm^3, or >10% immature forms.

Sepsis

The systemic response to infection. Definition as for SIRS but as a result of infection.

Severe sepsis

Sepsis associated with organ dysfunction or hypoperfusion. These may include, but are not limited to, lactic acidosis, oliguria, or an acute alteration in mental status.

Septic shock

Sepsis with hypotension, despite adequate fluid resuscitation, plus presence of perfusion abnormalities.

Multi-organ dysfunction syndrome (MODS)

Presence of altered organ function in an acutely ill patient such that homeostasis cannot be maintained without intervention. Multiple organ failure (MOF) has not achieved worldwide uniformity of definition.

See also:
Acute respiratory distress syndrome (1), p360; Acute renal failure—diagnosis, p400; Abdominal sepsis, p422; Pancreatitis, p424; Infection—diagnosis, p552; Pyrexia—causes, p602.

Systemic inflammation/multi-organ failure—management

Treatment is largely supportive though the cause should be removed/treated, if at all possible. Treatment includes antibiotics, drainage of pus, fixation of femoral/pelvic fractures, and debridement of necrotic tissue. An important facet of organ support is to minimise iatrogenic trauma. It is sufficient to maintain survival with relative homeostasis until recovery takes place rather than attempting to achieve normal physiological or biochemical target values. An example of this is permissive hypercapnia.

International guidelines for sepsis management are produced and updated regularly. A 'bundle' approach is also advocated for early and late aspects of management. Consensus is far from complete due to a lack of definitive outcome studies or prospective validation of the recommendations. However, opinion is unanimous on the need for early recognition and intervention of sepsis. Local policies may favour eclectic therapies based on small trials/case series/anecdotal success or a reasonable theoretical basis for administration. Examples include antioxidants, protease inhibitors, immunonutrition, plasmapheresis, vasodilators, and immunoglobulin. It is generally agreed that rapid resuscitation and restoration of oxygen delivery, glycaemic control, and prompt removal of any treatable cause is desirable in preventing the onset of SIRS or progression of organ failure.

Because of non-standardisation of definitions, outcome data are conflicting; single organ 'failure' carries 20–30% mortality while ≥3 organ 'failures' lasting ≥3 days carries >40–50% mortality. Recovery is often complete in survivors, though recent studies reveal long-term physical and psychological sequelae in a significant proportion.

Principles of management
The following represent the authors' current practice.

Respiratory	SaO$_2$ >90–95% (may have to settle for lower)
	Permissive hypercapnia
Cardiovascular	Maintain cardiac output/oxygen delivery and blood pressure compatible with adequate organ perfusion (e.g. no metabolic acidosis)
Renal	Maintain adequate metabolic and fluid homeostasis by intravascular filling, diuretics, vasoactive agents, and/or haemo(dia)filtration
Haematological	Maintain haemoglobin >7g/dL, platelets >20–40 x 10^9/L, INR <1.5–2.5
Gastrointestinal	Stress ulcer prophylaxis (consider stopping once enteral nutrition is established)
Infection	Antibiotics, pus drainage, good infection control
Nutrition	Preferably started early and by enteral route
DVT prophylaxis	LMW heparin ± thromboembolic stockings
Pressure area/mouth/joint care	Frequent turns, low pressure support surfaces, nursing care, and physiotherapy
Psychological	Support to both patient and family

Key paper

Dellinger RP Levy MD, Carlet JM, et al. (2008) Surviving Sepsis Campaign: International guidelines for management of severe sepsis and septic shock. *Crit Care Med* **36**: 296–327.

See aslo:

Ventilatory support—indications, p44; Enteral nutrition, p128; Tight glycaemic control/intensive insulin therapy, p132; Acute respiratory distress syndrome (2), p362; Hypotension, p380; Acute renal failure—management, p402; Infection—treatment, p554; Sepsis and septic shock—treatment, p560; Pyrexia—management, p604.

Sepsis and septic shock—treatment

Principles of treatment

As for other causes of multi-organ dysfunction syndrome, outcome in sepsis improves with:

1. Prompt diagnosis and treatment of the underlying cause.
2. Rapid resuscitation to prevent prolonged tissue hypoxia.
3. Good glycaemic control.
4. Strict infection control.
5. Recognition and appropriate treatment of secondary infections.
6. Adequate nutrition.
7. Recognition that 'normal' physiological/biochemical levels do not necessarily need to be attained while the patient is critically ill, provided he/she is not compromised. For example, a mean BP of 55–60mmHg is often acceptable unless evidence of poor perfusion or ischaemia suggests higher levels should be sought.
8. Avoidance of preventable mishaps, e.g. prolonged hypotension, pressure sores, thromboembolism.
9. Temperature control in the range 36–38.5°C.
10. Prevention of contractures, early mobilisation, etc.
11. Specific treatments (see below).

Specific treatments for severe sepsis/septic shock

1. Activated protein C significantly improved outcome in patients with ≥2 organ dysfunctions if commenced <48h of onset. Issues about safety and efficacy, particularly in less severely septic patients, has prompted a repeat study that is currently in progress.
2. 'Low-dose' hydrocortisone (50mg 6-hourly) + fludrocortisone (50mcg daily) given for 7 days improved survival in 'pressor-unresponsive' shock if commenced <8h of presentation, though only in the subset with an abnormal cortisol response to synthetic ACTH. The recent CORTICUS trial (5 days' hydrocortisone 50mg 6-hourly, reducing over the next 6 days in all patients with septic shock <48h) failed to confirm the utility of Synacthen testing and the overall benefit of steroid use.
3. The VASST study found 'low-dose' vasopressin (0.01–0.03U/min) produced survival benefit over norepinephrine in less severe shock (defined as requiring <15mcg/min norepinephrine) and equivalent outcomes in more severe cases.
4. No overall difference was shown between epinephrine and norepinephrine (± dobutamine). Our current practice is based on the pharmacological rationale of epinephrine (inotrope + pressor) for low output shock and norepinephrine (pressor) for high output shock.
5. For pressor-resistant septic shock, i.e. high-output severe hypotension not responding to adequate fluid loading, norepinephrine >0.4mcg/kg/min, and hydrocortisone, we consider use of terlipressin (or methylthioninium chloride (methylene blue)). Until more data are forthcoming, these agents should be viewed as rescue therapies rather than a straight alternative for norepinephrine.
6. For continuing resistant shock, we consider plasmapheresis, glucose-insulin-potassium infusion (for low output shock) or high output haemofiltration. The evidence base for these therapies is weak.

Sepsis resuscitation bundle

More details are available at <http://ssc.sccm.org>

Complete within 6h:

1. Measure serum lactate.
2. Obtain blood cultures prior to antibiotic administration.
3. Administer broad-spectrum antibiotic within 3h of Emergency department admission and within 1h of non-emergency department admission.
4. In the event of hypotension and/or serum lactate >4mmol/L: (i) deliver initial minimum of 20mL/kg of crystalloid or an equivalent volume of colloid, and (ii) give vasopressors to keep mean BP >65mmHg if not responding to fluid.
5. If still hypotensive despite fluid resuscitation and/or lactate >4mmol/L, achieve CVP >8mm Hg and $ScvO_2$ >70% or SvO_2 >65%.

Complete within 24h:

1. Give low-dose steroids for shock according to local policy.
2. Administer activated protein C according to local policy.
3. Maintain glucose control between 70–150mg/dL (3.9–8.3mmol/L).
4. Maintain median inspiratory plateau pressure <30cmH$_2$O.

Key papers

Bernard GR, Vincent JL, Laterre PF, et al. for the PROWESS study group. (2001) Efficacy and safety of recombinant human activated protein C for severe sepsis. *N Engl J Med* **344**: 699–709.

Annane D, Sébille V, Charpentier C, et al. (2002) Effect of treatment with low doses of hydrocortisone and fludrocortisone on mortality in patients with septic shock. *JAMA* **288**: 862–71.

Annane D, Vignon P, Renault A, et al. for the CATS Study Group. (2007) Norepinephrine plus dobutamine versus epinephrine alone for management of septic shock: a randomised trial. *Lancet* **370**: 676–81.

Sprung CL, Annnane D, Keh D, et al. for the Corticus Study Group. (2008) Hydrocortisone therapy for patients with septic shock. *N Engl J Med* **358**: 111–24.

Russell JA, Walley KR, Singer J, et al. for VASST Investigators. (2008) Vasopressin vs norepinephrine infusion in patients with septic shock. *N Engl J Med* **358**: 877–87.

Dellinger RP, Levy MD, Carlet JM, et al. (2008) Surviving Sepsis Campaign: International guidelines for management of severe sepsis and septic shock. *Crit Care Med* **36**: 296–327.

See also:

Ventilatory support—indications, p44; Enteral nutrition, p128; Tight glycaemic control/intensive insulin therapy, p132; Bacteriology, p224; Virology, serology, and assays, p226; Lactate, p236; Inotropes, p264; Vasopressors, p268; Antimicrobials, p326; Corticosteroids, p328; Immunomodulatory therapies in sepsis, p332; Basic resuscitation, p338; Abdominal sepsis, p422; Infection—diagnosis, p552; Infection—treatment, p554; Systemic inflammation/multi-organ failure—causes, p556; Pyrexia—causes, p602; Pyrexia—management, p604.

Multi-resistant infections

Background to multi-resistance

A major problem worldwide is the increasing incidence of infections caused by multi-resistant organisms. These include:

- Gram-positive organisms, notably methicillin-resistant *S. aureus* (MRSA) and vancomycin-resistant *Enterococcus* (VRE).
- Gram-negative bacteria, e.g. multi-resistant *Acinetobacter* and *Pseudomonas*, carbapenem-resistant *Klebsiella pneumoniae*.
- Fungi, e.g. non-albicans *Candida* species that are increasingly fluconazole-resistant.
- Atypical organisms, including multi-resistant *M. tuberculosis*, malaria, *Pneumocystis jiroveci* (previously *Pneumocystis carinii*).

The predominant factor underlying this worrying rise is the widespread and often inappropriate use of antibiotics.

Prevention

Prevention is key so concerted and maintained efforts must be made to minimise antibiotic use:

- Is sepsis/infection a likely diagnosis? If not, do not give antibiotics.
- Is antibiotic prophylaxis needed? Increasingly, surgery can be performed without the need for prophylaxis or with only 1–3 doses. Prolonged courses should be avoided.
- If antibiotics are prescribed for presumed infection/sepsis, consider the need for their continuation daily. Sadly, optimal duration for a course of antibiotics remains poorly defined.
- Antibiotics should be stopped promptly if the diagnosis turns out to be non-infective; there is no point in finishing a full course. For infection, antibiotics should be stopped 1–2 days after resolution of clinical symptoms. UK practice tends towards 3–7 day courses for 'uncomplicated' infections (e.g. without bone or heart valve involvement). Course duration tends to be longer in mainland Europe and North America.
- If an organism is isolated and sensitivities known, consider changing from broad-spectrum combinations to targeted monotherapy

Management

When prescribing antibiotics consider the likelihood of multi-resistance in the following patients:

- Inpatient for ≥3 days.
- Recently hospitalised.
- Recently in an area with known high resistance rates, e.g. penicillin-resistant meningococcus from Spain.

Patients colonised/infected with multi-resistant organisms should, in general, be placed in source isolation to protect other patients. However, strong evidence for efficacy is lacking. Source isolation is probably more relevant for airborne (aerosolised) organisms spread by coughing and organisms producing diarrhoeal illnesses. Strict hand hygiene, glove and gown wearing, and other local infection control policies should be observed.

Decolonisation regimens may be considered for MRSA, e.g. chlorhexidine bodywashes and topical antibiotics (e.g. mupirocin) nasally and/or orally. Again, the evidence base for efficacy is not very strong.

See also:

Bacteriology, p224; Virology, serology, and assays, p226; Antimicrobials, p326; Infection control—general principles, p544; Infection control—dangerous pathogens, p546.

Necrotising fasciitis

This is a rapidly spreading and often lethal soft tissue infection caused predominantly by group A β-haemolytic *Streptococci*, but also by other Gram-positive bacteria, e.g. Panton–Valentine Leukocidin *S. aureus*, *Clostridium* species (e.g *C. novyi* in skin poppers), Enterococci, and Gram-negative bacteria such as *E. Coli* and *Klebsiella*. Two thirds are polymicrobial. It can involve any layer within the soft tissue compartment (dermis, subcutaneous tissue, superficial or deep fascia, muscle) and is associated with tissue necrosis. Though not usually associated with abscess formation, it can originate from untreated/inadequately drained abscesses.

Risk factors
- Intramuscular/subcutaneous drug injection (especially illicit).
- Chronic comorbidities, e.g. diabetes, immunosuppression, obesity.
- Recent surgery.

Diagnosis
- Can be difficult initially so have a high index of suspicion.
- Swelling, erythema, pain over affected area.
- As infection progresses, tense oedema (appears around the area of compromised skin), degree of pain disproportionate to clinical appearance, skin discoloration, subcutaneous bruising, blisters/bullae, necrosis, crepitus, and/or subcutaneous gas.
- Fever, tachycardia, hypotension, shock.
- Elevated creatine kinase, markers of inflammation (CRP, procalcitonin), hyponatraemia, hyperglycaemia, neutrophilia.
- CT/MRI (shows subcutaenous gas and inflamed fascia) or X-ray (identifies subcutaenous gas) have high sensitivity but low specificity.

Treatment
- Source control—urgent and complete debridement is crucial by an experienced surgeon (ideally, a plastic surgeon) to ensure adequate debridement has been performed. After surgery, the patient's condition is often considerably worse. Frequent repeat debridements are needed until it is clear the fasciitis is not spreading.
- Antibiotics—this is an important adjunct to source control. High-dose clindamycin, a potent protein synthesis inhibitor, inhibits toxin production, particularly in *Streptococcus* and *Clostridium* infection. This is given in combination with high-dose benzylpenicillin (or a carbapenem if penicillin allergic) ± an aminoglycoside (if Gram-negative infection suspected) ± a glycopeptide or linezolid (if MRSA suspected). Continue until no further debridements are needed.
- Critical care support—such patients are often very sick requiring multiple organ support, correction of coagulopathy, blood transfusion to replace blood loss from the debrided area, and consideration of activated protein C.
- Intravenous immunoglobulin (IV Ig) has been used successfully in small randomised studies, particularly for toxin-related infection due to group A *Streptococcus* or *Clostridium*. Current UK recommendations support its use in patients who do not respond to standard measures.
- Hyperbaric oxygen has been advocated in some small series, but this should not delay or prevent surgical debridement.

See also:
Bacteriology, p224; Antimicrobials, p326; Immunomodulatory therapies in sepsis, p332; Infection—diagnosis, p552; Infection—treatment, p554; Sepsis and septic shock—treatment, p560.

HIV-related disease

Patients with HIV-related diseases may present to critical care electively after surgical procedures, including diagnostic biopsies of brain or lung. Other cases present with complications of HIV-related disease, especially pulmonary infection (e.g. *Pneumocystis jiroveci*, CMV, TB) or seizures (e.g. cerebral lymphoma, cerebral abscess, meningitis). HIV-related disease is now considered to be a chronic manageable condition with a good short-term prognosis. It is reasonable to offer critical care support.

As a group, IV drug abusers are at high risk for HIV-related disease. However, they tend to present to critical care more commonly as a result of the drug abuse (e.g. drug withdrawal syndromes, overdose, sepsis, endocarditis, hepatitis, rhabdomyolysis).

An HIV specialist should be consulted about continuing or commencing antiretroviral drugs in patients with known or newly diagnosed HIV infection. Risks of resistance, difficulties in administration of oral medications, possible contraindicated use of proton pump inhibitors and H_2 blockers, delayed renal and/or hepatic clearance, drug interactions and toxicity (e.g. acute hypersensitivity reactions, immune reconstitution syndrome (IRS), Stevens–Johnson syndrome, pancreatitis, lactic acidosis) should all be considered. Recent evidence suggests antiretrovirals are not responsible for improved critical care outcomes.

Pneumocystis jiroveci (carinii) pneumonia

- The commonest respiratory disorder affecting HIV patients. Prognosis has improved considerably in recent years, even in those requiring mechanical ventilation. Intensive, early support with CPAP and appropriate chemotherapy may avert the need for ventilatory support.
- Diagnosis is made clinically without waiting for laboratory confirmation.
- First-line drug treatment is with high dose co-trimoxazole or pentamidine plus adjuvant high dose steroids. The onset of effect of co-trimoxazole is quicker and it has a broader spectrum of antibacterial activity covering common secondary pathogens. Pentamidine is usually used where co-trimoxazole fails or cannot be taken (e.g. allergy).
- Methylprednisolone is used to suppress peribronchial fibrosis and alveolar infiltrate. There may be an initial deterioration on treatment.
- Respiratory support is provided initially with CPAP (5–10cmH$_2$O) if hypoxaemic despite high FIO$_2$ (or BiPAP if the patient is tiring). Lower CPAP pressures should be used where possible since such patients carry a considerable risk of developing pneumothorax.
- Mechanical ventilation is reserved for those who have a rising respiratory rate with deteriorating gas exchange and fatigue despite NIV.
- Chest X-ray changes respond very slowly.
- Avoid excessive fluid as considerable capillary leak can occur.

Immune reconstitution syndrome (IRS)

Occurs days to weeks after initiation of antiretroviral therapy. Characterised by paradoxical worsening of symptoms. It results from an exaggerated inflammatory response to *Pneumocystis*, *Mycobacterial*, viral, or other antigens. It can lead to fever, lymphadenopathy, respiratory failure, hepatitis, CNS, and skin manifestations. Diagnosis is by exclusion of other causes. Management includes treatment of infection and corticosteroids. Continue antiretroviral therapy unless life-threatening.

Drug Dosages

Co-trimoxazole	120mg/kg/d in divided doses IV for 10–14 days, then PO to complete 21 days
Pentamidine	4mg/kg/d IV
Methylprednisolone	1g/d for 3 days

Key paper

Huang L, Quartin A, Jones D, et al. (2006) Intensive care of patients with HIV infection. *N Engl J Med* **355**: 173–81.

See also:

Ventilatory support—indications, p44; Continuous positive airway pressure, p70; Non-invasive respiratory support, p76; Antimicrobials, p326; Corticosteroids, p328; Infection control—general principles, p544; Infection control—HIV, p546.

Malaria

Malaria should be suspected in any patient returning from endemic areas with a febrile illness which may have cerebral, abdominal, lung, or renal features. Rarely, people living near airports may be bitten by a transported *Anopheles* mosquito. There may be considerable delay (weeks to months) between the mosquito bite and signs of infection. It is caused by protozoal infection with the *Plasmodium* genus. The most severe form is *P. falciparum* which causes malignant, tertian malaria. Other forms (*P. malariae, P. vivax, P. ovale*) rarely cause life-threatening disease.

Pathophysiology

P. falciparum invades erythrocytes regardless of age. High levels of parasitaemia >5% are considered severe in non-immune travellers. The cells may haemolyse or be destroyed in liver or spleen. Anaemia may be severe. Increased vascular permeability, cytokine release, red cell agglutination, and intravascular coagulation (DIC) may also occur.

Clinical features

- Symptoms include headache, fever with rigors, myalgia, abdominal pain, vomiting, and diarrhoea. Signs include splenomegaly, jaundice, tender hepatomegaly, and anaemia. Hyponatraemia is common.
- A minority have paroxysms of fever with 'cold' and 'hot' stages.

If >5% parasitaemia, features include:
- Cerebral malaria, causing coma, delirium, seizures, or focal deficits.
- Cough and haemoptysis or acute respiratory distress.
- Blackwater fever is associated with massive intravascular haemolysis, jaundice, haemoglobinuria, collapse, and renal failure.
- Acute renal dysfunction occurs in a third of adult ICU patients.
- Acute cardiovascular collapse ('algid malaria') and metabolic acidosis.
- Thrombocytopaenia, DIC, and spontaneous bleeding.

Diagnosis

- Plasmodia are seen in RBC in thick or thin smears of peripheral blood. Parasitaemia intensity may vary from hour to hour and may be scanty. Carefully scrutinise the smear and repeat if doubt persists.
- Leucocytosis is not a feature of malaria.
- Splenomegaly is almost invariable during the second week of illness.

Treatment

1. Early IV quinine infusion is the mainstay of treatment of severe malaria. Complications include hypoglycaemia and tinnitus. Artemether should be considered in cases of likely quinine resistance, or as first-line treatment for uncomplicated cases.
2. Consider a 2–3L exchange transfusion if the patient is severely ill and parasitaemia levels >10–20%.
3. Pay careful attention to fluid and electrolyte balance. Excess fluid should be avoided as these patients have increased capillary leak.
4. Treatment of hypoglycaemia, renal failure, coagulopathy, metabolic acidosis, seizures, etc. follow conventional lines.
5. Steroids are not recommended for cerebral oedema.
6. Malaria patients are immunosuppressed and prone to atypical infection. Suspect Gram-negative infection with circulatory collapse.

Drug dosages

First-line	
Quinine	20mg quinine salt/kg IV over 4h, then 10mg/kg infusion over 4h, repeated 8-hourly until the patient can swallow, then tablets (10mg quinine salt/kg 8-hourly) to complete a 7-day course.
	Halve maintenance dose to 5mg salt/kg 8-hourly if continuing parenteral therapy for >48 h.
Artemether	3.2mg/kg IM followed by 1.6mg/kg daily
Second-line after asexual parasites eliminated	
Sulfadoxine 500mg / pyramethamine 25mg	3 tablets once
Doxycycline	200mg, then 100mg daily for 7 days

See also:
Acute respiratory distress syndrome (1), p360; Acute respiratory distress syndrome (2), p362; Oliguria, p398; Acute renal failure—diagnosis, p400; Acute renal failure—management, p402; Jaundice, p428; Coma, p438; Generalised seizures, p444; Anaemia, p472; Haemolysis, p476; Pyrexia—causes, p602; Pyrexia—management, p604.

SARS, VHF, and H5N1

SARS

SARS is a severe respiratory disease caused by a coronavirus. It was first recognised in China in November 2002 and spread worldwide before being contained by July 2003. Further outbreaks were recognised over the following year. The possibility of SARS re-emergence remains. Treatment is supportive with source isolation. Various treatments, including ribavirin, corticosteroids, interferon, and intravenous immunoglobulin, have not shown confirmed outcome benefit.

Viral haemorrhagic fever (VHF)

VHF is a group of viral infections that cause a severe haemorrhagic disease. They include Lassa, Ebola, and Marburg fevers. Treatment is supportive and mortality high for these highly contagious pathogens. In some countries, such patients are managed in a high-risk Infectious Diseases Unit with personal protective equipment for staff. These units generally have restricted access, lobbied entrance to isolation rooms, negative pressure with HEPA filtration for exhaust air, en suite facilities, and staff shower and change facilities. Protective suits limit the time staff can work to four hours. In other countries, these patients are managed in bed isolator tents (Trexler units) with the provision of all care via invaginated sleeves into the tent. The provision of intensive care within a Trexler tent is nearly impossible.

H5N1

H5N1 is an avian influenza A virus that has caused illness in humans. There is evidence of limited human-to-human transmission and transmission of the virus to those handling of infected poultry. Around 60% of humans known to have been infected with the recent Asian strain have died. H5N1 may mutate into a strain capable of efficient human-to-human transmission. Treatment is supportive although oseltamivir may inhibit the virus from spreading within the body.

See also:
Infection control—general principles, p544; Infection control—dangerous pathogens, p548.

Rheumatic disorders

Rheumatoid arthritis

A debilitating arthritis that may present to critical care through pulmonary involvement or through complications of treatment (e.g. renal failure, immunosuppression, bleeding disorders). Pleuro-pulmonary involvement may precede arthritic symptoms and is more common in those with active rheumatoid disease and middle-aged men. Care is required when intubating patients with rheumatoid arthritis since the neck joints may sublux. Advice should be sought from a rheumatologist about starting/continuing treatment with steroids or other disease modifiers such as methotrexate, anti-TNF antibody, or rituximab.

Rheumatoid pleurisy

Often presents with effusion and can be asymptomatic. Effusions may be recurrent or chronic and may impede respiratory function. The effusion is an exudate, low in glucose, and often high in cholesterol.

Rheumatoid lung

A diffuse interstitial pneumonitis with bibasal fibrotic changes on chest X-ray or CT. It produces a restrictive pulmonary defect. The mainstay of treatment is early systemic corticosteroid therapy.

Systemic lupus erythematosis (SLE)

A non-organ specific autoimmune disease characterised by anti-nuclear antibodies with high titres of anti-double stranded DNA antibodies. Vasculitis is prominent though cutaneous and CNS involvement are not vasculitic. SLE may present to intensive care through pulmonary, renal, or central nervous system involvement.

Renal failure

Renal failure is vasculitic in origin and may progress to end-stage renal failure requiring long-term dialysis. Early treatment with systemic steroids and immunosuppressives may halt the disease progress.

Lupus pleurisy and pericarditis

Unlike rheumatoid pleurisy, pleural involvement in SLE is often painful and associated with large pleural effusions.

Pulmonary haemorrhage

This is associated with renal failure and may be life-threatening. Plasma exchange may be helpful.

Interstitial pneumonitis

Interstitial pneumonitis is uncommon. Parenchymal infiltrates are more likely to be infective in origin, secondary to immunosuppressive therapy.

Pulmonary thromboembolic disease

Patients typically have a prolonged APTT due to circulating lupus anticoagulant but are more prone to thrombotic episodes. Lupus anticoagulant is associated with anticardiolipin antibodies. Recurrent pulmonary emboli may be associated with chronic pulmonary hypertension. Treatment is long-term anticoagulation.

Vasculitis

See also:
Respiratory imaging, p158; Anticoagulants, p318; Corticosteroids, p328; Rituximab, p334; Pulmonary embolus, p376; Acute renal failure—diagnosis, p400; Acute renal failure—management, p402; Vasculitis, p574.

Vasculitis

Vasculitis should be suspected in any patient with multisystem disease, especially involving the lungs and kidneys.

Wegener's granulomatosis

A systemic vasculitis characterised by necrotising granulomas of the upper and lower respiratory tract, glomerulonephritis, and small vessel vasculitis. Wegener's granulomatosis is associated with positive core anti-neutrophil cytoplasmic antibodies (c-ANCA), particularly granular with central attenuation on immunofluorescence. Intensive care admission is usually because of renal and pulmonary involvement.

Renal failure

Focal necrotising glomerulonephritis leads to progressive failure. Treatment with steroids and cyclophosphamide may give complete remission.

Upper airway disease

Nasal symptoms include epistaxis, nasal discharge, and septal perforation. Critical care admission may be required for severe epistaxis. Ulcerating lesions of the larynx and trachea may cause subglottic stenosis. This is usually insidious but may present problems on attempted intubation.

Pulmonary involvement

Usually associated with haemoptysis, dyspnoea, and cough with rounded opacities ± cavitation on chest X-ray/CT. Nodules may be solitary. Alveolar haemorrhage may be life-threatening. The mainstay of treatment is steroids and cyclophosphamide which may produce complete remission. Plasma exchange may be helpful.

Polyarteritis nodosa (PAN)

PAN is a necrotising vasculitis affecting small and medium-sized muscular arteries. Intensive care admission may be provoked by renal failure, ischaemic heart disease, hypertensive crisis, and bronchospasm although true pulmonary involvement is uncommon. Diagnosis may be confirmed by mesenteric angiography or renal biopsy. Treatment involves renal replacement therapy, high dose steroids, and cyclophosphamide.

Goodpasture's syndrome

Anti-glomerular basement membrane (anti-GBM) antibodies bind at the glomerulus and alveolus. Patients present with a proliferative glomerulonephritis and haemoptysis. Diagnosis is confirmed by positive anti-GBM antibodies and renal biopsy. Treatment is with immunosuppressive therapy and plasma exchange.

See also:

Plasma exchange, p114; Corticosteroids, p328; Airway obstruction, p348; Haemoptysis, p372; Acute renal failure—diagnosis, p400; Acute renal failure—management, p402; Rheumatic disorders, p572.

Toxic epidermal necrolysis

Toxic epidermal necrolysis (TEN) is an acute onset, potentially life-threatening, idiosyncratic mucocutaneous reaction, usually occurring after starting a new drug, e.g. antibiotics, non-steroidal anti-inflammatory drugs, anticonvulsants, allopurinol or, less commonly, immunisation. It is often complicated by infection and multi-organ dysfunction. Mortality is 25–75%, often from secondary sepsis.

Clinical features

- There is often a flu-like prodrome for 2–3 days.
- Macular rash that may become confluent, with desquamation of skin and mucosae leaving raw, moist, denuded surfaces.
- Conjunctivitis may precede skin changes by 1–3 days.
- More common in women patients with HIV disease.
- Relevant drugs will have been started within the previous four weeks.

Management

- Clinical diagnosis is usually sufficient; skin biopsy may be needed for atypical cases.
- Stop all potential causative drugs.
- Intravenous catheters should avoid involved skin, if possible.
- A SCORTEN assessment should be made. Patients with SCORTEN ≥2 or significant comorbidity should be managed in a critical care facility.
- Fluid loss from desquamation mandates careful assessment and replacement of fluid. Requirements approach those needed for an equivalent burn injury.
- Give oral or intravenous analgesia.
- Give thromboprophylaxis.
- Regularly assess for infection and sepsis. Hypothermia may indicate the onset of sepsis. Since TEN patients are susceptible to infection, they should be managed in protective isolation.
- Manage patients on a pressure-relieving mattress in a humidified environment.
- Early attention to eye care is essential. Apply chloramphenicol eye ointment 6-hourly (unless chloramphenicol is a possible causative agent).
- Desquamation may obstruct the tracheobronchial tree or urethra.
- Avoid adhesive tapes and do not debride skin. Detached skin should be left in place and protected with 50:50 white soft paraffin.

SCORTEN indicators of prognosis

Age more than 40
Heart rate more than 120/min
Malignancy
>10% body surface area blistered at day 1
Urea >10mmol/L
Bicarbonate <20mmol/L
Glucose >14mmol/L

Mortality up to 10% for 1 indicator, 10–19% for 2, 20–39% for 3, 10–59% for 4, and >60% for >5.

Key Paper

Bastuji-Garin S, Fouchard N, Bertocchi M, et.al. (2000) SCORTEN: a severity-of-illness score for toxic epidermal necrolysis. *J Invest Dermatol* **115**: 149–53.

See also:

Wound and pressure sore management, p134; Wound management principles, p136; Dressing techniques, p138; Special support surfaces, p140; Basic resuscitation, p338; Fluid challenge, p342; Infection—diagnosis, p552; Infection—treatment, p554; Pain, p618.

Anaphylactoid reactions

Minor reactions to allergens (itching, urticaria) are common before a severe reaction occurs; any such history should be taken seriously and potential allergens avoided. Most reactions are acute in onset and clearly related to the causative allergen. However, some complement-mediated reactions may take longer to develop.

Clinical features

- Respiratory—laryngeal oedema, bronchospasm, pulmonary oedema, pulmonary hypertension.
- Cardiovascular—hypotension, tachycardia, generalised oedema.
- Other—urticaria, angio-oedema, abdominal cramps, rigors.

Management

1. Stop all infusions and blood transfusions, and withhold any potential drug or food allergen. Blood and blood products should be returned to the laboratory for analysis.
2. Give appropriate oxygen to maintain normoxaemia. If hypoxaemia persists, consider urgent intubation and mechanical ventilation.
3. If there is laryngeal obstruction, bronchospasm, or facial oedema, give IM or nebulised adrenaline and IV hydrocortisone. If there is no rapid relief of airway obstruction, consider urgent intubation or, *in extremis*, emergency cricothyroidotomy or tracheostomy. Persistent bronchospasm may require epinephrine ± salbutamol ± aminophylline infusion, or assisted expiration (manual chest compression).
4. Treat hypotension with adrenaline IV/IM and rapid colloid infusion. Large volumes of colloid may be required to replace the plasma volume deficit in severe anaphylaxis.
    - Severe oedema may coexist with hypovolaemia.
    - Plasma volume has not been adequately replaced if the haemoglobin is higher than normal.
5. Treat persistent hypotension with further epinephrine, hydrocortisone, and colloid infusion guided by CVP ± cardiac output monitoring. Use norepinephrine in high output vasodilatory shock to divert blood centrally and increase peripheral resistance.
6. Urticaria requires chlorphenamine IV or PO, depending on the severity of the reaction.
7. After control of the anaphylactoid reaction, advice should be sought from the immunology laboratory and appropriate samples taken for confirmation.
8. Reactions to long-acting drugs or fluids will require continued support (perhaps for many hours).

Drug dosages

	Initial dose	Continued treatment
Laryngeal oedema and bronchospasm		
Epinephrine	0.3–0.5mg IM or 0.5mg nebulised	Start at 0.05mcg/kg/min
Hydrocortisone	200mg IV	
Hypotension		
Epinephrine	0.5–1.0mg IM or 0.05–0.2mg IV	Start at 0.05mcg/kg/min
Colloid	500mL	According to response
Hydrocortisone	200mg IV	200mg IV qds
Chlorphenamine		10mg IV tds
Urticaria		
Chlorphenamine		10mg IV tds or 4mg PO tds
Hydrocortisone		50–100mg IV tds
Prednisolone		20mg PO daily

See also:
Endotracheal intubation, p42; Bronchodilators, p254; Inotropes, p264; Corticosteroids, p328; Basic resuscitation, p338.

Trauma and burns

Multiple trauma (1)

Such patients are admitted either after surgery or for close observation and medical management. The principles of management are to:

• Maintain or quickly restore adequate tissue perfusion and gas exchange.
• Control pain.
• Secure haemostasis and correct any coagulopathy.
• Provide adequate nutrition.
• Monitor closely and deal promptly with any complications.

Circulatory management

• Patients are often cold and vasoconstricted on admission. This can camouflage concurrent hypovolaemia and compromise perfusion.
• Institute adequate monitoring at an early stage.
• Development of a persisting tissue oxygen debt has been shown to lead to subsequent multiple organ dysfunction which may not become clinically apparent for 3–7 days. Therefore, adequate perfusion must be restored promptly by repeated fluid challenges. Addition of a vasodilating agent, e.g. glyceryl trinitrate, may be beneficial.
• An early increasing metabolic acidosis should prompt suspicion of inadequate resuscitation, covert haemorrhage, or tissue necrosis. Myocardial depression or failure may also be implicated.

Respiratory management

• If ventilated, ensure haemodynamic stability, removal of any metabolic acidosis, adequate rewarming, and satisfactory gas exchange before attempting to wean. If the patient remains unstable, it is advisable to delay extubation in case urgent surgery is required.
• If spontaneously breathing, give supplemental oxygen to provide adequate arterial oxygenation, encourage deep breathing to prevent atelectasis and secondary infection, and ensure sufficient analgesia albeit not too much to suppress ventilatory drive.

Haematological management

• Initially maintain haemoglobin >9–10g/dL to assist oxygen transport and provide a buffer for any sudden onset new haemorrhage. Crossmatched blood should be readily available.
• Correct coagulopathy as appropriate with fresh frozen plasma ± platelets, and, occasionally, other blood products (e.g. cryoprecipitate) or activated factor VII. Seek advice from a haematologist.
• Surgery or arterial embolisation may be needed for ongoing blood loss.

Peripheries

Injury to the limb may result in nerve injuries, obstruction of the vascular supply, or muscle damage which may lead to compartment syndrome and rhabdomyolysis. A high level of suspicion should be held and corrective surgery undertaken promptly if necessary. Ensure plaster casts do not compromise peripheral limb perfusion.

See also:
Trauma score, p34; Ventilatory support—indications, p44; Wound management principles, p136; Dressing techniques, p138; Blood transfusion, p248; Blood products, p250; Multiple trauma (2), p584; Head injury (1), p586; Head injury (2), p588; Spinal cord injury, p590; Coagulants and antifibrinolytics, p322; Basic resuscitation, p338.

Multiple trauma (2)

Analgesia

- Adequate analgesia is imperative to avoid circulatory instability and decreased chest wall excursion, especially following chest, abdominal, or spinal trauma.
- Increased use of regional techniques (depending on absence of infection and coagulopathy) and patient-controlled analgesia have facilitated pain relief and weaning.
- Opiates are recommended for initial analgesia. Non-steroidals are particularly effective for bony pain though may occasionally precipitate coagulopathies, stress ulceration, and renal failure.
- Agitation may be due to causes other than pain, e.g. infection, intracranial lesion, alcohol, or recreational drug withdrawal.

Nutrition

Early nutrition has been shown to reduce post-operative complications. This should ideally be enteral, an approach which has been demonstrated as safe even after abdominal laparotomy for trauma.

Infection

- Depending on the site of trauma, the type of wound (open/closed, clean/dirty), and the need for surgery, prophylactic tetanus, and antibiotic cover varying from 1 dose to 1–2 weeks may be needed.
- The trauma patient is at high risk of developing secondary infection, in particular, chest, wound sites, intravascular catheter insertion sites and, post-abdominal trauma, intra-abdominal abscesses. Preventive measures and strict infection control should be undertaken.
- Replace intravascular catheters inserted during emergency resuscitation under non-sterile conditions.

Prophylaxis

- Attention should be paid to pressure areas; this may involve the use of specialised mattresses or support beds.
- Clear instructions should be obtained from the surgeon regarding care of the wound and drain sites.
- Deep venous thrombosis is common after trauma, especially after orthopedic procedures on the pelvis and lower limb. Discuss with the surgeon when to commence low molecular weight heparin in view of any ongoing bleeding risk.

Review

- Regular review of the patient is necessary to ensure complications are detected and dealt with promptly. This may require repeat laparotomy, angiography, ultrasound, or CT/MRI scanning.
- Later complications include pancreatitis, acalculous cholecystitis, and multiple organ dysfunction (including ARDS).

Head injury (1)

The head may be injured with or without significant trauma to other parts of the body. Priority in management of the multiply injured patient must be placed on securing adequate gas exchange and circulatory resuscitation, and dealing with any life-threatening injury, e.g. an arterial injury, before definitive treatment for head injury.

The patient will usually be admitted to critical care after CT scanning has identified the extent of injury. The neck should also be imaged by CT, particularly if the patient is ventilated. It is also likely that surgery will already have been undertaken for any significant space-occupying lesion or for elevation of a depressed fracture.

General management

- See http://www.nice.org.uk/Guidance/CG56/Guidance/pdf/English.
- Assume an unstable neck fracture until excluded by an expert opinion and appropriate investigations.
- Most head injury patients admitted to non-neurosurgical Critical Care Units will have diffuse or local brain injury for which a non-operative approach has been adopted. The regional Neurosurgery centre should be contacted if raised intracranial pressure is present as local policy may encourage early bone flap decompression or referral for invasive monitoring (e.g. intracranial pressure, jugular venous bulb O_2 saturation).
- If a basal skull fracture is suspected (e.g. X-rays, rhinorrhoea, otorrhoea), avoid nasal insertion of feeding or endotracheal tubes.
- Deterioration in conscious level, developing neurological deficits or focal signs (e.g. unilateral pupillary dilatation) should prompt urgent repeat CT scanning for late complications, e.g. subdural haematoma.

Complications

- Actively manage raised intracranial pressure.
- Actively treat seizures with anticonvulsants to prevent further hypoxaemic cerebral damage, reduce cerebral oxygen requirements, and ICP. Load with IV phenytoin as prophylaxis against further fits. Consider additional causes such as hypoglycaemia, development of a new space-occupying lesion, recreational drugs (or withdrawal), and infection.
- Diabetes insipidus suggests hypothalamic injury and carries a poor prognosis. Desmopressin 1–4mcg IV should be given daily to maintain urine outputs of 100–150mL/h.
- Actively manage hyperpyrexia. Some studies show long-term benefit from induced hypothermia; this needs to be aggressively instituted as early as possible after the injury to be most effective.
- Ensure good glycaemic control with insulin as needed. Avoid hypoglycaemia.

Key papers

Rovlias A, Kotsou S. (2000) The influence of hyperglycemia on neurological outcome in patients with severe head injury. *Neurosurgery* **46**: 335–42.

Clifton GL, Miller ER, Choi SC et al. (2001) Lack of effect of induction of hypothermia after acute brain injury. *N Engl J Med* **344**: 556–63.

See also:

Head injury (2)

Analgesia

- Adequate analgesia (usually opiates) must be given to the head-injured patient as pain and agitation will increase intracranial pressure, thereby causing a secondary insult.
- Short-acting sedation should be used as this enables rapid assessment of the underlying conscious level and any focal neurological deficit.

Respiratory management

- Aggressive hyperventilation is no longer recommended apart from short-term management of raised intracranial pressure. If ventilated, aim to maintain $PaCO_2$ at 3.5–4kPa.
- Face or neck injuries may have required emergency cricothyroidotomy or tracheostomy to obtain a patent airway. If orotracheally intubated, ensure local swelling has subsided (nasendoscopy, air leak around deflated cuff) before extubation.
- Severe agitation and confusion may last for several weeks; this will often delay weaning and extubation. Judicious sedation, e.g. with haloperidol, may be necessary.

Circulatory management

- Avoid hypotension with adequate fluid resuscitation ± vasopressor.
- Elevated blood pressures may be tolerated unless excessive.
- β-blockers are useful in reducing the myocardial and immunosuppressive effects of excessive catecholamine levels.

Other drug therapy

- Antibiotic prophylaxis is not routinely recommended.
- High-dose steroid therapy has not been shown to be beneficial.
- Trials of other neuroprotective agents, e.g. free radical scavengers, have also failed to show benefit.

Indications for consideration of intracranial pressure monitoring

Indications

- Glasgow coma score ≤8 and any abnormality on CT scan.
- GCS ≤8 and a normal CT scan, but any two of the following: (i) age >40y, (ii) hypotension, (iii) decerebrate posturing.
- GCS >8, but requiring general anaesthesia for treatment of other injuries or requiring treatment likely to increase ICP, e.g. high levels of PEEP.

ICP monitoring should be continued as long as the ICP is elevated, during active management of ICP, or for up to 3 days in the absence of significant elevation.

Contraindications

- Coagulopathy.
- Infection.

See also:
Ventilatory support—indications, p44; Tracheotomy, p80; Intracranial pressure monitoring, p200;
Non-opioid analgesics, p302; Opioid analgesics, p304; Sedatives and tranquilisers, p308; Head injury
(1), p586; Pain, p612.

Spinal cord injury

Spinal injury, with or without damage to the cord, may be apparent soon after admission to hospital. However, deterioration may occur, requiring a high index of suspicion and careful monitoring.

Immobilisation

- Immobilise the spine until a senior surgical/orthopaedic opinion has confirmed that no unstable fracture is present.
- Place a hard cervical collar and immobilise head with lateral supports. This does not stabilise the spine; either skull traction or operative stabilisation will be needed for an unstable fracture.
- Move the patient by 'log-rolling' or straight-lifting, using at least four staff members. Exercise care with neck manipulation; intubation should be performed by an experienced operator.

Circulatory instability

- So-called 'spinal shock' may occur with marked hypotension due to sympathetic outflow disturbance. Hypovolaemia should be excluded first. Consider damage to other organs/vessels, e.g. spleen, aorta.
- Vasopressor therapy may be necessary if evidence of tissue hypoperfusion persists, e.g. oliguria, metabolic acidosis.
- Postural hypotension and circulatory instability (including symptomatic bradycardia) is commonplace for the first few weeks. Autonomic dysfunction affects 50% of cervical and high thoracic cord injuries.

Respiratory management

- High cervical cord injury above C5 results in loss of diaphragmatic function. Injury above C8 can result in loss of intercostal function. This may compromise or prevent breathing and weaning from IPPV.
- When able, the patient should be managed in an upright posture.
- Atelectasis is common and requires regular physiotherapy.
- Early tracheostomy may facilitate support and comfort.

General measures

- Carefully monitor neurological function to enable early detection of spinal cord compression and referral for urgent remedial surgery.
- Give LMW heparin SC for thromboembolism prophylaxis.
- The incidence of stress ulceration is high. Use enteral nutrition at an early stage. Drugs (e.g. H$_2$-blockers) may be needed.
- Enteral feeding may be difficult to institute initially as gastric distension and paralytic ileus are common. An NG tube should be inserted for gastric decompression. An enterostomy may be needed for feeding.
- Bowel and bladder function may be deranged. Insert a silastic bladder catheter. Regular laxative and enema therapy should be started early.
- Special care is needed to prevent pressure sores.
- Institute regular exercises to prevent contractures.
- Psychological support for patient and family is crucial, particularly if long-term disability is likely.
- High-dose steroid therapy may be beneficial if started within 8h, though this still remains controversial.
- Hyperbaric oxygen therapy is of unproven benefit.
- After spinal injury, muscle relaxants may cause severe hyperkalaemia.

Key papers

Bracken MB, Shepard MJ, Holford TR, et al. (1997) Administration of methylprednisolone for 24 or 48 hours or tirilazad mesylate for 48 hours in the treatment of acute spinal cord injury. Results of the Third National Acute Spinal Cord Injury Randomised Controlled Trial. National Acute Spinal Cord Injury Study. *JAMA* **277**: 1597–604.

Morris CG, McCoy W, Lavery GG. (2004) Spinal immobilisation for unconscious patients with multiple injuries. *BMJ* **329**: 495–9.

See also:

Ventilatory support—indications, p44; Tracheotomy, p80; Chest physiotherapy, p90; Enteral feeding and drainage tubes, p122; Wound and pressure sore management, p136; Special support surfaces, p140; Vasopressors, p268; H_2 blockers and proton pump inhibitors, p286; Anticoagulants, p318; Corticosteroids, p328; Multiple trauma (1), p582; Multiple trauma (2), p584.

Burns—fluid management

Major thermal injuries (i.e. >20% body surface area) are admitted to an Intensive Care Unit, usually specialised in the management of burns, for meticulous attention to fluid resuscitation, prevention of infection, and the frequent need for mechanical ventilation.

Monitoring

- Fluid loss from major burns requires careful assessment of intravascular volume status. Traditional markers of fluid resuscitation such as CVP, urine output, and haematocrit are often inadequate.
- Either invasive or non-invasive cardiac output monitoring is needed for accurate titration of fluid. This is particularly applicable in the presence of a hyperdynamic, vasodilated circulation which often commences within 1–2 days. Although infection is not necessarily present, vasopressors may be needed to maintain an adequate systemic BP.
- Intravascular catheters should not be inserted through affected skin areas, if at all possible.
- Insertion of intravascular catheters, urinary catheters, and NG tubes should be carried out soon after admission as rapid onset swelling within a few hours may make these procedures impossible.

Fluid management

- The extent of injury will have been estimated by plastic surgeons who will also determine the proportion of full thickness dermal injury to calculate the approximate fluid resuscitation required.
- Fluid resuscitation in the UK often follows the Mount Vernon (albumin-based) formula while the Parkland (crystalloid-based) formula is often used in the US. Colloids may reduce oedema at non-burn sites and restore blood volume faster than crystalloids.
- These formulae only provide an approximate guide and frequently underestimate losses both into the interstitial spaces and through the lost skin barrier. Evaporative losses are approximately 2mL/kg/h. Water losses may be increased if wounds are not covered. Losses increase further with inhalation injury.
- Overzealous fluid infusion should be avoided to minimise oedema.
- The increased permeability and fluid leak phase lasts approximately 1–2 days. After 2–5 days, a diuretic phase usually commences when excess tissue fluid is lost and the body swelling reduces.
- Electrolyte levels (especially K^+ and Mg^{2+}) can fluctuate widely in both periods, requiring monitoring and replacement as necessary.
- Though some haemolysis may occur, blood transfusion requirements are usually low, but debridement will result in major blood loss often requiring major transfusion (>8–10U). A coagulopathy will often occur, in part due to a dilutional effect of the albumin infusion.

Fluid resuscitation regimens

These regimens should be used as a guide only. In the Critical Care Unit, haemodynamic monitoring gives a better guide to fluid requirements.

Adapted from Parkland formula

- Total volume of Ringer's lactate for the first 24h = 4mL Ringer's lactate solution × bodyweight [kg] × % burn.
- Half the volume is administered in the first 8h, the rest is delivered over the next 16h.

Adapted from Mount Vernon formula

- Divide first 36h from the time of burn into six consecutive periods of 4, 4, 4, 6, 6, and 12h.
- For each period, give 0.5mL 5% albumin × bodyweight [kg] × % burn.
- Give 1.5–2mL/kg/h 5% glucose.

With either formula, give blood as necessary to maintain Hb >10g/dL. Reassess cardiorespiratory variables and urine output at frequent intervals to determine whether volume replacement is inadequate or excessive; adjust fluid input accordingly.

See also:

Central venous catheter—use, p170; Pulmonary artery catheter—use, p176; Cardiac output—central thermodilution, p178; Cardiac output—peripheral thermodilution, p180; Cardiac output—indicator dilution, p182; Cardiac output—Doppler ultrasound, p184; Cardiac output—pulse contour analysis, p186; Cardiac output—other techniques, p188; Pressure and stroke volume variation, p190; Crystalloids, p242; Colloids, p246; Blood transfusion, p248; Basic resuscitation, p338; Fluid challenge, p342; Burns—general management, p594.

Burns—general management

Surgery

- Escharotomy may be needed on hospital admission to affected limbs as well as the neck and/or chest if a circumferential burn is present.
- Debridement of necrotic tissue is often begun within the first few days as early grafting is associated with improved outcome. Coverage is obtained using either split skin grafts from the patient's own unaffected skin, donor skin grafts, or even experimental 'skin'. Blood loss may be rapid and massive, e.g. 100mL per 1% of body surface grafted.

Wound care

- Early application of dressings and Flamazine (silver sulphadiazine) cream, which has antibacterial properties against Gram-negative bacteria, may usefully prevent secondary infection.
- Early grafting often takes place within the first 2–3 days to provide a skin protective barrier.

Nutrition

- Enteral nutrition should be commenced soon after admission as studies have shown that early enteral nutrition improves outcome.
- Target intake is protein of 1g/kg + 2g per % burn, and a calorie intake of 20Cal/kg + 50Cal per % burn.

Infection

- Prophylactic antibiotics are often not given to burn patients.
- Body temperature rises on days 1–2 as high as 40°C may persist for several days and does not indicate secondary infection.
- Likely infecting agents include *Streptococci*, *Staphylococci*, and Gram-negative bacteria such as *Pseudomonas*. Appropriate antibiotic treatment should be given as indicated.

Other considerations

- Diagnose and treat any suspected inhalation injury.
- Ensure adequate analgesia (opiates). Ketamine is a useful anaesthetic as it also has analgesic properties.
- Tetanus toxoid should be given soon after hospital admission.
- Reduce heat and fluid losses by placing the patient on a heated air-fluidised bed and by early coverage of burnt skin through application of occlusive dressings and placing affected limbs in transparent plastic bags.
- Stress ulceration can usually be avoided through prompt resuscitation and early enteral nutrition.
- Prevent pressure sores and contractures by careful nursing and physiotherapy.
- Avoid suxamethonium from 5–150 days post-burn because of the risk of rapid and severe hyperkalaemia.
- Increasing resistance to non-depolarising muscle relaxants may occur.
- β-blockade has been associated with outcome improvement in children sustaining burn injury.

See also:
Enteral nutrition, p128; Wound and pressure sore management, p136; Wound management principles, p136; Dressing techniques, p138; Special support surfaces, p140; Non-opioid analgesics, p302; Opioid analgesics, p304; Infection control—general principles, p544; Infection—diagnosis, p552; Infection—treatment, p554; Systemic inflammation/multi-organ failure—causes, p556; Burns—fluid management, p592.

Blast injury

Pathophysiology

Blast injuries are traditionally divided into four categories: primary, secondary, tertiary, and quaternary (or miscellaneous) injuries.

- Primary blast injury is caused by the direct effect of blast overpressure on tissue. Unlike water, air is easily compressible so air-filled structures such as lung, ear, and the gastrointestinal tract are frequently affected. Tympanic membrane rupture indicates high-pressure wave ($\geq$40kPa) injury and suggests (but does not confirm) the presence of vital organ injury.
- Secondary blast injury is ballistic trauma related to flying objects. The severity of a ballistic wound is determined by the kinetic energy of the projectile. Therefore, velocity has more impact than mass of the object.
- Tertiary blast injury occurs with high-energy explosions when people fly through the air and strike other objects.
- Quaternary injuries cover all other injuries, e.g. burns, crush injuries, and toxic gas/smoke inhalation.

Investigations (as indicated)

Assessment should be as for any trauma with focus on airway, breathing, and circulation followed by a primary assessment of injuries.

- Lung—X-ray or CT scan for lung contusion, pneumothorax, ARDS, flail chest. Contusion may evolve over several hours.
- Heart—ECG, echocardiography, and troponin for myocardial contusion and to exclude pericardial tamponade.
- Abdomen—CT scan to exclude injury to both solid and hollow organs, including penetrating objects, perforation, cavitation, and occult haemorrhage. Intestinal haematoma can take up to 36h to develop. Intestinal perforation is more common with underwater blast injury.
- X-ray or CT to other injured areas—for fractures, shrapnel, gas embolus, etc.
- Blood tests for diagnosis of DIC, rhabdomyolysis.

Management

- Standard surgical management of fractures, burns, wounds, etc.
- If possible, avoid positive pressure ventilation and PEEP due to the risk of alveolar rupture and air embolus. If IPPV is necessary, use low tidal volumes and minimise airway pressure.
- For patients with arterial gas embolism (AGE), give 100% O_2 by tight-fitting face mask, and if possible, place the patient in the left lateral position to minimise risk of further air emboli leaving the heart. If the lung responsible for the air emboli can be identified, single lung ventilation may prevent further air entry into the vasculature during IPPV. Hyperbaric oxygen treatment is the definitive treatment for AGE, especially cerebral AGE where blood vessels in brain or spinal cord are occluded.
- Myocardial depression usually self-reverses within minutes to hours.
- Consider and treat as appropriate: (i) DIC, (ii) carbon monoxide, smoke and other toxic inhalation, (iii) rhabdomyolysis and compartment syndrome, and (iv) peripheral compression injuries.
- Follow local protocols for biological, chemical, or radiation contamination if a 'dirty' bomb is implicated in the blast injury.

See also:

Respiratory imaging, p158; ECG monitoring, p162; Echocardiography, p192; Cardiac function tests, p216; Pneumothorax, p368; Inhalation injury, p374; Multiple trauma (1), p582; Multiple trauma (2), p584; Rhabdomyolysis, p612; Raised intra-abdominal pressure, p614.

Physical disorders

Hypothermia

Clinical features

- >33°C—shivering in an attempt to correct body temperature.
- <33°C—neurological signs of dysarthria and slowness appear.
- <31°C—hypertonicity and sluggish reflexes with cardiovascular dysfunction become life-threatening.
- <28°C—arterial pulses often impalpable. Hypothermic rigidity is difficult to distinguish from death.

Prognosis depends on the degree and duration of hypothermia.

ECG changes

Sinus bradycardia is followed by atrial flutter and fibrillation with ventricular ectopics. The PR interval, QRS complex, and QT interval are prolonged. Atrial activity eventually ceases. 'J' waves most often seen <31°C; ventricular fibrillation is common <30°C, with asystole <28°C.

Complications

Hypoxaemia is common due to hypoventilation and ventilation perfusion mismatch. Hypovolaemia and metabolic acidosis are common. Renal tubular damage may result from renal blood flow reduction. Acute pancreatitis, rhabdomyolysis, and gastric erosions are common.

Management

1. Oxygen to maintain SaO_2 >95%.
2. Fluid replacement with careful monitoring.
3. Rewarming—all hypothermic patients with no evidence of other fatal disease should be assumed fully recoverable. In the event of cardiac arrest, full resuscitation should continue until normothermia is achieved. VF is resistant to defibrillation between 28–30°C. The technique used for rewarming depends on core temperature (measured with a low-reading rectal thermometer) and clinical circumstances.

Rapid central rewarming

For core temperature <28°C (<33°C with acute exposure hypothermia) or where there is cardiac arrest, rapid rewarming should be instituted. This may be achieved by continous arterio-venous rewarming circuits, peritoneal dialysis, gastric or bladder lavage with warmed fluids. Cardiopulmonary bypass is an effective rewarming strategy for patients with cardiac arrest resistant to defibrillation. These techniques may achieve rewarming rates of 1–5°C/h. Active surface rewarming with a heated blanket or warm air blanket can achieve rates of 1–7°C/h and is less invasive. Haemodynamic changes and fluid shifts may be dramatic during active rewarming, requiring careful monitoring and support. If extracorporeal rewarming is available, rates of 3–15°C/h may be achieved with the addition of cardiovascular support.

Spontaneous rewarming

Spontaneous rewarming proceeds at a rate inversely proportional to the duration of hypothermia. With good insulation (space blanket), rewarming rates of 0.1–0.7°C/h can be achieved. Core temperature may fall during spontaneous rewarming as cold blood is returned from the periphery to the central circulation.

Causes of hypothermia

- Coma and immobility.
- Cold water immersion.
- Exposure.
- Hypothyroidism.
- Hypopituitarism.
- Sepsis.
- Erythroderma.

See also:
Electrical cardioversion, p94; ECG monitoring, p162; Basic resuscitation, p338; Cardiac arrest, p340; Tachyarrhythmias, p384; Bradyarrhythmias, p386; Pancreatitis, p424; Thyroid emergencies, p514; Rhabdomyolysis, p612.

Pyrexia—causes

Pathophysiology

Mechanisms underlying temperature rise are poorly understood. It reflects the balance between heat loss and heat production. There may be inability to lose heat (e.g. high ambient temperature), 'thermostat' dysregulation within the hypothalamus, and increased heat generation (e.g. due to mitochondrial uncoupling). There is some laboratory evidence that a raised temperature may be beneficial in terms of white cell response, heat shock protein activation, and mitochondrial protection. Prognosis is worse in septic patients presenting with a low temperature.

An excessive temperature may be unpleasant to the patient (e.g. rigors). It will increase metabolic rate and therefore, oxygen demand, induce excessive vasodilatation, and increase salt and water loss. At very high temperatures, biochemical function is disrupted with altered enzyme function and increased cell breakdown (e.g. rhabdomyolysis).

Causes

Infection

The commonest cause in the ICU patient, though over-diagnosed. Main sites are chest and intravascular catheter sites. Urinary tract infections are difficult to diagnose in the presence of a urethral catheter. Similarly, the respiratory tract is routinely colonised with bacteria within a few days of ICU admission; differentiation between colonising and pathogenic bacteria is difficult. Seek malaria in patients who have visited endemic areas. Antibiotic therapy may itself be a cause of pyrexia.

Inflammation

Inflammation unrelated to infection will usually generate a pyrexic response, e.g. systemic inflammatory response syndrome, post-cardiac surgery, post-burns, post-myocardial infarction, vasculitis, glomerulonephritis, hepatitis, acalculous cholecystitis. Management is generally symptom-orientated; this includes cooling.

Adverse drug reaction

Numerous drugs induce an idiosyncratic pyrexia, including antibiotics, sedatives, paralysing agents, and amphetamines. The neuroleptic malignant syndrome (NMS) is a rare, life-threatening, idiosyncratic reaction to neuroleptics (e.g. haloperidol) and central dopamine blockers (e.g. metoclopramide). It is characterised by fever, muscular rigidity, altered mental status, and autonomic dysfunction. Usually, removal of the offending drug ± anti-pyretics are sufficient, but more aggressive measures may have to be taken, including active cooling. Dantrolene is not recommended.

Adverse reaction to blood transfusion

May be an immunological reaction to a cellular constituent or contamination with an organism, bacterial cell product, or other pyrogen.

Ambient heating

Excessive heating or prevention of heat loss may cause pyrexia. Consider strong sunlight, temperature settings on specialised beds, and heat-retaining clothing.

Miscellaneous

Other causes of pyrexia include neoplasm and cerebral insult.

Key paper
Circiumaru B, Baldock G, Cohen J. (1999) A prospective study of fever in the intensive care unit. *Intensive Care Med* **25**: 668–73.

Pyrexia—management

At present, the optimal temperature to target in disease states is not known, other than cerebral insults where normo- or (preferably) hypothermia offers neuroprotection by reducing cerebral metabolic rate. In other conditions, it seems reasonable to accept mild pyrexia provided this is tolerated by the patient.

Principles of management

1. Diagnose, then remove or treat the offending cause. For example, seek and treat infection, stop blood infusion, and send discontinued bag to laboratory for analysis, discontinue administration of any causative drug, use anti-inflammatory ± immunosuppressive agents for vasculitis.
2. Cooling aids symptomatic recovery, reduces metabolic rate, and lowers pressor requirements.
   - Increase evaporative losses, e.g. tepid sponging, wet sheets, ice packs in groin and axilla.
   - Increase convective losses, e.g. fanning to improve air circulation.
   - Cooled intravenous fluids.
   - Cooling blankets.
   - Antipyretics, e.g. paracetamol.
   - More aggressive cooling if temperature >41°C, e.g. irrigation of bladder/peritoneum with ice-cool fluids, ice-cool baths.
   - Aim to lower temperature <38.5°C, then reassess.
3. Paralysis and mechanical ventilation may be needed if the patient is shivering excessively.
4. Seek and treat concurrent rhabdomyolysis, DIC, seizures.

See also:
Therapeutic hypothermia, p100; Infection—treatment, p554 Sepsis and septic shock—treatment, p560; Pyrexia—causes, p602.

Hyperthermia

Hyperthermia is defined as a core temperature above 41°C.

Clinical features

- Delirium and seizures are associated with temperatures of 40–42°C.
- Coma is associated with temperatures >42°C.
- Tachycardia.
- Tachypnoea.
- Salt and water depletion.
- Rhabdomyolysis.
- Disseminated intravascular coagulation.
- Heart failure with ST depression and 'T' wave flattening.

Causes

- Hyperthermia may be an extreme form of pyrogen-induced fever associated with infection, inflammation, neoplasm, or CVA.
- Heat stroke is associated with severe exercise in high environmental temperatures and humidity. Excess clothing, hypovolaemia, or recent alcohol intake reduces the body's ability to dissipate heat production.
- Malignant hyperthermia is a drug-induced myopathy associated with a hereditary calcium transfer defect in patients receiving volatile anaesthetics, muscle relaxants, antidepressants, alcohol, or Ecstasy. Heat production is increased by muscle catabolism, spasm, and peripheral vasoconstriction.
- The neuroleptic malignant syndrome is a drug-induced hyperthermic syndrome usually secondary to phenothiazines or butyrophenones. It is associated with muscle rigidity, akinesia, impaired consciousness, and autonomic dysfunction, and continues for 1–2 weeks.

Management

1. Institute rapid cooling for patients with temperatures >41°C.
2. Supportive treatment includes fluid replacement and seizure control.
3. Remove clothing and nurse in a cool environment.
4. Surface cooling can be achieved with a fan, tepid sponging, wet sheets, ice packs in groin and axillae, or a cool bath.
5. Handling should be minimised and active cooling measures should be stopped when the core temperature is <39°C.
6. Consider internal cooling using cooled IV fluid, and bladder lavage or peritoneal lavage using cooled fluids.
7. Phenothiazines may be used to reduce temperature and prevent shivering (do not give in neuroleptic malignant syndrome).
8. Consider muscle relaxants if the patient is ventilated.
9. For malignant hyperthermia, stop any offending drug.
10. Monitor and treat hyperkalaemia.
11. Treat the neuroleptic malignant syndrome by stopping the offending drug ± dopamine agonists (e.g. L-dopa or bromocriptine). Dantrolene is no longer recommended as recovery is delayed and mortality may be increased.

See also:

Ventilatory support—indications, p44; Coagulation monitoring, p222; Basic resuscitation, p338; Heart failure—assessment, p392; Heart failure—management, p394; Coma, p438; Delirium, p442; Thyroid emergencies, p514; Amphetamines and ecstasy, p530; Pyrexia—causes, p602; Pyrexia—management, p604; Rhabdomyolysis, p612.

Electrocution

The effects of electrocution are due to the effects of the current and the conversion of electrical energy to heat energy on passage through the tissues. Important factors are:

- Energy delivered—heat = amperage^2 x resistance x time, i.e. the amperage is the most important determinant of heat production.
- Resistance to current flow—tissues are resistant to current flow in the following decreasing order: bone, fat, tendon, skin, muscle, blood vessels, nerves. A high skin resistance and short duration of contact concentrate the effects locally. However, skin contaminants, moisture, and burning reduce resistance.
- Type of current—alternating current is more dangerous than direct current. Tetanic muscle contractions may prevent the victim from releasing the current source whereas the single, strong muscle contraction with direct current often throws the victim clear. Alternating current is more likely to reach central tissues with consequent sustained apnoea and ventricular fibrillation (with as little as 50–100mA for 1–10ms).
- Current pathway—cardiorespiratory arrest is more likely the closer the contact is with the chest and heart.

Lightening strike differs from contact electrocution in that high intensity, ultra-short duration of current may produce cardiac arrest with little tissue destruction.

Clinical features

- Tachyarrhythmias—including ventricular tachycardia and fibrillation.
- Asystole—more likely with high current (>10A).
- Myocardial injury—heat injury, coronary artery spasm, arrhythmias, myocardial spasm.
- Respiratory arrest—tetanic contraction of the diaphragm, arrhythmias, cerebral medullary dysfunction.
- Trauma—tetanic muscle contraction, falling or being thrown clear.
- Burns—to skin and internal tissues.

Management

Most severe electrical injuries require urgent field treatment prior to hospital admission.

1. Ensure the source of the electrical injury is not a hazard to rescuers.
2. Manage cardiorespiratory arrest.
3. Prevent further injury, e.g. spinal protection, removal of smouldering clothes.

After hospital admission and restoration of the circulation, management is directed towards the complications.

1. Ventilatory support.
2. Management of hypovolaemia associated with burn injury. Fluid requirements are usually greater than for victims of thermal burns and require close monitoring.
3. Check cardiac enzymes for degree of myocardial injury. Treat heart failure and/or arrhythmias as indicated.
4. Management of rhabdomyolysis and covert compartment syndrome.
5. Surgical debridement of necrotic tissue and fixation of bony injury.

Near-drowning

Pathophysiology

Management

See also:
Endotracheal intubation, p42; Ventilatory support—indications, p44; Electrical cardioversion, p94; Cardiac function tests, p216; Basic resuscitation, p338; Cardiac arrest, p340; Tachyarrhythmias, p384; Burns—fluid management, p592; Burns—general management, p594; Rhabdomyolysis, p612.

Near-drowning

The major complications of near-drowning are lung injury, hypothermia, and effects of prolonged hypoxia. Although hypothermia bestows protective effects against organ damage, rewarming carries particular hazards.

Pathophysiology

Prolonged immersion usually results in inhalation of fluid. However 10–20% of patients develop intense laryngospasm leading to so-called 'dry drowning'. Traditionally, fresh water drowning was considered to lead to rapid absorption of water into the circulation with haemolysis, hypo-osmolality, and possible electrolyte disturbance whereas inhalation of hypertonic fluid from seawater drowning produced a marked flux of fluid into the alveoli. In practice, there seems to be little distinction between fresh and seawater as both cause loss of surfactant and severe inflammatory disruption of the alveolar-capillary membrane leading to an ARDS-type picture. Initially, haemodynamic instability is often minor. A similar picture often develops after 'dry drowning' and subsequent endotracheal intubation.

Acute hypothermia often accompanies near-drowning with loss of consciousness and haemodynamic alterations.

Management

1. Oxygen—give sufficient to increase SaO_2 >92%. Comatose patients should be intubated. Early CPAP or PEEP may be useful.
2. Bronchospasm is often present and may require nebulised β_2 agonists, and either nebulised or SC epinephrine.
3. Fluid replacement should be directed by appropriate monitoring. Inotrope therapy may be necessary if hypoperfusion persists after adequate fluid resuscitation. Intravascular fluid overload is uncommon and the role of early diuretic therapy with a view to lowering intracranial pressure is controversial. Haemolysis may occur and require blood transfusion.
4. Arrhythmias may arise from myocardial hypoxia, hypothermia, and electrolyte abnormalities, and should be treated conventionally.
5. Metabolic acidosis may be profound. However, bicarbonate therapy is rarely indicated as the acidosis usually corrects on restoration of adequate tissue perfusion.
6. Electrolyte abnormalities are usually minor and can be managed conventionally.
7. Rewarming follows conventional practice; cardiopulmonary bypass may be considered if core temperature is <30°C. Cardiopulmonary resuscitation, including cardiac massage, should be continued until normo-thermia is achieved.
8. Cerebral protection usually follows raised intracranial pressure protocols though, as mentioned above, the role of diuretic therapy and fluid restriction is controversial. Signs of brain damage such as seizures may become apparent and should be treated as they arise.
9. Antibiotic therapy (e.g. clindamycin or cefuroxime plus metronidazole) should be given if strong evidence of aspiration exists. Otherwise, take specimens and treat as indicated.
10. Decompress the stomach using a nasogastric tube to lessen any risk of aspiration. Enteral feeding can be initiated afterwards.

See also:

Endotracheal intubation, p42; Ventilatory support—indications, p44; Positive end expiratory pressure (1), p66; Positive end expiratory pressure (2), p68; Continuous positive airway pressure, p70; Bronchodilators, p254; Antiarrhythmics, p272; Basic resuscitation, p338; Cardiac arrest, p340; Hypothermia, p600.

Rhabdomyolysis

Breakdown of striated muscle that may result in compartment syndrome, acute renal failure, and electrolyte abnormalities (hyperkalaemia, hypocalcaemia, hyperphosphataemia).

Causes
- Trauma, especially crush injury.
- Prolonged immobilisation, e.g. after fall, drug overdose.
- Drugs, e.g. opiates, cocaine, Ecstasy.
- Hyperpyrexia.
- Vascular occlusion (including lengthy vascular surgery).
- Infection.
- Burns/electrocution.
- Severe hypophosphataemia.
- Congenital myopathy (rare).

Diagnosis
- Suggested by disproportionately high serum creatinine compared to urea (usual ratio is approximately 10μmol:1mmol).
- Raised creatine kinase (usually >2000IU/L).
- Myoglobinuria produces a positive urine dipstick to blood. Urine is usually red or black, but may be clear despite significant rhabdomyolysis.

General management
- Admit for careful monitoring and adequate fluid resuscitation.
- Do not treat hypocalcaemia unless the patient is symptomatic; calcium may form crystals with the high circulating phosphate.
- Hyperkalaemia may be resistant to medical management and require urgent haemodialysis or haemodiafiltration.

Compartment syndrome
- Suspect if limb is tender or extremely painful and peripheries are cool. Loss of peripheral pulses and tense muscles are late signs.
- Manometry in muscle compartments reveal pressures >20–25mmHg.
- Arm, legs, and buttock compartments may be affected.
- Management involves either prophylactic fasciotomies if at high risk or close monitoring (including regular manometry) with decompression if pressures exceed 20–25mmHg.
- Fasciotomies may result in major blood loss.

Renal failure
- Renal failure is thought to be produced by a combination of free radical injury, hypovolaemia, hypotension, and possibly, myoglobin blocking the renal tubules.
- Renal failure may be prevented by prompt rehydration and urinary alkalinisation with 1.26% sodium bicarbonate solution for 3–5 days. The urinary pH should be ≥6 and blood pH <7.5. Urinary alkalinisation increases urinary excretion of myoglobin.
- Potassium, sodium, calcium, and magnesium levels should be monitored regularly and managed as appropriate.
- If renal failure is established, dialysis, or filtration techniques will be required, usually for a period of 6–8 weeks.

Key paper

Better OS, Stein JH. (1990) Early management of shock and prophylaxis of acute renal failure in traumatic rhabdomyolysis. *N Engl J Med* **322**: 825–9.

See also:

Raised intra-abdominal pressure

Intra-abdominal pressure is normally <6mmHg at rest. A healthy individual may increase intra-abdominal pressure to 25mmgHg with defaecation, 45mmHg with vomiting, and 60mmHg with coughing.

A sustained increase in intra-abdominal pressure >15mmHg affects organs both within and outside the abdomen. The effects of raised intra-abdominal pressure are known as the abdominal compartment syndrome. Left untreated, a raised intra-abdominal pressure is associated with high mortality.

Transmission of pressure to the pleural space reduces lung compliance, altering the ventilation/perfusion ratio with resulting hypoxaemia and hypercapnia. Higher inspiratory pressures are required during mechanical ventilation. The resulting increase in both abdominal and intrathoracic pressures reduces venous return, leading to a fall in cardiac output and rise in intracranial pressure.

Despite the reduction in venous return, raised intra-abdominal pressure will increase measured CVP. As a result of reduced cardiac output and venous congestion reducing capillary blood flow, perfusion of the intra-abdominal organs is reduced. Oliguria and renal failure, splanchnic hypoperfusion, and decreased liver metabolism may result.

Causes
- Bowel or abdominal wall oedema, e.g. large volume resuscitation.
- Intestinal obstruction.
- Intra- and retroperitoneal haemorrhage, e.g. ruptured aneurysm.
- Morbid obesity.
- Ascites.
- Peritoneal dialysis.

Measuring intra-abdominal pressure
The classical technique is to measure pressure in the relaxed bladder via a Foley catheter. With the patient supine, the catheter tubing is clamped distal to the sampling bung. A pressure manometer is connected to a three-way tap and needle which is inserted into the sampling bung. The bladder should be partially filled via the three-way tap with 50mL 0.9% saline. The transducer should then be zeroed at the level of the symphysis pubis. The bladder pressure measurement is assumed to be equivalent to intra-abdominal pressure. Manometers for measuring the bladder pressure are now available commercially.

Management
- Removal of cause if possible.
- Restoration of cardiac output with fluid resuscitation.
- Consider surgical decompression (laparostomy) or tube decompression for pseudo-obstruction if intra-abdominal pressure >25mmHg.

See also:
IPPV—failure to deliver ventilation, p54; Respiratory failure, p350; Oliguria, p398; Acute renal failure—diagnosis, p400; Intra-abdominal bowel perforation and obstruction, p418; Abdominal sepsis, p422; Pancreatitis, p424; Rhabdomyolysis, p612.

See also:

Pain and post-operative critical care

Pain

Pain results from many insults, e.g. trauma, invasive procedures, specific organ disease, and inflammatory processes. Pain relief is necessary for physiological and psychological reasons:

- Anxiety and lack of sleep.
- Increased sympathetic activity contributing to an increased metabolic demand and adrenergic stress.
- The capacity of the circulation and respiratory system to meet this increase in metabolic demand may not be adequate.
- Myocardial ischaemia is a significant risk.
- The endocrine response to injury is exaggerated with consequent salt and water retention.
- Physiological attempts to limit pain may include immobility and muscle splinting, and consequent reductions in ventilatory function and cough.

Pain perception

The degree of tissue damage is related to the magnitude of the pain stimulus. The site of injury is also important; thoracic and upper abdominal injury is more painful than injury elsewhere. However, the perception of pain is dependent on other factors, e.g. simultaneous sensory input, personality, cultural background, and previous experiences of pain.

Management of pain

Systemic analgesia

- Opioid analgesics form the mainstay of analgesic drug treatment.
- Small, frequent IV doses, or a continuous infusion provide the most stable blood levels. Since the degree of analgesia is dependent on blood levels, it is important that they are maintained.
- Higher doses are required to treat rather than prevent pain.
- The dose of drug required for a particular individual depends on their perception of pain and whether tolerance has built up to previous analgesic use.
- The use of non-opioid drugs may avoid the need for or reduce the dose required of opioid drugs. This includes paracetamol and non-steroidals, ketamine, and α_2-agonists such as clonidine.

Regional analgesia

- Regional techniques reduce respiratory depression, but require experience to ensure procedures are performed safely.
- Epidural analgesia may be with local anaesthetic agents or opioids.
- Opioids avoid the vasodilatation and hypotension associated with local anaesthetic agents, but do not produce as profound analgesia.
- The combination of opioid and local anaesthetic is synergistic.
- Intravenous opioids should be avoided or close monitoring should continue for 24h after cessation of epidural opioids due to the potential for late respiratory failure. Sample regimens are shown opposite.
- Local anaesthetic agents may be used to block superficial nerves, e.g. intercostal nerve block with 3–5mL 0.5% bupivacaine plus adrenaline.

Non-pharmacological techniques

Adequate explanation, positioning and physical techniques may all reduce drug requirements.

Regimens for epidural analgesia

Lumbar	10–15mL 0.5% bupivacaine, followed by an infusion of 5–20mL/h 0.125% bupivacaine
Thoracic	4–6mL 0.5% bupivacaine followed by an infusion of 6–10mL/h 0.125% bupivacaine
Opioid	5mg morphine gives up to 12h analgesia.
Combined	An infusion of 3–4mL/h 0.125% bupivacaine with 0.3–0.4mg/h morphine or 25–50mcg/h fentanyl

See also:

Non-opioid analgesics, p302; Opioid analgesics, p304; Epidural analgesia, p306; Multiple trauma (2), p584; Blast injury, p596; Post-operative critical care, p620; Pain and comfort, p624.

Post-operative critical care

Patients may be admitted to critical care after surgery, either electively (see table opposite) or after unexpected peri-operative complications.

General care

- Ensure surgical and anaesthetic plan has been agreed, e.g. overnight ventilation, special precautions (e.g. wire cutters if mandible wired), movement restriction, haemodynamic targets, etc.
- Provide adequate analgesia.
- Ensure adequate rewarming.
- Maintain euglycaemia.
- Provide appropriate thrombosis prophylaxis.
- Blood gas, electrolyte, and haemoglobin monitoring.

Post-operative respiratory problems

Common in those with pre-existing respiratory disease, especially with a reduced vital capacity or peak flow rate. Problems include:
- Exacerbation of chronic chest disease.
- Retained secretions.
- Basal atelectasis.
- Pneumonia.
- Upper airway problems, e.g. laryngeal oedema.

Anaesthesia and surgery (especially upper abdominal surgery) reduce functional residual capacity, thoracic compliance, and cough. There is reduced macrophage function and systemic inflammatory activation with infection and acute lung injury as possible consequences.

Therapeutic aims

Preoperative preparation may help avoid some of the problems:
- Cessation of smoking for >1 week.
- Bronchodilatation.
- Respiratory muscle training.
- Chest physiotherapy.
- Avoidance of hypovolaemia in the nil-by-mouth period.

Post-operative clearance of secretions and maintenance of basal lung expansion are very important. These require effective analgesia and chest physiotherapy. Mechanical ventilation assists basal expansion and secretion clearance where anaesthetic recovery is expected to be prolonged or surgery ± pre-existing disease increases the risk of secretion retention and atelectasis. Ensure a patent airway prior to extubation.

Post-operative circulatory problems

- Prevention of hypovolaemia is crucial in avoiding inflammatory activation and, therefore, many post-operative complications.
- Haemorrhage is usually obvious and managed by resuscitation, correction of coagulation disturbance, and surgery.
- Sub-clinical hypovolaemia is common. Hypothermia and high catecholamine levels help to maintain CVP and BP despite continuing hypovolaemia. Avoiding a reduced stroke volume, metabolic acidosis, and a low $ScvO_2$ are the best indicators of adequate resuscitation.
- Fluid challenges with colloid should be used to confirm and treat hypovolaemia where there is any circulatory disturbance, metabolic acidosis, or oliguria.

Reasons for elective critical care admission

- Airway monitoring, e.g. major oral, head, and neck surgery.
- Respiratory monitoring, e.g. cardiothoracic surgery, upper abdominal surgery, prolonged anaesthesia, previous respiratory disease.
- Cardiovascular monitoring, e.g. cardiac surgery, vascular surgery, major abdominal surgery, prolonged anaesthesia, previous cardiovascular disease.
- Neurological monitoring, e.g. neurosurgery, cardiac surgery with circulatory arrest, spinal surgery.
- Flap monitoring, e.g. major plastic, and head and neck surgical procedures.
- Elective ventilation, e.g. cardiac surgery, major abdominal surgery, prolonged anaesthesia, previous respiratory disease.

See also:

Critical Care Unit admission criteria, p10; Oxygen therapy, p38; Airway maintenance, p40; Ventilatory support—indications, p44; Continuous positive airway pressure, p70; Non-invasive respiratory support, p76; Chest physiotherapy, p90; Blood transfusion, p248; Fluid challenge, p342; Airway obstruction, p348; Respiratory failure, p350; Atelectasis and pulmonary collapse, p352; Hypotension, p380; Oliguria, p398; Vomiting/gastric stasis, p406; Abdominal sepsis, p422; Bleeding disorders, p468; Electrolyte management, p482; Infection control—general principles, p544; Pyrexia—causes, p602; Pain, p618.

Oncological critical care

Pain and comfort

Patients with oncological disease may complain of pain or discomfort related to the neoplasm itself or as a consequence or complication of the treatment. Approximately 90% of patients with advanced cancer experience severe pain that is often under-treated. Pain management may be further complicated by a chronic dependency on analgesia, necessitating high doses for managing acutely painful episodes.

Patients may complain of persistent or continuous pain and/or breakthrough pain (brief, rapid-onset flare-ups of severe pain that can occur despite regular pain medication). A personalised approach is essential as effective strategies will vary between patients and some will be more affected by side effects, e.g. excessive drowsiness from opiates. Advice should be sought from palliative care or pain teams who are highly experienced in dealing with all aspects of cancer pain.

Cancer pain/discomfort may arise from:
- Post-operative pain.
- Organomegaly with stretching of the capsule and pressure discomfort (e.g. splenomegaly).
- Occluded blood vessels causing distal tissue ischaemia.
- Bone fracture(s) from metastases.
- Infection.
- Inflammation (e.g. pleurisy, peritonitis).
- Side effects from cancer therapy (e.g. chemo- or radiotherapy).
- Neuropathy (compression, infiltration, chemotherapy-related).
- Psychological or emotional problems.

Analgesia

Post-operative pain should be managed in standard fashion, i.e. oral analgesics ± dermal patches graduating to IV infusions/boluses of opiates and/or NSAIDS, epidurals, and patient-controlled analgesia.

In addition to opiate and non-opiate treatment, specific conditions may warrant directed adjunctive therapy. For example, neuropathic pain may respond to antidepressants, anticonvulsants, oral or cutaneous lidocaine, and/or corticosteroids. Local or regional nerve blocks may be useful for somatic or visceral pain. Transcutaneous electric nerve stimulation (TENS) may block pain transmission by low-level stimulation of nerve endings.

Alternative medicine therapies (e.g. acupuncture, therapeutic massage, homeopathy) may also prove effective in some patients.

Psychological support

Many psychological and emotional factors can contribute to suffering. These vary between individuals, and reflect underlying personality and degree of family support. Many patients manifest signs of clinical depression, especially those at advanced stages of the disease. Admission to critical care may be very frightening for mentally competent patients. Psychotherapy is an important part of cancer pain management. Provision of emotional support and stability can help patients to cope. Assistance can be sought from oncology and palliative care teams. Treatments such as hypnosis and relaxation techniques may prove useful. Adequate provision of information regarding critical care management and prognosis is an important means of allaying anxiety for both patient and family. Care must be taken not to distress the patient further.

See also:

Communication, p18; Non-opioid analgesics, p302; Opioid analgesics, p304; Epidural analgesia, p306; Anticonvulsants, p312; Corticosteroids, p328.

Effects of chemo- and radiotherapy

Bone marrow suppression

Neutropaenia, thrombocytopaenia, and anaemia can be expected with most therapeutic regimens. The patient is at increased risk of infection from bacterial, fungal, viral, and atypical infections, and from bleeding that may be relatively minor (e.g. petechiae, cannula sites) or catastrophic (e.g. cerebral haemorrhage).

Low platelet counts are generally well tolerated; transfusions are given to keep counts >10 x 10^9/L though higher levels will be targeted for active bleeding, for elective procedures, and in the presence of sepsis. Frequent platelet transfusions greatly increase the risk of antiplatelet antibody formation with consequent risk of adverse reactions and a failure to increment the platelet count adequately. Excess transfusion should thus be avoided, if possible. Single donor pools may also be used to increase the increment.

Anaemia is generally managed by red cell transfusion. In general, haemoglobin levels ≥7g/dL are acceptable though higher levels may be needed for active bleeding or cardiorespiratory impairment. Supplementation of haematinics such as folate and B12 should not be overlooked.

Impaired gas exchange

The lung is often compromised by infection (pneumonia, pneumonitis), non-infective pneumonitis, pleural effusion, high or low pressure pulmonary oedema (i.e. ARDS or left heart failure), haemorrhage, bronchiolitis obliterans with organising pneumonia (BOOP), or fibrosis (especially after busulphan or radiotherapy). Fluid overload is common following renal dysfunction and/or large fluid volumes used for chemotherapy and multiple antibiotics.

- Treat the underlying cause, e.g antibiotics for infection, steroids for pneumonitis, and BOOP.
- High FIO$_2$ should be avoided with suspected 'busulfan lung'. Aim for PaO$_2$ 90–92%.
- Avoid fluid overload as excess capillary leak will worsen gas exchange.
- Mortality is high (>60%) if mechanical ventilation is necessary. CPAP and BiPAP can prove highly effective in avoiding the need for intubation, especially if used early to avoid fatiguing the patient.

Cardiomyopathy

Certain chemotherapeutic agents (e.g. doxorubicin, mitoxantrone) can cause cardiomyopathy. Secondary sepsis can also cause myocardial depression. This may be dose-related or idiosyncratic. Treatment is based on standard heart failure regimens. Fluid overload should be avoided. Heart failure should be considered if such patients fail to wean.

Renal dysfunction

Tumour lysis syndrome (hyperkalaemia, hyperuricaemia, and acute renal failure) may follow rapid destruction of a large white cell mass. Prevent with good hydration, a maintained diuresis, and rasburicase (recombinant urate oxidase) or allopurinol. Once established, haemo(dia)filtration and other measures to lower serum potassium levels may be necessary.

See also:

Continuous positive airway pressure, p70; Non-invasive respiratory support, p76; Dyspnoea, p346; Respiratory failure, p350; Acute chest infection (1), p356; Acute chest infection (2), p358; Acute respiratory distress syndrome (1), p360; Acute respiratory distress syndrome (2), p362; Heart failure—assessment, p392; Heart failure—management, p394; Bleeding disorders, p468; Anaemia, p472; Platelet disorders, p478; Infection—diagnosis, p552; Neutropaenia, p628.

Neutropaenia and infection

Though defined as a neutrophil count <2 x 10^9/L, neutropaenic patients are not generally placed in protective isolation until counts fall <0.5–1 x 10^9/L. Adequate functionality is not guaranteed even despite restoration of a 'normal' count. Many studies show equivalent outcomes between neutropaenic and non-neutropaenic haematological oncology patients admitted to critical care. The patient is usually asymptomatic until infection supervenes, but they may deteriorate very rapidly.

Causes in the oncology patient
- The neoplasm itself (e.g. leukaemia, myeloma) or as a consequence of chemotherapy or radiation causing marrow suppression.
- Systemic inflammation, infection, and sepsis.
- Nutritional deficiencies, e.g. folate, vitamin B_{12}, malnutrition.
- Adverse drug reaction, e.g. sulphonamides.
- Part of an aplastic anaemia, e.g. idiopathic, drugs, infection.
- Hypersplenism.

Infections
- Initial infections are with common bacterial organisms such as pneumococci, staphylococci, and coliforms.
- With recurrent infections or after repeated courses of antibiotics, more unusual and/or multi-resistant organisms may be responsible, e.g. fungi (NB. *Candida* spp.), *Pneumocystis jiroveci*, CMV, TB.

Management
1. In the absence of chemotherapy, any implicated drug should be discontinued.
2. If the neutrophil count is low, consider protective isolation, ideally in a cubicle equipped with laminar flow air conditioning.
3. Adopt strict infection control procedures.
4. Minimise invasive procedures and avoid PR examination.
5. Maintain good oral hygiene. Apply topical treatment as necessary, e.g. nystatin mouthwashes for oral fungal infection.
6. Clotrimazole cream for fungal skin infection.
7. For suspected sepsis, start parenteral antibiotics within 2h of fever ≥38°C (broad-spectrum if no organism has been isolated). Seek cause, including CT scan and bronchoalveolar lavage, as indicated. Haematology units have their own regimens, frequently escalating antibacterial cover with antifungals ± antivirals ± treatment of atypicals (e.g. *Pneumocystis jiroveci*). A balance must be reached between adequate treatment of infection versus problems related to resistance, bacterial overgrowth (e.g. *C. difficile*), liver, renal and gut toxicity, and fluid overload. The pyrexia may be due to the antibiotic treatment itself.
8. Remove vascular catheters, if possibly implicated, including Hickman-type catheters.
9. Avoid uncooked foods (*Pseudomonas* risk) and bottled pepper (*Aspergillus*).
10. Granulocyte-colony stimulating factor (G-CSF) is frequently given to stimulate a bone marrow response.
11. Neutrophil infusions are short-lived, expensive, and often induce a pyrexial response. Their role remains controversial.

See also:
Full blood count, p220; Bacteriology, p224; Virology, serology, and assays, p226; Antimicrobials, p326; Infection control—general principles, p544; Infection—diagnosis, p552; Infection—treatment, p554; Pyrexia—causes, p602; Effects of chemo- and radiotherapy, p626.

Leukaemia/lymphoma

Such patients may present acutely to critical care with complications arising from either the disease or the therapy.

Complications arising from the disease

- Decreased resistance to infection.
- Hyperviscosity syndrome—drowsiness, coma, focal neurological defects.
- Anaemia, thrombocytopaenia, bleeding tendency, DIC.
- Weight loss, lethargy, fever, night sweats.
- Central nervous system involvement.

Management

1. The raised white cell mass may be reduced rapidly by leucophoresis if a hyperviscosity syndrome is present.
2. Frequent blood transfusions to maintain Hb levels >7g/dL.
3. Platelet transfusions if counts remain <10 x 10^9/L, or if <50 x 10^9/L and remaining symptomatic, or undergoing an invasive procedure.
4. Fresh frozen plasma and other blood products as needed.
5. Neutropaenia management, including protective isolation, appropriate antibiotic therapy ± granulocyte-colony stimulating factor.
6. Psychological support for both patient and family is vital.

Graft versus host disease (GVHD)

An immune response following allogenic stem cell transplantation. Features include mucositis, pneumonitis, hepatitis, jaundice, diarrhoea, abdominal pain, rash, and blistering.

Treatment includes steroids ± ciclosporin, tacrolimus, alemtuzumab, infliximab, rituximab, anti-lymphocytic, or anti-thymocytic globulin and symptomatic relief. Parenteral nutrition may be needed if diarrhoea is severe.

Grades of GVHD

Grade	Skin	Liver	Gut
1	Rash <25% body	Bilirubin 35–50µmol/L	Diarrhoea <1L/d
2	Rash 25–50% body	Bilirubin 51–100µmol/L	Diarrhoea 1–1.5L/d
3	Rash >50% body	Bilirubin 101–250µmol/L	Diarrhoea >1.5L/d
4	Desquamation or bullae	Bilirubin >250µmol/L	Pain or ileus

Obstetric emergencies

Pre-eclampsia and eclampsia

The hallmark of pre-eclampsia is hypertension with proteinuria. It is considered mild if proteinuria is 0.25–2g/L and severe if >2g/L. Eclampsia is the same condition associated with seizures, but this only affects 1 in 100 pre-eclamptics. Both are associated with cerebral oedema and, in some cases, haemorrhage. A reduced plasma volume, raised peripheral resistance, and disseminated intravascular coagulation all impair tissue perfusion, with possible renal and hepatic failure. Pulmonary oedema may occur secondary to increased peripheral resistance and low colloid osmotic pressure. Pre-eclampsia and eclampsia are responsible for a fifth of deaths in pregnant women.

Management

Hypertensive crises and convulsions may continue for 48h post-partum, during which time close monitoring in a high dependency or intensive care area is essential.

Circulatory management

- High blood pressure in (pre-)eclampsia is due to arteriolar vasospasm and reduced plasma volume so controlled plasma volume expansion is essential as the first-line treatment.
- A standard fluid challenge regimen carries little risk of fluid overload.
- Oliguria often coexists with reduced plasma volume; controlled volume expansion is usually more appropriate than diuretic therapy.
- If plasma volume expansion fails to control hypertension, anti-hypertensives such as labetalol, nifedipine, or hydralazine may be used.

Seizures

- Seizures are best avoided by good blood pressure control.
- Initial seizure control may be achieved with small doses of benzodiazepines.
- Magnesium sulphate is the treatment of choice for eclamptic seizures. Magnesium levels should be monitored and kept between 2.5–3.75mmol/L. Above 3.75mmol/L, toxicity with possible cardiorespiratory arrest may be seen.
- Prophylactic anticonvulsant therapy with magnesium is often given in severe pre-eclampsia, and may be considerd in mild to moderate cases.
- Excess sedation should be avoided due to the risk of aspiration although continued seizures may require elective intubation, mechanical hyperventilation, and further anticonvulsant therapy.

Early fetal delivery

The definitive treatment for (pre-)eclampsia is fetal delivery, but the needs of the fetus must be balanced against those of the mother. The mother's life takes priority. If fetal maturity has been reached, immediate delivery after control of seizures and hypertension is necessary.

Drug dosages

Labetalol	Start at 2mg/min IV or quicker if a rapid response is required. Labetalol is usually effective once 200mg has been given after which a maintenance infusion of 5–50mg/h may be continued.
Nifedipine	10mg SL is an often effective alternative, given every 20min if necessary.
Hydralazine	5–10mg by slow IV bolus, repeat after 20–30min. Alternatively, by infusion starting at 200–300mcg/min and reducing to 50–150mcg/min.
Magnesium	4g over 20 min, followed by 1–1.5g/h by intravenous infusion until seizures have stopped for 24h.

Key papers

Magpie Trial Collaboration Group. Do women with pre-eclampsia, and their babies, benefit from magnesium sulphate? (2002) The Magpie Trial: a randomised placebo-controlled trial. *Lancet* **359**: 1877–90.

Which anticonvulsant for women with eclampsia? (1995) Evidence from the Collaborative Eclampsia Trial. *Lancet* **345**: 1455–63.

See also:

Blood pressure monitoring, p164; Hypotensive agents, p270; Hypertension, p382; Generalised seizures, p444; Raised intracranial pressure, p454.

HELLP syndrome

HELLP syndrome is a pregnancy-related disorder associated with haemolysis, elevated liver function tests, and low platelets.

- Microangiopathic haemolysis results from destruction of red cells as they pass through damaged small vessels.
- Hepatic dysfunction is characterised by periportal necrosis and hyaline deposits in the sinusoids. In some cases, hepatic necrosis may proceed to hepatic haemorrhage or rupture.
- Thrombocytopaenia results from increased platelet consumption, although prothrombin time and activated partial thromboplastin time are normal, unlike DIC. It rarely falls below 20×10^9/L.

Nearly 10% of women with severe pre-eclampsia and 30–50% of eclamptics are affected though the exact relationship is unknown. Approximately half have complete HELLP (all components present) while half have incomplete HELLP (1–2 components present). The maternal mortality is 1%, resulting from ruptured subcapsular liver haematoma, haemorrhage, and stroke. Major haemorrhage is uncommon, but wound site oozing or subcutaneous haematoma may occur.

Clinical features

- Epigastric or right upper quadrant pain with malaise.
- Nausea and vomiting, headache.
- Generalised oedema is usual though 15% have diastolic BP <90 mmHg.
- Presentation may not occur until post-partum. The lowest platelet count usually occurs at 24–48h post-partum.

Criteria for diagnosis of HELLP syndrome

Haemolysis	Abnormal blood film
	Hyperbilirubinaemia
	LDH >600U/L
Elevated liver enzymes	AST >70U/L
Thrombocytopaenia	Platelets <100 × 10^9/L

Management

- Priorities for management include basic resuscitation and exclusion of hepatic haemorrhage or ruptured liver. In the latter case, an early Caesarean section and definitive urgent surgical repair are required.
- Magnesium prophylaxis is given to prevent seizures.
- Microangiopathic haemolysis and thrombocytopaenia may respond to plasma exchange and fresh frozen plasma infusion.
- Platelet transfusions should be avoided unless there is active bleeding.
- Corticosteroids increase platelet count but do not affect outcomes.

Key paper

Fonseca JE, Mendez F, Catano C, Arias F. (2005) Dexamethasone treatment does not improve the outcome of women with HELLP syndrome: a double-blind, placebo-controlled, randomised clinical trial. *Am J Obstet Gynecol* **193**: 1591–8.

See also:

Liver function tests, p218; Full blood count, p220; Jaundice, p428; Haemolysis, p476; Platelet disorders, p478.

Post-partum haemorrhage

Usually due to incomplete uterine contraction after delivery, but may be due to retained products. The magnitude of haemorrhage may be severe and life-threatening. It is the leading cause of maternal mortality.

Resuscitation

The principles of resuscitation are the same of those applying to any haemorrhagic condition. Blood transfusion requirements may be massive and therefore, there may be a need to replace coagulation factors. There may be significant retroplacental bleeding which may lead to underestimation of blood volume loss. Large bore intravenous access must be established. It is safer to manage major fluid and blood replacement with haemodynamic monitoring.

Stimulated uterine contraction

Begin fundal massage and administer uterotonic drugs such as oxytocin (5U IV bolus or 10–20U in 1L of normal saline infused quickly). Prostaglandin F2α, injected locally into the uterus or IM, is an effective method of stimulating uterine contraction and may avoid the need for surgery.

Aortic compression

Temporary reduction of haemorrhage may be achieved by compressing the aorta with a fist pushed firmly above the umbilicus, using the pressure between the fist and vertebral column to achieve compression. This manoeuvre may buy time while definitive surgical repair is organised.

Arterial occlusion

Angiographic embolisation or internal iliac artery ligation may avoid the need for hysterectomy in some cases. The disadvantages of these procedures include a significant delay in organisation and, in the latter case, a high failure rate.

See also:
Full blood count, p220; Blood transfusion, p248; Blood products, p250; Basic resuscitation, p338.

Amniotic fluid embolus

- An uncommon, but dangerous, complication of childbirth that presents with a precipitous onset of hypoxaemic respiratory failure, disseminated intravascular coagulation, and shock, or even cardiac arrest. Tonic clonic seizures are seen in 50% of cases.
- High early mortality is associated with acute pulmonary hypertension.
- The initial response of the pulmonary vasculature to the presence of amniotic fluid is intense vasospasm, resulting in severe pulmonary hypertension and hypoxaemia.
- Right heart function is initially compromised severely, but returns to normal with a secondary phase during which there is severe left heart failure and pulmonary oedema.
- Amniotic fluid contains lipid-rich particulate material which stimulates a systemic inflammatory reaction. In this respect, the progress of the condition is similar to other causes of multiple organ failure with associated capillary leak and disseminated intravascular coagulation.
- Diagnosis is usually based on clinical features alone. It may be supported by amniotic fluid and fetal cells in pulmonary artery blood and urine, though this finding is not specific for embolus.

Management

Management is entirely supportive. If amniotic fluid embolism occurs prior to delivery, perform urgent Caesarean section to prevent further embolisation.

Respiratory support

Provide oxygen to maintain SaO_2 of 92–98%. CPAP or mechanical ventilation may be required.

Cardiovascular support

Standard resuscitation principles apply with controlled fluid loading and inotropic support being started as required.

Haematological management

Management of the coagulopathy requires blood product therapy guided by laboratory assessment of coagulation times. In addition, some cases improve after treatment with cryoprecipitate, possibly due to the effects of fibronectin replacement.

See also:
Ventilatory support—indications, p44; Continuous positive airway pressure, p70; Coagulation monitoring, p222; Blood products, p250; Basic resuscitation, p338; Fluid challenge, p342; Systemic inflammation/multi-organ failure—causes, p556; Systemic inflammation/multi-organ failure—management, p558.

Transport of the critically ill

Intra-hospital transport

Critically ill patients frequently have to be moved out of the Critical Care Unit for investigation or operative procedures. Although much of the equipment used in the Critical Care Unit has battery back-up power supply, many items are too large to consider moving safely with the patient. Therefore, transport within hospital requires provision of suitably portable equipment. A hospital critical care trolley should be of fixed height with an equipment shelf and other fixed anchorage points below the level of the patient to enable such equipment to be clamped for safe transportation.

Specification of transport equipment

The critical care transport trolley must accommodate:
- Portable ventilator.
- Oxygen cylinder.
- Monitor including ECG, NIBP, facility for direct BP, SpO_2, $ETCO_2$, temperature, FIO_2.
- Syringe drivers.
- Volumetric pumps.
- Suction.
- Back-up batteries.
- Anchorage for a 5-point patient harness.

Patient preparation for intra-hospital transport

In addition to the usual requirements for provision of bedside critical care medicine, the following are required:
- Assessment of the risk:benefit ratio for the move.
- Assessment of degree of stabilisation required before movement.
- Assessment of security equipment and tubes.
- Safe storage and stowage of equipment on the transport trolley.
- Transfer is associated with an increased likelihood of arrhythmias so PaO_2 should ideally be normalised.

Required competencies of accompanying staff

Accompanying staff must be competent in the following:
- Airway device insertion and management.
- Chest drain insertion and management.
- Cardiovascular monitoring.
- Sedation/paralysis.
- Mechanical ventilation with transport ventilators.
- Lifting and handling.
- Managing access in confined spaces.
- Management during imaging, e.g. special issues relating to ventilation during MRI.

See also:
Endotracheal intubation, p42; Pulse oximetry, p144; CO_2 monitoring, p146; ECG monitoring, p162; Blood pressure monitoring, p164; Inter-hospital transport—road, p646; Inter-hospital transport—air, p648.

Inter-hospital transport—road

Many critically ill patients are transported between hospitals on a daily basis, mainly by ambulance. Staff may be unfamiliar with the ambulance environment and may suffer from motion sickness. There should be at least two attendants, one of whom should be a critical care medical practitioner, ideally with previous experience of transport in a supernumerary capacity. They must be familiar with the transport equipment and communication systems. Transport services should be organised and co-ordinated to deliver safe, efficient, and timely inter-hospital transfer.

Patient preparation

The steps in preparation for transport are Assessment, Control, Communication, Evaluation, Preparation and Packaging, and Transportation (ACCEPT).

The decision to move a patient between hospitals must be taken jointly by the most senior clinicians available at the referring and receiving hospitals. Evaluate the risk:benefit ratio of transport, staffing, and equipment needs based on the nature of the illness, urgency, vehicle availability, geographical factors, traffic and weather conditions. Patients should be properly resuscitated and stabilised prior to transport. Hypovolaemia is poorly tolerated. Intubate if GCS ≤8. Intubated patients should normally be paralysed and sedated. Chest drains can be placed on Heimlich-type valves. Patients should be covered in an insulating blanket.

Required staff competencies for road transport

In addition to the competencies required for intra-hospital transport:
- Ability to assess patients remotely.
- Understanding the limitations of resource and power in an ambulance.
- Understanding physiological effects of acceleration and deceleration.
- Familiarity with chains of communication and command.
- Use of diverse modes of communication and associated protocols.
- Handling emergencies on the road; when to stop and when to divert.
- Understanding ambulance emergency drills.
- Understanding the law relating to blue light use etc.

Vehicle design

Guidance covering design, specification, and equipment requirements for road ambulances are contained within European Committee for Standardisation CEN 1789. A type C ambulance is a mobile ICU designed and equipped for transport, advanced treatment, and monitoring of patients. To ensure that critical care can be continued throughout the journey, these vehicles need to have a 240V AC generator capable of providing 2.2kVA, with a back-up inverter fitted. There should be six 240V outlets, positioned to allow equipment in use to be safely connected without creating trip hazards. The vehicles should also have three 12V jack sockets, a pair of 12V switched screw terminals, and one 12V cigar-lighter size socket. The vehicle should provide secure, CEN-compliant anchorage fixings for essential equipment, e.g. a portable ventilator, up to 6 syringe drivers, volumetric pumps, gas cylinders etc. There must be CEN compliant provision for the fixing of critical care trolleys of different design. The vehicles must carry a minimum of two HX oxygen cylinders and have storage for D size spares for the stretcher trolley.

Transport preparation (ACCEPT)

Assessment	Be aware of the full patient history and current problems.
Control	Identify the leader and allocate tasks.
Communication	Make sure all communication is clear, source identified, and involves all staff involved with patient dispatch and receipt.
Evaluation	Assess risks and benefits of transport, equipment needed, and urgency.
Preparation and packaging	Prepare patient, equipment, and staff.
Transportation	Having identified the mode of transport and completed the preparation, transport the patient.

See also:

Endotracheal intubation, p42; Pulse oximetry, p144; CO_2 monitoring, p146; ECG monitoring, p162; Blood pressure monitoring, p164; Sedatives and tranquilisers, p308; Muscle relaxants, p310; Intra-hospital transport, p644; Inter-hospital transport—air, p648.

Inter-hospital transport—air

Aircraft are preferred for longer distance transfers with fixed wing aircraft preferred for distances >150 miles. Time to organise air transport should be taken into account when judging any advantage of speed over longer distances. Helicopters are generally less comfortable, and provide a more cramped environment than either ambulance or fixed wing aircraft.

Particular problems of air transport

A lower barometric pressure reduces alveolar partial pressure of oxygen (leading to hypoxaemia) and increases the volume of gas filled cavities. Noise and vibration may increase pain and discomfort or contribute to nausea.

Patient preparation

Patient assessment to calculate risk:benefit ratio of air transport and staffing and equipment needs based on the nature of the illness, urgency of transfer, availability of transport, mobilisation times, geographical factors, traffic and weather conditions.

An increased FIO_2 is mandatory for all aeromedical transfers where the cabin is not pressurised to sea level barometric pressure. Pneumothoraces must be drained. Nasogastric tubes should be inserted and placed on free drainage. Pneumoperitoneum and intracranial air are relative contraindications to air transport. Tissues may also swell and plaster casts should be split. Nausea and pain must be adequately controlled.

Required staff competencies for air transport

In addition to the competencies required for road transport the following are required:
- Understanding the limitations of resource and power in aircraft.
- Understanding the effects of altitude, vibration, and noise on physiology and monitoring.
- Understanding emergency drills for helicopters and fixed wing aircraft.

See also:
Endotracheal intubation, p42; Chest drain insertion, p84; Enteral feeding and drainage tubes, p122; Pulse oximetry, p144; CO_2 monitoring, p146; ECG monitoring, p162; Blood pressure monitoring, p308; Sedatives and tranquilisers, p310; Muscle relaxants, p312; Intrahospital transport, p644; Interhospital transport—road, p646.

Death and the dying patient

Brain stem death

- Correct diagnosis allows discontinuation of futile ventilation and enables potential retrieval of organs for donation.
- Diagnosis is usually followed by asystole within a few days.
- Before brain stem function testing can be performed to confirm the diagnosis, the patient must have an underlying irreversible condition compatible with brain stem death. There must be no evidence that coma is due to hypothermia, depressant drugs, significant metabolic abnormality, or muscle relaxant effect.
- Performance of brain stem death tests should not proceed until relatives, and medical and nursing staff have had a chance to take part in discussions. The test itself does not require consent.
- Cessation of mechanical ventilation is seen, incorrectly, by many lay people as the final point of death.
- If considering organ donation, involve the transplant coordinator early.

Brain stem death testing

Procedures vary internationally. In the UK, assessment of brain stem reflexes must be performed by two doctors registered for >5 years, competent in the field of brain stem death testing, and not members of the transplant team. At least one should be a consultant. An EEG is required in other countries.

Pupillary light reflex

Pupils should appear fixed in size and fail to respond to a light stimulus.

Corneal reflexes

These should be absent bilaterally.

Pain response

There should be no cranial or limb response to supraorbital pain.

Vestibulo-ocular reflexes

After confirming that the tympanic membranes are clear, unobstructed, and non-perforated, 20mL iced water is syringed into the ear. The eyes would normally deviate toward the opposite direction. Absence of movement to bilateral cold stimulation confirms an absent reflex.

Gag or cough reflex

The gag reflex is absent in brain stem death. However, the gag reflex is often lost in patients who are intubated. In these patients, cough reflex in response to bronchial stimulation must be absent.

Apnoea test

While the reflex assessments are being performed, the patient should be pre-oxygenated with 100% oxygen. Disconnect the ventilator and pass 6L/min oxygen into the trachea via a catheter. Apnoeic oxygenation can sustain SaO_2 for prolonged periods, but there is an inevitable rise in $PaCO_2$ which should stimulate respiratory effort. After 3–15min of disconnection, blood gas analyses are performed until $PaCO_2$ >6.65kPa. Any respiratory effort negates the diagnosis of brain stem death.

Time of death

Death is not pronounced until the second test has been completed, but the legal time of death is when the first test indicates brain stem death.

See also:
Blood gas analysis, p154; EEG/CFM monitoring, p204; Electrolytes (Na^+, K^+, Cl^-, HCO_3^-), p212; Toxicology, p224; Hypoglycaemia, p600; Hypothermia, p606; Care of the potential organ/tissue donor, p656.

Withdrawal and withholding treatment

This is arguably the most difficult and stressful decision that has to be made for the critically ill patient.

- Withdrawal involves reduction or cessation of vasoactive drugs and/or respiratory support. In some Critical Care Units, the patient is heavily sedated and disconnected from the ventilator.
- Withholding involves non-commencement or non-escalation of treatment, e.g. applying an upper threshold dose for an inotrope, not starting renal replacement therapy.

Discussion with patient and/or family

Before approaching the patient/family, there should be a consensus among medical and nursing staff that quantity and/or quality of life are significantly compromised and unlikely to recover. Often, the patient's viewpoint is very well-defined and carers may rue the fact that the discussion was not initiated earlier.

Ethnic, cultural, and religious factors will influence both doctor and patient/family in the timing and frequency of such decisions. In some societies, doctors have a more paternalistic approach with little involvement of patient and/or family in the decision-making process. Others are overly inclusive, sometimes to the point of excessively acquiescing to the family's demands despite obvious futility in continuing care. Clearly, a balance needs to be struck that serves the best interests of the patient.

Although potentially awkward, the mentally competent patient should be involved as this is the most important decision affecting their life. This should be done as considerately as possible, avoiding unnecessary distress. A series of discussions may be needed over several days, allowing time to contemplate. Consensus is reached with >95% of patients/families by the third discussion.

It should be stressed that care is not being withdrawn/withheld; pain relief, comfort, hydration, and general nursing care will be continued. Likewise, decisions are not final, but can be amended depending on the patient's progress, e.g. moving from withholding to withdrawal or re-institution of full treatment. A 'negotiated settlement' is often a useful interim compromise for families unable to accept a withdrawal decision, whereby limitation of treatment is instituted and subsequently reviewed.

Relatives can sometimes be very distraught and, occasionally, irrational on discussing withdrawal/withholding. For many, this will be their first experience of the dying process in a loved family member. A number of other factors, including guilt, anger, and within-family disagreements may also surface. It should be stressed that the withdraw/withhold decision is a medical recommendation and their passive agreement is being sought. The emphasis of the discussion is to inform them of the likely outcome and to seek their view of what the patient would want. They need to be dealt with both sensitively and honestly, and they should not feel pressured to give instant decisions.

Discussions should involve the patient's nurse and other involved carers as appropriate. It should be accurately documented in the case notes to ensure good communication between caregivers and act as source data should subsequent complaints surface.

Key paper

Sprung CL, Cohen SL, Sjokvist P et al for the Ethicus Study Group. (2003) End-of-life practices in European intensive care units: the Ethicus Study. *JAMA* **290**:790–7.

See also:

Communication, p18.

Care of the potential organ/tissue donor

Patients with suspected brain stem death should be considered candidates for organ or tissue donation. Tissue donation is excluded if there is:
- Systemic malignancy (other than for eye donation).
- HIV, HTLV, or hepatitis B or C positive or behavioural risk.
- Syphilis.
- Creutzfeldt–Jacob disease (CJD) or family history of CJD.
- Progressive neurological disease of uncertain pathophysiology.
- Previous transplantation.

There are few absolute contraindications to solid organ donation:
- HIV positive.
- CJD or suspected CJD.

The transplant coordinator should be contacted early (before the family is approached) to confirm likely suitability. If the family is amenable, the transplant coordinator will then initiate organ donation procedures. Do not reject brain dead potential donors who, for example, have fully treated infections or acute renal failure without consultation with the transplant coordinator.

Management
1. Confirm brain stem death with appropriate testing.
2. Laboratory tests for blood group, HIV and hepatitis status, and electrolytes.
3. Confirm organ donation is permissible by the coroner (or equivalent).
4. Maintain optimal cardiorespiratory status with fluid ± inotropes and vasopressin, optimal ventilation, low PEEP, and physiotherapy.
5. Diabetes insipidus should be treated with DDAVP.
6. Maintain haemoglobin >9g/dL and correct coagulation disturbance.
7. Maintain body temperature with warmed fluids and heated blankets.
8. Contact surgical and anaesthetic teams.

Organ suitability
- Kidneys.
- Heart.
- Lungs.
- Liver.

The transplant coordinator will advise on other organ and tissue suitability, e.g. pancreas, trachea, bowel, skin.

Non-heart beating donation
Solid organs suitable for transplantation from non-heart beating donors include kidneys, livers, and lungs. Tissue donation (e.g. corneas, etc.) should also be considered in asystolic cadaveric donors. Contraindications are similar to those for brain stem dead heart-beating donors. Consideration of non-heart beating donation should be made in all patients in whom treatment is to be withdrawn.

Index

Please note the use of **bold** type indicates major coverage of a subject.